D1030346

the broader implications of the research, chapters address such compelling topics as:

- Differences between ostracism and other forms of discipline or punishment
- How situational and individual differences make people more or less vulnerable to ostracism
- Consequences for targets' coping responses, self-esteem, and sense of belonging, control, and meaningful existence
- How the effects of being ostracized evolve over days, months, and years
- What individuals and groups have to gain (and lose) by engaging in ostracism

Marshaling an impressive body of original data and identifying vital directions for future investigation, this book will be read with interest by students, researchers, and practitioners in a wide range of psychological disciplines. It may also serve as an ancillary text in advanced undergraduate and graduate-level courses on interpersonal relationships, close relationships, and psychology research methods.

About the Author

KIPLING D. WILLIAMS, PHD, is currently Professor of Psychology at Macquarie University in Sydney, Australia. He has taught previously at Drake University, the University of Toledo, and the University of New South Wales. He received his doctorate in social psychology from The Ohio State University. The coeditor of several books, Dr. Williams has written numerous articles and book chapters on social influence, group dynamics, and psychology and law.

OSTRACISM

EMOTIONS AND SOCIAL BEHAVIOR

Series Editor: Peter Salovey, Yale University

OSTRACISM

The Power of Silence

KIPLING D. WILLIAMS

Series Editor's Note by Peter Salovey

2001

THE GUILFORD PRESS
New York   London

© 2001 The Guilford Press
A Division of Guilford Publications, Inc.
72 Spring Street, New York, NY 10012
www.guilford.com

Printed in the United States of America

This book is printed on acid-free paper.

Last digit is print number: 9 8 7 6 5 4 3 2 1

Library of Congress Cataloging-in-Publication Data

Williams, Kipling D.
  Ostracism : the power of silence / Kipling D. Williams.
      p. cm. — (Emotions and social behavior)
  Includes bibliographical references and index.
  ISBN 1-57230-689-0 (hardcover : alk. paper)
    1. Social isolation. I. Title. II. Series.
  HM1131 .W55 2001
  302.5′45—dc21   2001045132

About the Author

Kipling D. Williams, PhD, is currently Professor of Psychology at Macquarie University in Sydney, Australia, and has taught previously at Drake University, the University of Toledo, and the University of New South Wales. Dr. Williams received his PhD in social psychology from The Ohio State University. The coeditor of several books in the Sydney Symposium on Social Psychology, he has written numerous articles on social influence, group dynamics, and psychology and law.

Series Editor's Note

About 10 years ago, I heard Kipling Williams give a presentation concerning his work on social ostracism. His presentation was marvelous, with examples ranging from students at military academies to marital partners shunned by spouses. He even described an ostracism analogue used in his laboratory experiments in which participants tossed a ball to each other but deliberately neglected one of the other participants. All of this work pointed to the profound emotional and social consequences of being ignored, left out, and isolated.

I realized, as I listened to Dr. Williams, that he might be one of the only psychologists in the world studying this powerful social process. With this in mind, I conveyed to Seymour Weingarten, Editor-in-Chief at The Guilford Press, that we should invite Dr. Williams to contribute a volume to the Emotions and Social Behavior series. It took a little while to convince Dr. Williams to write this book, but we are pleased we persisted because what he has produced here is a fascinating and captivating account of the psychology of ostracism. The book is remarkable in synthesizing what research is available in this area and integrating it in a way that sheds light on educational, workplace, marital, and other social problems. In fact, I would go so far as to say that I believe this volume represents the most important writing in the social and behavioral sciences on the causes and consequences of ostracism. I am delighted and proud that it is part of this series.

PETER SALOVEY, PHD
Chris Argyris Professor and Chair of Psychology
Yale University

Preface

A few years ago, I was on sabbatical at the University of Queensland in Brisbane, Australia, and my wife and I traveled north to Rockhampton where I was to give a talk. While there, I met a psychologist who worked at a nearby prison. She had just gotten home from work. She reported that an Aboriginal inmate at the prison had been apprehended for trying to escape. She really didn't think he'd tried to escape, however, because the guards found him between two sets of barbed-wire fences, and instead of climbing the fence or running from the guards, he was picking up litter. When the guards got to him, he did not struggle. In fact, she said, he seemed relieved, almost happy that they handcuffed him. Asked why he tried to escape, he said he wasn't really trying to escape—it was just that no one paid any attention to him in prison; no one talked to him, looked at him, or even made the effort to address racist comments at him. He said he went between the fences to see if he really existed. And he was happy that the guards bothered to catch him, because now he knew he existed and that he mattered.

This example is one of many that illustrates the power and complexity of ostracism. The word *ostracism* has been used to mean everything from ignoring and excluding individuals or groups to killing them. In this book, I adopt a moderately liberal definition of ostracism. For my purposes, it means any act or acts of ignoring and excluding of an individual or groups by an individual or group. I stop short, however, of including any acts of verbal or physical abuse. I am interested in the immediate, short-term, and long-term effects of being ignored and excluded, how both the source and the target interpret it, and the reasons for using it. Individuals and groups can ostracize and can be ostracized. Ostracism spans species, crosses cultures, traverses time, and ranges from formal declarations of exile by governmental institutions and religious orders, to short time-outs given in the schoolroom, to unannounced and unexplained silences and averted eye contact issued by one's partner in close interpersonal relations.

In this book, I present a research program that examines the complexities, causes, and consequences of ostracism. I do so by using a multimethod approach that is guided by an overarching model (presented in Chapter 3; see also Williams, 1997; Williams & Zadro, 2001). All methods have their own unique sets of advantages and disadvantages. My belief is that by using a variety of methods, the particular disadvantages of one method can be offset by the advantages of another. For instance, short-term effects of ostracism can be studied experimentally, such that pertinent factors can be manipulated while others are held constant. Here, cause and effect can be inferred. Even within the experimental paradigm a variety of approaches are used, including role play, Internet-based research, and field and laboratory experimentation.

We use surveys, narrative accounts, and in-depth interviews to examine naturally occurring instances of ostracism. Surveys allow us to estimate the frequency with which individuals ostracize others and are ostracized by others. Narratives are typically used to obtain detailed descriptions of single incidences of ostracism. In-depth interviews are reserved for sources and targets of long-term ostracism. Whereas cause-and-effect inferences cannot be made from such accounts, they do provide us with a remarkably powerful and rich data set that communicates the experience of ostracism in ways that cannot be reproduced in the laboratory. They also allow us to test the long-term effects proposed by my model.

Arguably, the motives behind interpretation of ostracism make it the powerful and aversive thing that it is, and this is probably true for both sources and targets. For the source, depending upon how it is done (and the motives behind it), the act of ignoring may or may not be effortful, aversive, or empowering. For the target, the act of being ignored may, at times, mean little and result in virtually no psychological effects; other times, however, being ignored may symbolize one's nonexistence and can be more devastating than the sharpest word or hardest punch.

Acknowledgments

Many people have directly or indirectly influenced my interest and thinking about ostracism. I have had the pleasure of working with a large number of undergraduate and graduate students who have served as experimenters or confederates, or who have chosen to work with me on ostracism for their honors theses, master's theses, or dissertations, or for extracurricular research. In this regard, I am indebted to Michele Bogle, Marty Bourgeois, Christopher Cheung, Shellene Cheung, Wilma Choi, Vanessa Croker, Maggie Cruickshank, Rima El-Hajje, Kate Elliot, Alla Ezrakovich, Sonja Faulkner, Cassandra Govan, Jon Grahe, Joel Harvey, Rob Hitlan, Neha Jain, Anita Jerrems, Amy Kaylor, Amanda Kerr, Se Kang Kim, Tina Ko, Alby Lam, Helen Lawson Williams, Marek Moldowski, Chris Nadasi, Sherri Ondrus, Steve Predmore, Barth Reilly, Melissa Samolis, Kristin Sommer, Bill Taylor, Daniel Tynan, Carla Walton, and especially Lisa Zadro.

I have had several colleagues who have been incredibly supportive, willing to talk long hours into the night, or e-mail me continually throughout the day, to hammer out rough ideas or rework inconsistencies within my thinking. Thank you Frank Bernieri, Julie Fitness, Joe Forgas, Steve Harkins, Mike Hogg, Irv Horowitz, Robert Josephs, John Levine, Dick Moreland, Steve Nida, John Pryor, Rick Richardson, Ren Sloan, Ladd Wheeler, and Paul White. And thanks to Scott Plous, whose Social Psychology Network webpage allowed us to reach many participants in our cyberostracism studies.

One friend and colleague in particular has been responsible for much of the theoretical development of my model through hours of lively face-to-face and computer-mediated discussions, so I would like to specifically thank Wendelyn Shore for her constant support and constructive criticism throughout the writing of this book.

I am indebted to the Australian Research Council, which funded much of this research; to the University of Toledo, for supporting my emerging interest in ostracism; to the University of New South Wales, which surrounded me with excellent colleagues, students, and resources; and finally, to Macquarie University, for providing me with additional resources and supportive colleagues to continue my research.

I would also like to express my gratitude to two mentors: Denis Mitchell, who gave me my first taste of empirical research and the exciting process of discovery through careful and controlled experiments, and Bibb Latané, who opened my eyes to the advantages of employing multiple and psychologically engaging methods.

I am very grateful to The Guilford Press, in particular Seymour Weingarten and Carolyn Graham, who were especially patient with me, and to the editor of the Emotions and Social Behavior series, Peter Salovey, who gave me invaluable advice to make the book more reader-friendly.

Finally, I would like to thank my children, Kory and Kitty, who mean more to me than they can imagine; Cooper and Dylan, whose arrival may have slowed the progress of this book, but who made it all worthwhile; my parents, who have always encouraged me; and my lovely wife, Cindy, for believing in me.

Contents

OSTRACISM

Ostracism

Ubiquitous and Powerful

My girlfriend gives me the "silent treatment" whenever we argue. I spilled some pop on her roommate's pillow and she blew up and we argued. She then didn't talk to me. It made me feel mad, because I *hate* to be ignored. I have a bad temper and I would pick on her, hitting her sunburn to release my anger. She then got real mad and started hitting me and I *hate* it when people hit me and I walloped her and continued to do so until she was crying. The ultimate consequences of being ignored are that I lose my temper and it eventually leads to a fight.
—MALE UNDERGRADUATE STUDENT, 1993

Few events in life are more painful than feeling that others, especially those whom we admire and care about, want nothing to do with us. There may be no better way to communicate this impression than for others to treat you as though you are invisible—like you didn't exist. Maybe at first glance this doesn't seem as intolerable as I suggest. But recall for a moment a situation in which your friends, family, coworkers, or relationship partners acted as though you did not exist. Remember feeling as though you were invisible, yet you could see the others going about their lives as though nothing unusual was happening. What did you do? Did you try talking to them to find out what was going on? But what if they didn't talk back, but instead acted as though they had not heard you? Maybe you waved your hands in front of their faces? If you did, what did it feel like when they looked right through them and you? What did you think when they even refused to make eye contact with you? Were you able to carry on as though everything was normal? Did you start to withdraw? Or did you reciprocate their actions? Remember the time your family or friends made plans and everyone was included

1

except you? Did you ask to be involved anyway, or did you disengage, wondering if you really belonged with these people after all?

Notice that I did not ask if you could *imagine* these events, but instead asked if you *remembered* them. The odds are very high that you have experienced episodes of ostracism, particularly in the form of "the silent treatment," which can occur in groups and in dyads (Faulkner, Williams, Sherman, & Williams, 1997). The silent treatment is one of many forms of ostracism, but it is the one that most of us have experienced. We are less likely to have encountered other forms of ostracism, such as solitary confinement or banishment. Still, even these sorts of physical ostracism are not totally unknown to most of us. Have you ever locked yourself in a room during an argument? Were you ever placed in a time-out room in school for misbehaving? Have you ever had a friend who stopped visiting your home after an argument? Many of us have even experienced ostracism in situations other than face-to-face interactions. For instance, how many times has someone hung up on you during a telephone conversation? Were letters you sent not reciprocated? If you are experienced using the Internet, have you ever stopped receiving routine e-mail messages from a friend?

In a few well-chosen words, William James captured the terror and emptiness that an individual would feel in such situations:

> A man's Social Self is the recognition which he gets from his mates. We are not only gregarious animals, liking to be in sight of our fellows, but we have an innate propensity to get ourselves noticed, and noticed favorably, by our kind. No more fiendish punishment could be devised, were such a thing physically possible, than that one should be turned loose in society and remain absolutely unnoticed by all the members thereof. If no one turned round when we entered, answered when we spoke, or minded what we did, but if every person we met "cut us dead," and acted as if we were nonexisting things, a kind of rage and impotent despair would ere long well up in us, from which the cruelest bodily tortures would be a relief; for these would make us feel that, however bad might be our plight, we had not sunk to such a depth as to be unworthy of attention at all." (1890, pp. 293–294)

This phenomenon of feeling invisible, of being excluded from the social interactions of those around you, of being ostracized, is the subject matter of this book. So, too, are the psychological effects on individuals who use ostracism. We are just as likely to have been the sources of ostracism as its targets. What is gained (and lost) by ignoring and excluding others? What do you feel like when you use the silent treatment on a loved one, friend, or colleague? Is it easy or difficult to do?

Narratives written by young and returning college students; interviews with long-term sources of ostracism, some of whom were in their

80s; and even offhand remarks made by my assistants in the laboratory who ostracize participants for only 5 minutes—all indicate that the act of ostracism is psychologically costly. It takes energy and depletes cognitive resources. And it can cause irreparable damage to close relationships. Clearly, ostracism is a two-edged sword, cutting not only the target but also the source. But, as we shall see, ostracism also affords the user certain benefits, which undoubtedly ensures its reuse on other people in other situations.

I first became interested in ostracism in 1977 when I watched a made-for-TV movie about a young cadet at the U.S. Military Academy at West Point. In 1969, Lieutenant James J. Pelosi had failed to immediately put his pencil down at the end of an exam in one of his classes. He was brought up on cheating charges, and the honor committee found him guilty of disobeying West Point examination rules. The superintendent eventually dismissed the charges, and Pelosi was reinstated in good standing. Nevertheless, the honor committee did not exonerate him. Because he defied the internal structure of West Point, his peers "silenced" him. For 19 months, Pelosi was forced to live alone and to eat alone. No other cadet socialized with him or spoke to him—not even his former best friends. His mail was frequently torn up and his possessions were vandalized. The silencing was intended to force Pelosi to quit West Point, but he would not budge. Cadet Pelosi endured the ostracism and graduated. During those 19 months, he worked out in the gymnasium, kept a journal, and struck up conversations with the military police. He also lost 26 pounds (Steinberg, 1975).

The power and simplicity of the act of silencing entranced me. Although Pelosi stuck it out, it was clear that he endured a living hell for those 2 years, and probably even after that, when he was stationed overseas. I learned later that silencing had been used at West Point on the man who eventually became the first black brigadier general in the U.S. Army, Benjamin O. Davis Jr. (Davis, 1991). He was silenced for his entire 4 years at West Point. He had no roommate; no one talked with him, ate with him, or voluntarily interacted with him throughout his time at West Point because he was black. Despite the fact that these 4 years presented one of the toughest challenges in his life to that point, or perhaps because of it, Davis persevered and succeeded.

I was fascinated by these ordeals and realized that the psychological assumption behind many well-established social phenomena was that people feared precisely this sort of treatment: being ostracized, excluded, rejected, treated as though one did not belong with the others or even exist. Asch (1956) demonstrated that young men would change their perception of an unmistakably correct judgment about the length of a line simply to conform to the opinion of the unanimous majority of peers. Why? The presumption was that they did not want to be excluded and rejected by this group of strangers. Milgram (1974) found that people would obey an authority who ordered them to shock another person, even when they could hear that the person was in pain and wanted the experiment to stop. Why? Presumably because the participants did not want to be thought of badly by the authority and were willing to hurt another person so as not to be rejected. Countless studies have shown that people comply with others' requests, purchase items they do not need or want, or donate money, time, or blood to organizations or causes that they had not initially intended to help (Cialdini, 1993). Why? Presumably because they did not want to risk exclusion and rejection by the salespeople and donation seekers.

The list is endless. We resist the urge to take free coupons for cheeseburgers in the presence of strangers (Petty, Williams, Harkins, & Latané, 1977); we decline to seek help to report a broken computer terminal while taking an exam (Williams & Williams, 1983); we are slow to help others in distress (Latané & Darley, 1970)—all because we do not want others (typically strangers) to look askance at us, to berate us, and effectively to exclude us from their potential connection.

Clearly, fears of rejection and exclusion that are presupposed in these other areas of research are not unfounded. Schachter (1951) conducted research that demonstrated what could happen to group members who did not conform to the majority. Groups of students signed up to have weekly discussions on a variety of topics. During the first discussion, Schachter planted a "deviate" who argued eloquently but in opposition to the majority. Was this enthusiastic and reasoned contribution to the group discussion rewarded? Hardly. Over and over again, groups rejected the deviate, after they first tried and failed to change his mind. When group members were asked to pare down who they would like to have in their discussion group in the following weeks, they rarely chose the deviate. Group members who agreed with their fellows, but who contributed far less to the discussion, were more likely to be chosen. However, if the group believed it had succeeded in changing the deviate's mind (the "slider" condition), then this "reformed deviate" was one of the most popular choices for inclusion in the group.

This is as far as our knowledge of ostracism took us. Yes, we fear exclusion and rejection, enough to alter our perceptions, attitudes, and behaviors, but what happens when others ostracize us? What do we do then? How does ostracism affect our innermost states and our outward expression of them? Schachter (1959) again shed some light on this issue, but only a glimmer. He attempted to study humans in isolation. If we fear exclusion so much, what happens when we are physically isolated from our fellows? Schachter isolated five volunteers, who were put alone in a windowless room for as long as they could manage. They were, of course, fed and could avail themselves of bathroom facilities. He noted considerable individual differences in tolerance of this isolation. One participant demanded to be removed within 2 hours ("almost hammering on the door to get out"; p. 9). Three others remained isolated for 2 days: two appeared unaffected, but one individual expressed uneasiness. The fifth volunteer lasted 8 days and did not appear to suffer any adverse consequences. This preliminary research was disappointing, time-consuming, costly, and ethically questionable. Schachter terminated this line of inquiry and redirected his interests by examining the effects of fear on desire to affiliate. But regarding his isolation research, Schachter mused about how fascinating it would be to study the effects of isolation on individuals' propensity to be vulnerable to social influence.

The research program I present in this book is, in part, an attempt to readdress Schachter's questions about isolation and social influence. After watching the TV movie about Cadet Pelosi, I realized that psychological isolation need not require physical isolation. We can and do experience isolation even when there are others around us . . . even if we are in a crowd, even if we are surrounded by loved ones. If the people who are around us ignore us, or as James put it, "cut us dead," then psychologically, we are isolated. We are ostracized, or more precisely, we are "socially ostracized." I reasoned that if we could ostracize individuals in this manner for a short time in a controlled setting, we could then answer the questions posed by Schachter, and a lot more. Not only could we examine vulnerability to social influence, but we could also examine physiological responses, self-reported anxiety, mood, and other emotions, and subsequent desires and behaviors of the ostracized individual alone and in groups. We could ask whether certain types of ostracism (like, say, physical isolation) affect us differently than other types (like social ostracism).

Are all acts of ignoring perceived and reacted to similarly? Let's take a single instance of ignoring and consider the plethora of motives that could be attributed to it. Picture yourself walking down the hallway at work. Your boss walks right past you. You nod, but your boss looks through you, showing no signs of recognition. What are the possible motives that you could infer? One possibility is that your boss was simply preoccupied with important decisions and was not ostracizing you at all. Another possibility is that it is normative in your workplace not to repeatedly "say hi" after the first encounter of the day. Or perhaps your boss felt badly about giving a promotion you sought to another worker and feared your derision. Maybe your boss ignored you because your boss was angry with you (maybe she overheard something critical you said about her to one of your coworkers). Even worse, maybe she thinks so little about you that she did not even recognize you. Deciding upon which of these explanations is plausible and which is most likely will probably determine the magnitude and nature of your reaction.

Are there important individual differences that make some of us relatively immune to the effects of ostracism, whereas for others even imagined ostracism can be debilitating and horrific? If our self-esteem is already low, are we especially vulnerable to ostracism, perhaps believing it is happening even when it is not? Does our adult attachment style, which some would argue is determined in infancy to be primarily secure, avoidant, or anxious/ambivalent, affect the likelihood or intensity of experiencing ostracism (Bartholomew & Horowitz, 1991; Hazan & Shaver, 1987)? Because extroverts seek more stimulation, is deprivation of stimulation (e.g., attention) more aversive for them than it is for introverts?

What fundamental human needs are especially threatened or thwarted when one is ostracized? Being cut off, cut loose, cut down, and cut dead is perhaps the worst thing that can happen to us. I argue that the simple act of being ignored simultaneously attacks four fundamental human needs. Our sense of connection and belonging is severed; the control we desire between our actions and outcomes is uncoupled; our self-esteem is shaken by feelings of shame, guilt, or inferiority; and we feel like a ghost, observing what life would be like if we did not exist. How do we cope with these needs threats?

I will investigate answers to this question via two lines of research. One examines the short-term consequences of ostracism, the other focuses on long-term consequences. In the short term, the general hypothesis is that after the initial hurt and anger of being ostracized, individuals will seek to regain or reestablish the very needs that were threatened. For example, if one's sense of belonging is endangered, then one will attempt to reestablish a bond, either with the source(s) who ostracized or with another person or group. In the long term, if people are exposed to repeated or long-lasting episodes of ostracism, their attempts to restore what they have lost will eventually give way to feelings of alienation, helplessness, depression, and despair.

To investigate long-term ostracism, different methods must be used. With proper precautions and thoughtful debriefing, we can examine the effects of short-term episodes of ostracism by ignoring individuals for short periods of time in the laboratory, the field, or even over the Internet. It would be impractical and unethical, however, to subject individuals to long-term episodes of ostracism. How can long-term consequences be studied? I take a variety of approaches. Participants have provided rich narratives of single memorable ostracism experiences (both giving and getting) that I have carefully content analyzed (see

Chapters 2 and 4). My colleagues and I agreed to ostracize one person in our group per day over a period of a week and keep a diary of our feelings (see Chapter 5). Volunteers have been armed with event-contingent self-recording diaries to document and report their responses to naturally occurring ostracism episodes over a period of 2 weeks (see Chapter 10). Although these methods allow us to look at both naturally occurring and longer term episodes, they still do not give us much insight into experiences with chronic ostracism. How would people feel if they were exposed to ostracism over a period of months, years, or decades? In structured interviews (see Chapters 2 and 10), we talked with employees who had been ostracized by their coworkers for months or years, students shunned and excluded by their peers for several semesters, and spouses who were given the silent treatment by their partners for up to 4 decades.

We also break new ground by examining the other side of the ostracism coin: How does ostracism affect the ostracizers (or "sources," as I will call them)? What individual differences and situational factors cause us to ostracize rather than to confront? Is ostracism easier to carry out than arguing? After all, it can be characterized as a nonbehavior, requiring no speech or eye contact by the source, so perhaps it is effortless and efficient. And what benefits, if any, do ostracizers accrue?

Before I begin to describe, explain, and predict the causes and consequences of ostracism, I first review the existing research on ostracism and related phenomena that has been conducted in a variety of disciplines. These include history, anthropology, sociology, political science, and such subdisciplines in psychology as developmental, clinical, and social animal behavior.

OSTRACISM: A REVIEW OF THE LITERATURE

The pervasiveness of ostracism is such that it transcends time and is evident in almost all civilizations and known cultures (Gruter & Masters, 1986a). The term itself comes from the Greek *ostrakismos,* a practice originating in Athens circa 488–487 B.C. to remove those with dictatorial ambitions from the democratic state (Zippelius, 1986). Citizens would cast their vote to exile the individual in question by writing their preference on *ostraca*, shards of pottery (a similar practice was used by the Syracusans, but they wrote their preferences on olive-leaf petals. If not for the more potent Athenian culture, perhaps this book would have been called *Petalism* [Abbott, 1911]).

The ubiquity of ostracism is also reflected in the many terms used to describe it: "the cold shoulder," "avoiding," "shunning," "treat with ig-

nore," "being sent to Coventry," "the silent treatment," "exile," "banishment," "expulsion," "time-out," and "silencing." Forms of ostracism
are evident throughout institutions in our society such as schools (e.g.,
time-outs, expulsion) and the workplace (e.g., ostracism of whistleblowers by coworkers [Faulkner, 1998]). Almost all religions punish noncom-
pliance with ecclesiastical law with some form of excommunication, bar-
ring the deviate member from the congregation and from any privileges
that membership holds in the afterlife, such as ascension to heaven
(Zippelius, 1986).

Governments, cultures, religions, military institutions, tribes, small
groups, and even individuals practice ostracism as a response to individuals or groups who deviate from acceptable expectations. Sometimes the
decision to ostracize is formal and explicit. The South African government, for instance, exiled outspoken anti-apartheid newspaper editor
Donald Woods within his own country, preventing him from speaking to
those within and without his country. Other times ostracism occurs
spontaneously without laws, explicit rules, or public proclamation, as
was the case with Benjamin O. Davis Jr., mentioned earlier. Nothing
official was proclaimed; he was silenced simply because he was black
(Davis, 1991, p. 21).

Tribal civilizations such as the Pathan tribes located in the North-
western Frontier Province of Pakistan, and the Slavic tribes of Montenegro both exile deviate individuals for the purpose of protecting the
remaining members of the group (Boehm, 1986; Mahdi, 1986). In Western Apache culture, when sons come home from boarding school and
are reunited with their mothers, they are met not with joy and celebra-
tion but with silence (for fear that the sons no longer value the Apache
way of life). Widows are not consoled but are ignored (they are feared to
be crazy during the period soon after their husband's death). Courting is
characterized by hours of silence (for fear that the courting couple may
say something stupid [Basso, 1972]). "Voodoo death," the idea that
those subjected to spells or sorcery may be brought to death, has also
been attributed to ostracism. Cannon (1942) discussed tribal taboo in
the Aboriginal people of the Northern Territory of Australia, and suggested that once the taboo was announced, the family and community
withdrew their support of and attention to the unfortunate individual. In
some cases, a person closely related to the victim would conduct the
fateful ritual of mourning declaring the individual dead. Often, death resulted.

The Amish practice *Meidung* (translated as shunning) as a means of
disciplining members of the faith (Gruter, 1986). The Amish view
Meidung as being a "slow death" because it demands that friends, community members, and even close family can not speak to the perpetrator

at risk of being similarly ostracized. In such exclusion, the perpetrator would be unable to carry out necessary interactions that would give him or her goods and essential services, rendering them and their families vulnerable to destitution.

In a compelling account of one man's experience with Meidung, Gruter (1986) documents a civil trial in which the plaintiff, Andrew Yoder, sued the elders of his Amish church. Yoder was a 33-year-old father of seven children who lived in an Amish community in Ohio. His 1-year-old daughter Lizzie had a physical ailment that required pro-longed medical treatment twice a week in a town 15 miles distant from Yoder's farm. Fearing for her health, he bought a car, which violated Amish law. His church elders imposed Meidung. At the trial, after 5 years of shunning, Yoder was described as frail and pale, acting like a "whipped dog." One year after the trial, his daughter died. Perhaps the costs involved in ostracism were also high: The two elders who issued the Meidung proclamation, as well as one of their wives, died a few months after the child's death.

Developmental psychologists have documented the use of shunning and exclusion behaviors in children, used among other techniques as a form of peer rejection (Asher & Coie, 1990; Asher & Parker, 1989; Dodge, Pettit, McClaskey, & Brown, 1986). Barner-Barry (1986) reports a case where a preschool class systematically ostracized a bully (i.e., ig-nored him and excluded him from games and conversation) without adult prompting, with apparent success. This case study suggests that the use of ostracism as a means of controlling the behavior of others is both innate and adaptive (Barner-Barry, 1986). Adolescent girls tend to favor ostracism as a tactic during conflicts; adolescent boys, however, prefer to resort to physical violence as a means of resolving conflict (Cairns, Cairns, Neckerman, & Ferguson, 1989). Recently, researchers have begun to examine bullying (sometimes called *mobbing*, if done by a group) at work and in schools (Olweus, 1978, 1993; Schuster, 1996). Schuster notes the distinction between *rejected children*, those disliked by their peers, and *neglected children*, those not noticed by their peers. Rejected children are more likely to be bullied, whereas neglected chil-dren are not. Both types of children may feel victimized, but in different ways.

The pervasiveness of ostracism throughout society, institutions, and small groups is matched by the high frequency of ostracism in interper-sonal dyadic relationships. Indeed, the prevalence of ostracism is such that most individuals will be both a target and a source of ostracism in their close relationships, whether with loved ones, colleagues, or strang-ers. A survey of over 2,000 Americans conducted by Faulkner et al. (1997) found that 67% admitted to using the *silent treatment*, deliberately not speaking to a person in their presence, on a loved one. The percentage was slightly higher (75%) for those who indicated that they had been a target of the silent treatment by a loved one. As high as these numbers are, the natural desire to create a favorable impression on others (even telephone interviewers) probably makes these percentages underestimates of the actual incidence.

The silent treatment has been noted as a behavioral symptom of deteriorating marriages by Gottman and his colleagues (e.g., Gottman & Krokoff, 1992). Buss, Gomes, Higgins, and Lauterbach (1987) found that the silent treatment was a common tactic used by individuals on their relationship partners. They asked couples to answer the question, "When you want to get your partner to do something (or to stop doing something), what do you do?" Six tactics emerged, one of which was the silent treatment. They found that the silent treatment was just as likely to be used by males as females, and that it was used more often to terminate a partner's behaviors than to elicit them. They also found a positive correlation between the use of the silent treatment and measures of neuroticism. Moreover, their investigation revealed that couples who were less similar and less well matched were more likely to use the silent treatment and other tactics of manipulation than those who were similar and well matched.

Ostracism is evident not only in human interactions, but also as a behavior within several animal species, including primates, lions, and wolves. The different forms of ostracism that have been documented among primates include exclusion of a group member (generally male) after his unsuccessful attempt to take leadership, forced immigration due to insufficient resources, and ostracism of a member due to abnormal behavior or illness (de Waal, 1986; Goodall, 1986; Lancaster, 1986). Ostracism may be beneficial among animal groups because it reduces both demand on scarce resources and the chance of inbreeding. However, rejection from the group and thus from the protection of other members is often the first step toward starvation and death for the ostracized member (Goodall, 1986).

In Gruter and Master's (1986b) special issue on ostracism in *Ethology and Sociobiology*, the definitions of ostracism ranged from disparaging humorous remarks about individuals or groups (Alexander, 1986) to execution of tribal offenders (Boehm, 1986). The overarching theme of this compendium of articles was that ostracism is a phenomenon in which individuals are excluded in order to preserve the group's cohesiveness and survival. Nevertheless, it is difficult to imagine that humor, murder, and everything in between could be adequately understood as a unitary phenomenon. Ostracism is indeed complex and has multiple causes and multiple consequences, but it should be distinguished from other aversive interpersonal behaviors, including verbal and physical assault.

Those characteristics that appear to comprise a workable definition of ostracism include ignoring, excluding, and rejecting (Gruter & Masters, 1986b; Snoek, 1962). In real life, these three components often are naturally intertwined. But they can be disentangled, especially in experiments. For example, simply being ignored, even by strangers, without explicit rejection or exclusion, can be unpleasant. Zuckerman, Miserandino, and Bernieri (1983) found that elevator riders who were not given the usual "glance-and-nod" by another rider had significantly lower moods after exiting the elevator. Whether there were inferences of being rejected and excluded, however, is not known. Likewise, a person can be rejected, but included, at least within the time frame of the rejection. This might describe a heated argument in which a person is insulted and verbally attacked, yet continues to interact, albeit unpleasantly, with the source of rejection. We would expect (and, in fact, have found) that reactions to these different forms of aversive interpersonal behavior are predictably different. For instance, a target of anger still feels more included and connected to arguing others than to ignoring others (Zadro & Williams, 1998a).

Individuals who deviate from others' expectations are often the targets of ostracism (Gruter & Masters, 1986; Schachter, 1959). Consequently, it appears as though the primary function of ostracism is to bring the target back into the fold or to expel him or her altogether. Either outcome strengthens the ostracizing group's cohesiveness.

The existing research demonstrates convincingly that ostracism is an aversive interpersonal behavior to the targets of ostracism. Unlike other forms of aversive interpersonal behaviors, however, for instance, verbal or physical abuse, ostracism can be characterized as a nonbehavior. Because of this, its occurrence is enveloped in several layers of ambiguity. For instance, targets may notice that they are being ignored and think to themselves, "Is it actually happening or is it my imagination?" Or, if it is clear that ostracism is indeed happening, the target might wonder, "Why is it being done to me? Are they mad at me? Am I so unimportant to them that they don't even notice me?" It is precisely this ambiguity, I believe, that makes ostracism uniquely powerful and often used. One could conceivably ostracize another without having to admit doing it or ever having to apologize for it.

Whereas there is a consensus among social and biological scientists that ostracism has a strong negative impact on its targets, there is little discussion or agreement about the nature of this impact and the conditions under which it will or will not occur. Some biologists and physiologists claim ostracism causes general "physiological deregulation": it interferes with our immunological functioning and hypothalamic reactions that are related to aggression and depression (Kling, 1986; Raleigh & McGuire, 1986). Case studies report stomach ulcers (Gruter, 1986), fear of public gatherings, and loss of tribal leadership (Boehm, 1986) as a result of ostracism. Psychotic behaviors are more likely to occur in prisoners who are subjected to solitary confinement (McGuire & Raleigh, 1986).

The effects on the sources of ostracism are even less clear. Ostracism is believed to be an effective means of controlling contranormative behaviors, punishing deviance, and increasing in-group cohesion (Alexander, 1986; Barner-Barry, 1986; Basso, 1972; Boehm, 1986; Mahdi, 1986). Indeed, a short-term use of ostracism, time-out, is one of the most widely recommended and popular methods of disciplining children used by teachers and parents.

The efficacy of using time-outs in the schools and in special education programs has received considerable attention. *Time-out* is generally defined as time out from reinforcement, but this definition is controversial because no one has established that all forms of reinforcement are removed (O'Leary & O'Leary, 1976). It is assumed that being given a time-out is a punishment, but it is unclear whether that punishment consists of an aversive stimulus, inattention, or a negative reinforcer, that is, taking away a rewarding stimulus, attention. The common denominator of most forms of time-out is the reduction of social attention. But this can and is carried out in any number of ways, from physically relocating the child to a time-out room, to systematically ignoring the child who remains in the same social environment (Brooks, Perry, & Hingerty, 1992; Heron, 1987). Recently, an article advocated systematic ignoring over physical relocation because ignoring was "non-coercive and non-exclusionary" (Allerton, 1998). Researchers in this area appear to restrict their interest in time-out to a practical concern for the technique's short-term effectiveness in controlling undesired behaviors. Whereas the term "time-out" enjoys a generally positive reputation, it is by no means uniform in its procedures. Recently, an Australian couple from New South Wales (NSW) sued the NSW education department after discovering their 6-year-old son had been repeatedly locked in a cupboard for bad behavior in class. The school termed this punishment "behavior modification" and the cupboard the "sad corner" (Harris, 1998). Admittedly, this is an extreme case that would not be condoned by most educators. But ignoring a student in class, or sending a student to a nonstimulating room is typical, with the potential for unanticipated and undesirable consequences. Some therapists advocate using time-outs within families to ward off family violence (Veenstra & Scott, 1993). This idea, of course, appears to contradict the opening quotation in this chapter, in which a young man admits to becoming violent when ignored.

With adults, Miceli and Near (1992) have presented an excellent and programmatic analysis of the phenomenon of *whistleblowing*, in which employees disclose illegal, immoral, or illegitimate practices that took place within their organizations. Although Miceli and Near report that whistleblowers frequently mention being shunned by their coworkers and supervisors as a consequence of their whistleblowing, the researchers do not refer to this form of coworker punishment as retaliation. Rather, retaliation is operationally defined in terms of denied promotions, involuntary transfers, demotions, and other (easier to document) forms of punishment. In Chapter 9, I will present a program of research conducted by my former PhD student, Sonja Faulkner, specifically examining the effects of ostracism on whistleblowers.

Researchers in the diverse areas of organizational behavior and interpersonal relations have studied power tactics. Individuals use these tactics to achieve compliance from others. These research programs have produced theoretically useful taxonomies of tactics and their likelihood and frequency of being used by specific groups (Kipnis, Schmidt, & Wilkinson, 1980). Although ostracism is not mentioned by name, there are places within these taxonomies where forms of ostracism can be located. Some mention "disengagement" or "withdrawal." Falbo (1977) refers to explicit announcements of withdrawing verbal interaction if compliance is not forthcoming as "threats." Using the terminology of power tactic researchers, ostracism would typically be regarded as "indirect" (Falbo & Peplau, 1980) or "weak" (Kipnis, 1984), but it could also be "direct" if it was explicitly threatened (Falbo, 1977). It could also be categorized as "nonrational" because it does not appeal to logic or reason. Finally, it is likely to be "unilateral" because it is one-sided and prevents the target from being a participant in the interaction (Falbo & Peplau, 1980). Falbo and Peplau (1980) found that nonrational, unilateral power tactics are more commonly used by the individual who has less power in the relationship. This result was found in both heterosexual and homosexual relationships. For their heterosexual sample, withdrawal was much more likely to be used by females.

Other research in interpersonal attraction and close relationships is also relevant. Insko and Wilson (1977) instructed groups of three to take turns engaging in a sequence of consecutive two-person conversations. During each two-person conversation, the remaining member was excluded from social interaction, but was still physically present. Because of an ostensible time constraint, the sequence was ended after just two rounds, resulting in an inbalance in which one member interacted once with each of the other two, while the other two had not interacted with each other. Each person was then asked to rate the other two. Compared with ratings of the group members with whom they had interacted, participants rated the group member with whom they had not interacted as less likable and less interpersonally attractive on a variety of dimensions. Participants also surmised that that individual would not like them either.

Recently, Gada-Jain and Bernieri (1998) studied perceptions of interpersonal rapport within a job interview context. Interviewees were instructed to establish rapport with one of the two interviewers. Compared to the interviewer with whom synchrony was established, the nonsynchronized interviewer perceived the interviewee as more confident (less nervous, more arrogant, more dominant) and more knowledgeable (more competent, higher status, higher knowledge of occupation, very polite, very mature). Additionally, the nontarget was less likely to like the interviewee and to hire her.

Research on long-term relationships, especially in response to conflict, is also relevant. Rusbult, Verette, Whitney, Slovik, and Lipkus (1991) employed a response typology in their model of accommodation (inhibiting destructive reactions and engaging constructive reactions to bad behavior by one's partner). This typology involves two orthogonal dimensions: destructive–constructive and active–passive. These dimensions produce a matrix with four resulting classes of responses. One is *exit* which involves separating (moving out of the relationship), but also includes actively destroying the relationship with verbal or physical abuse. Another is *voice*, which is actively and constructively attempting to improve conditions. The third class is *loyalty*, which is passively staying in the relationship and hoping for improvement. Finally, there is neglect, which includes ignoring the partner or spending less time together, but also incorporates destructive criticisms and treatment. According to this typology, ostracism could be classified primarily as neglect, but would not include the destructive criticisms and treatment beyond being ignored. Ostracism could fall under exit with respect to physical separation, but would not include verbal and physical abuse. Rusbult, Johnson, and Morrow (1986) found that the primary marker for good functioning couples was avoiding destructive acts (exit or neglect) rather than maximizing constructive responses. This research did not extract the solely exclusionary forms of ostracism for the analyses, so questions regarding its frequency of use in functioning versus nonfunctioning couples, or its impact on the couple, were not addressed.

Two areas that one might expect to see recognition of and attention to the use of the silent treatment are clinical or counseling psychology. Recall our survey results (Faulkner et al., 1997) indicating that nearly three-quarters of the people in the survey used the silent treatment on their loved ones and two-thirds reported it having been used on them. With such high frequency of use in close relationships, we might expect that researchers in clinical psychology, counseling, or family therapy would have devoted at least some attention to the silent treatment. Yet little or no mention has been given to the silent treatment in these fields. Self-help books offer much advice to couples concerning what to say and what not to say when they are arguing, but surprisingly nothing is said about saying nothing. One exception occurs in the research on communication interaction patterns in marriages (particularly "at-risk" marriages) by Gottman and his colleagues (Gottman, 1979, 1980; Gottman & Krokoff, 1992). Gottman categorizes silence as withdrawal, notes its importance in triggering violence, and sees it as symptomatic of deteriorating relationships. It is interesting that, for Gottman, withdrawal includes both physical and social withdrawal, and distinctions between the two were apparently not considered.

PREVIOUS SOCIAL PSYCHOLOGICAL INVESTIGATIONS OF OSTRACISM

Over the years, only a few researchers in social psychology have investigated the effects of social behaviors that resemble ostracism. Usually, each researcher published a single article and did not follow it up with other studies. In these studies, the researchers varied in their manipulation and conceptualizations of rejecting, excluding, or ignoring.

For example, Dittes (1959) examined rejection by presenting participants with bogus ratings ostensibly made by members of their group concerning the participant's desirability as a group member. Participants were given ratings that signaled acceptance or rejection as a member of the group. Similarly, in a recent study, Nezlek, Kowalski, Leary, Blevins, and Holgate (1997) examined rejection by telling participants whether they had been chosen to work in a group (the inclusion condition) or alone (the rejection condition). Snoek (1962) varied the strength of rejection by explicitly telling targets that they were either not accepted into the group (strong rejection) or that the group did not mind whether they stayed or not (mild rejection).

Pepitone and Wilpizeski (1960) confounded explicit and implicit forms of rejection with ignoring. During a brief recess, two confederates ignored targets in the explicit condition as they engaged in conversation. The confederates were instructed to "present an unfriendly demeanor" when glancing at the target. In the implicit condition, the confederates did not speak to each other or to the target for the duration of the recess. Geller, Goldstein, Silver, and Sternberg (1974) examined the act of "being ignored," which they operationally defined as giving minimal attention to the target, responding only briefly to direct questions, and maintaining minimal eye contact. Mettee, Taylor, and Fisher (1971) examined "being shunned" in terms of physical avoidance and verbal abuse. Targets experienced two potential incidents of ostracism. In the implicit negative evaluation condition, one of the confederates moved away from the target to sit closer to the other confederate, whom they engaged in conversation. In the explicit negative evaluation condition, one of the confederates openly derogated the target's stance on a recent media issue.

Some of these studies provided evidence that being ignored or rejected had a negative effect on target's self-evaluations (Pepitone & Wilpizeski, 1960). Geller et al. (1974) found that females who were ignored by two female confederates during a conversation reported feeling more alone, withdrawn, shy, alone, dull, frustrated, anxious, nervous, and bored compared to included participants. Included participants felt more relaxed, friendly, and comfortable. Craighead, Kimball, and Rehak (1979) found that participants who simply imagined that they were ignored in a conversation produced fewer positive self-relevant statements than those individuals who imagined that they were included in a conversation. Their participants also reported that they felt more lonely, sad, frustrated, puzzled, rejected, and unworthy.

Other researchers investigated how individual differences moderated responses to ostracism. Nezlek et al. (1997) examined personality moderators (depression and self-esteem) for rejection. They found that individuals who had scored low on trait self-esteem and high in depression tended to be more accurate in perceiving rejection. They concluded that depressed and low-self-esteem individuals were more sensitive to interpersonal cues that were suggestive of rejection, and consequently they had more accurate perceptions of interpersonal feedback in general than those who were high in self-esteem or low in depression.

Several of the studies investigated how being rejected or ignored affected targets' thoughts and feelings toward the sources of ostracism. Pepitone and Wilpizeski (1960) found that participants who had been rejected rated the sources as less likeable. Similarly, Geller et al. (1974) reported that participants who had been ignored rated confederates less favorably than those who were not ignored. When participants were given the opportunity to reward the least liked confederate (as indicated by the participants' ratings) on an altruistic performance task, those who had been ignored rewarded confederates less than those who had not been ignored. Dittes (1959) found that male participants who were made to feel accepted by the group tended to be more attracted to the group. However, this relation was only significant for those with low self-esteem.

Many of the studies examined whether ostracism affected the desire to affiliate or continue working with the sources of ostracism. The findings in these studies are equivocal. In some studies, targets preferred to avoid, or not work with, the sources of ostracism in the future (e.g., Mettee et al., 1971; Pepitone & Wilpizeski, 1960; Predmore & Williams, 1983). Some found increased attraction to the ostracizing group only for targets who were low in self-esteem (Dittes, 1959) or high in public self-consciousness (Fenigstein, 1979). Still others reported a heightened desire to work with those who had ostracized them. For instance, Snoek (1962) found that when males were rejected for impersonal reasons (e.g., because the group was too large), their desire to remain with the group decreased. However, when the target was rejected for personal reasons (e.g., they were deemed unworthy of group membership), they desired to continue their membership in the group. Snoek concluded that personally rejected individuals possessed a "need for social reassurance" that could be fulfilled only by remaining in the group.

LIMITATIONS OF EARLY SOCIAL PSYCHOLOGICAL RESEARCH

Taken together, these studies present the view that ostracism is an aversive experience, producing a "socially unattractive environment" for targets (Snoek, 1962). In all of the research presented, the interest of the researcher was solely focused on the target's perspective. None of the studies attempted to examine the psychological effects of ostracizing. However, Geller et al. (1974) observed that the confederates in their study experienced considerable discomfort while ostracizing targets, noting that "being an ignorer may be almost as uncomfortable as being ignored" (p. 556). Yet neither Geller et al. nor any of the other researchers has examined the psychological discomfort associated with being a source of ostracism.

Examining the body of ostracism research reveals that none of the researchers attempted to define or acknowledge the complex varieties of ostracism. Many of the studies employed types of ostracism that may be phenomenologically different. Being ignored in a conversation (e.g., Geller et al., 1974) consists of many indicators of ostracism: the target's attempts to contribute to the conversation are repeatedly ignored, eye contact with the target will be avoided or not maintained, and other nonverbal gestures (such as body orientation) will be withheld from the target. In contrast to the multiple and enduring instances of being ostracized during a conversation, physically moving away from a target (Mettee et al., 1971) consists of a single gesture of rejection. Are both instances of ostracism equivalent? The early studies do not address whether such different types of ostracism prompt different thoughts, feelings, or physiological responses in the target.

It is evident, then, that the plethora of definitions, applications, and interpretations of ostracism in the literature have prevented in-depth investigation of both the ways in which people may be ostracized and the consequences of ostracism for targets as well as sources.

CONCLUSIONS

From this literature, we can draw several conclusions: (1) ostracism has been defined quite loosely and broadly; (2) most of the examinations of this phenomenon have been made outside psychology; and (3) previous studies conducted on ostracism within psychology have been neither programmatic nor theoretical. The aim of this book is to report a program of research, driven by qualitative and quantitative data, but also by an overarching theory. In the next chapter, I present themes and descriptions based on some qualitative approaches we have used to study ostracism. They provide us with a rich array of phenomenological accounts of the experience of ostracism from the perspectives of both targets and sources. Then, in Chapter 3, I present a model that was both informed by these qualitative studies and could be used to interpret them. More importantly, the model provides specific hypotheses that can be tested empirically. In Chapters 4 and 5, I present some qualitative approaches to our examination of ostracism. In Chapters 6–9, a series of experimental studies using multiple methods are presented that test predictions of short-term ostracism derived from the model. In Chapter 10, I examine the evidence we have of frequent and long-term exposures to ostracism. And finally, in Chapter 11, I summarize what we have discovered about ostracism, discuss future directions for what more we need to know about ostracism, and present some practical suggestions regarding the employment of and response to the varieties and complexities of what is a most fundamental, yet understudied, social behavior.

Forty Years of Solitude

Cases of Ostracism

W hen I learned about the two West Point instances of silencing, I thought I had stumbled upon the most unusual and long-lasting cases of social ostracism. After all, these were instances in which individuals had to coexist in the presence of others—important others—who treated them as though they did not exist. What could be more extreme than to be ignored and excluded by all of one's colleagues for up to 4 years? I have come to find out that there may indeed be worse cases—cases that lasted much longer than 4 years, and that involved not just colleagues, but sons, daughters, fathers, mothers, and spouses.

I became aware of these cases when I gave talks at universities, or gave interviews for television, radio, magazines, or newspapers. After my talks at universities, individuals from the audience would come up afterward and tell me their stories. After my interviews, I would receive many letters from people that provided excruciatingly rich details about what amounted for them to a "social death." In some cases, people who did the ostracizing would write me too. From these contacts, and from advertising in newspapers and magazines, I have now amassed over 120 letters, faxes, and e-mails, and over 50 interviews with people who have endured some form of ostracism. Most of these cases come from the targets of ostracism, but about a fifth are from the sources of it. Quite frequently, targets become sources, so that interviews that started off with targets detailing incredible stories of long-term ostracism ended with stories about how they have now become sources of ostracism for other people.

Many of these cases involve instances of the silent treatment, a term that appears to be reserved for punitive ostracism exacted within dyadic relationships (this is discussed more fully in Chapter 3; see Williams, Shore, & Grahe, 1998). Still other cases involve being ostracized by school peers, coworkers, and even people on Internet chat rooms.

In this chapter I present a sampling of cases as they have been relayed to me, not in terms of a psychological model, hypotheses, or experimental findings, and not even after being subjected to content analyses. Rather, they are the raw information that readers and listeners have volunteered to me and my colleagues (most notably Sonja Faulkner at the University of Toledo and Lisa Zadro at the University of New South Wales) in their own words (Faulkner & Williams, 1995; Williams & Zadro, 1999). Nevertheless, much of how I think about ostracism, including the development of a model and the hypotheses that stem from it, originates with these stories.[1]

I present these letters, faxes, e-mails, and excerpts from interviews in a way that brings attention to recurrent themes. All names and identifiers of the actual individuals have been changed for their protection. My goals for this chapter are threefold: (1) to expose you to the astounding stories of personally experienced ostracism—astounding not only in their frequency, but in their intensity and severity; (2) to provide you with a broad range of examples of ostracism episodes so that you can appreciate the need to develop a taxonomic structure to be used to understand how different types of ostracism can have different types of impact; and (3) to lay the groundwork for the goals that the other chapters will address.

FORTY YEARS OF SOLITUDE

The first case is the basis for the title of this chapter. Lee was in her 70s and lived in the Midwest. She answered a newspaper advertisement that disclosed our interest in talking with people who had experienced the silent treatment for a long period of time. Her now deceased husband silenced Lee for the last 40 years of his life. Lee wept when recounting the years of silence, but could not remember what caused them to start in the first place. The gist of her story is summarized in the following quote:

> "I wish he would've beaten me instead of giving me the silent treatment, because at least it would have been a response. This has ruined my life—I have no chance for happiness now. . . . The bottom line is that it's the meanest thing that you can do to someone, especially because it doesn't allow you to fight back. I should have never been born."

Several issues are raised in Lee's account that I explore further in this chapter. First, Lee could not recall the impetus for her treatment, and as we will see, other targets also express similar bewilderment. What effects might not knowing the reason for one's ostracism have on targets? Second, targets like Lee often indicate that they would have preferred other aversive forms of punishment, even physical abuse, to ostracism. I examine cases by those who claim this preference, even from individuals who have faced both types of abuse, to see why they say this. Third, Lee experienced a continuous long-term silent treatment from her husband, but others report that they received frequent shorter term episodes over many years. I examine several cases that vary on this continuity dimension. Fourth, whereas Lee was ostracized solely by her husband, other targets experienced ostracism by several family members or even by large groups of people. Might there be additional impact (either quantitatively or qualitatively) when targets endure ostracism by multiple sources? Fifth, Lee reported depression and feelings of worthlessness as a result of her treatment. I present several accounts in which targets report that they experience psychological and illness-related consequences that they attribute to being ignored for long periods of time. Finally, unlike Lee, some targets of long-term ostracism report methods they used to contend with their treatment that allowed them to minimize its effects on them. I explore some of these strategies in the hopes of providing individuals who experience similar treatment possible means with which to cope with it.

I end this chapter by examining the perspective of sources of ostracism. How do they explain what they do and how do they feel about it afterward? Do they offer any insights into methods that may get them to cease using such methods? And are there any negative side effects that impact upon the sources of ostracism?

TARGETS' PERSPECTIVES

Silence Often Comes with No Explanation

Lee could not remember what caused her husband to institute his long bout of silent treatment. Perhaps this is not so surprising given that more than 40 years had passed since its onset. But I have noticed a similar pattern of bewilderment from other targets, many of whom were recently on the receiving end. One of the peculiar features of ostracism is that because it is usually meted out through such acts as feigned ignoring, averted gazes, and silence, it is often not accompanied by an announcement of its onset or by explanations that justify its employment. This leaves targets of ostracism wondering why it is happening to them. Because of this, two things seem to happen. Targets claim that most often the ostracism episodes were caused for "no reason" or for trivial infractions. This is consistent with work by Roy Baumeister and Kathleen Catanese (2001) who examined narratives of victims and perpetrators. Victims often believe that there was no reason for perpetrators to act the way they did toward them. Undoubtedly, this provides victims with the ability to vilify perpetrators without taking any responsibility for what happened. But perhaps victims of ostracism are more justified in taking no responsibility than are other sorts of victims. After all, many targets seek out reasons for the silence, the averted gazes, the curt replies (if any) by asking, "What's wrong?," only to be told, "Nothing."

Being provided no explanation also seems to produce a more insidious effect: it leads targets to speculate endlessly on what they must have done wrong to deserve such treatment. In this regard, the absence of an explanation is worse than knowing the reason, because knowing the reason would narrow the list of shortcomings targets would have to generate and contemplate about themselves. Additionally, being told the reason would at least give the target a sense of "interpretive control." That is, just knowing helps them explain the situation and gives them a feeling of understanding, a first step toward perceiving control. A young woman who received the silent treatment from her husband wrote:

> "For me, the silent treatment was usually over something trivial. If I didn't do something right according to his weird beliefs, forgot to do something he wanted, refused to do something, or went against his wishes—the silent treatment would happen. . . . When I started thinking about the situation that instigated the silent treatment I realized that it was over trivial matters."

Still another woman who got the silent treatment from her mother wrote:

> "At one point, my mother did not speak to me for 2 years as a result of not getting her own way about something trivial and ultimately meaningless. I remember her totally ignoring me, or worse, adopting a look of . . . martyrdom!"

Another letter talked about how all the children were on the unexplained receiving end of the silent treatment from their mother. Reminiscing about her childhood, one member of that family (who also used the silent treatment in her adult life) wrote:

> "It [the silent treatment] was never explained. *What* was the crime that deserved this punishment? Mum didn't seem to know. It would last for a few days at most. A kind of thick unspoken question mark in the air. Then things returned to normal. No explanation as far as us kids were aware."

Other targets acknowledge some understanding as to what triggered the silent treatment, but considered it arbitrary or capricious nonetheless, as is indicated in the following excerpts from letters written by two different women (one who got the silent treatment from her mother, the other from her husband):

> "I am now 48 years old, but when I was young (12–17 years) my mother would always give me the silent treatment if for any reason I did anything to upset her. Sometimes it would last for weeks."

> "My husband was exactly the same [often giving the silent treatment]. . . . I am not referring to major situations or issues, all were over small insignificant incidents."

The search for reasons is evident in this next woman's letter about how her brother and sister have not talked to her for years:

> "There are two possible reasons as to why my sister is treating me like this, but my mother says this is not the reason. . . . I have no idea why my brother is like this to me."

Two consequences of not knowing for sure what one did to cause such treatment is being uncertain as to how to make things better and not knowing how to defend oneself against the attack. Ironically, unexplained ostracism leads many targets to apologize to the source of the ostracism, even though they are not sure what they are apologizing for. A middle-aged man discussing what he felt and did when his wife gave him the silent treatment exemplifies this problem:

> "I remember feeling terrible at these times and would end up apologizing to her (even if it wasn't my fault) for it all to end. However, even this sometimes failed to work."

More than likely, people are often subjected to verbal or physical abuse without the accompaniment of some explanation, no matter how inaccurate or irrational. Ostracism, because it is characterized by silence, is inextricably tied to the absence of explanations—strengthening its power over its targets.

Preference for Other Forms of Abuse

It is hard to imagine that anyone would prefer to be verbally or physically abused to being ostracized. Yet such a preference is one of the most recurrent themes in accounts by targets of long-term ostracism, many of whom also experienced verbal and physical abuse. What could possibly lead them to voice such a preference? There appear to be at least three reasons: (1) verbal and physical abuse is at least some sort of acknowl-edgment; (2) sources are less accountable for ostracism than they are for verbal or physical abuse; and (3) verbal and physically abusive incidents end (at least temporarily), whereas the silent treatment often goes on and on with no end in sight.

Lee and many others have indicated that they would prefer any-thing other than silence because other possible punishments indicate at the very least that they are important enough to warrant a response by the source. Recall the quotation from William James in Chapter 1:

> If no one turned round when we entered, answered when we spoke, or minded what we did, but if every person we met "cut us dead," and acted as if we were nonexisting things, a kind of rage and impotent despair would ere long well up in us, from which *the cruelest bodily tortures would be a relief*; for these would make us feel that, however bad might be our plight, we had not sunk to such a depth as to be unworthy of attention at all. (James, 1890, p. 294, emphasis added)

Apparently, it is better to get some response—even a negative response—than to get no response whatsoever. The feeling that one does not exist, if not in one's own mind at least in the minds of others, may be a uniquely aversive consequence of being ostracized. Of course, certain forms of ostracism send this message more than others. Demonstrable and "noisy" silent treatments that involve much stomping about and slamming of doors is likely to indicate to the target that he or she is at least worthy of all this wrath. But the types of ostracism that indicate disengagement (hiding behind the newspaper, going out with friends, grunting "Huh" whenever spoken to) are more likely to threaten the tar-get's sense of existence and worth, especially if the target is already suf-fering from feelings of self-doubt. A young woman who was the target of the silent treatment sums up these feelings:

> "If the recipient has low self-esteem to begin with, this [getting the si-lent treatment] surely augments that—'What?? Am I not even wor-thy of being spoken to? Am I invisible?' "

Another reason for preferring verbal or physical abuse stems from the desire to hold sources of ostracism accountable for their actions. One woman involved in a relationship in which both she and her partner use the silent treatment on each other noted:

> "It's a powerful weapon. No one can ever accuse you of attack, vio-lence, or harassment. But the wounds are still inflicted."

These sentiments are further expressed in the following two quotes by two different women:

"I wish I had been beaten so that I would have bruises to show others, including the police, that I was indeed being abused. No one would believe that my husband could be so unkind, and there was nothing I could point to to prove what he was doing."

"Everyone who meets him thinks he is prince charming so I have not confided in a lot of people. They would find it hard to believe."

Finally, verbal insults and beatings have discernable beginnings and endings; continuous silence signals no end. Individuals who receive long continuous episodes of the silent treatment seem to be worn down by its ceaseless and all-encompassing nature, as is evidenced in the following two quotes, one from a woman, the other from a man:

"I believe I would rather have received a belting every week than to endure the silent treatment as I believe it ate at my soul. It has been a long road for me. . . . "

"I recall asking her for a hiding at age 12 rather than endure another period of silence, and the shocking atmosphere it created."

People who voiced their preference for verbal or physical abuse over ostracism are not simply those who only experienced ostracism. Many people who have written us have experienced all forms of abuse, as is the case from a woman who wrote the following letter.

"My [husband]'s way of being the master of the house (so to speak) was to totally ignore, whenever your opinions differed to his. He walked around our home for weeks on end not uttering a word to anyone, and I personally learned to react in return, with this same cruel, unforgiving method. My husband not only used the 'silent treatment' by not speaking to me; he also used it by (1) avoiding any bodily contact, i.e., would walk past you sideways so as not to touch you; (2) slept on the lounge or in the car until you begged him not to; (3) refused to eat any meals; (4) took away all financial support, i.e., had bank accounts transferred into his own name and allowed you no access to them; (5) refused to let you use the car. This mental cruelty almost destroyed myself and my family and it wasn't until I suffered a breakdown and spent 8 weeks in a hospital undergoing psychotherapy that I came to realize the devastating effects this treatment had on my life and those I loved. *My second husband, who was an alcoholic, used to physically abuse me, but the bruises and scars healed very quickly and I believe that mental cruelty is far more damaging than a black eye,* although any type of violence to me now is unacceptable." (italics added)

Learning about such long-term experiences naturally raises the questions, "Why would she have stayed with him for so long if he didn't talk to her? What's wrong with her?" Of course, these questions are also asked about spouses who persist in remaining in physically abusive relationships. Perhaps one reason is that targets of long-term silent treatment still feel that they get something from their relationship. Lee revealed that she and her husband still had sexual relations with each other occasionally, though he still would not look at her or speak to her even during those intimate moments. Despite this peculiarity, she said for her it was the only time she was sure he knew she was there, that at least she could be comforted by his touch, if not by his words or gaze. But perhaps more importantly, the reasons for her staying in such a relationship were revealed in her comments that her life was ruined, that she had no chance for happiness, and that she should not have been born. Many of the people who have contacted us have voiced similar sentiments. They appear to have come to the conclusion that if they were not even important enough to be recognized by their husband (or wife, or father, or mother, or children), then perhaps they were not worthy individuals. They came to think that no one else would like them or find them worthy of attention either.

> "I interpreted [the silent treatment] as an effort to drive me out of the home; thus my husband could retire from his stressful job, having no further responsibility towards me. As I had nowhere to go, and no sufficient means of support, I hung on."

But, sometimes, as the saying goes, "Silence is golden." A few people indicated that they learned to prefer or even enjoy the silent treatment. After years of enduring the silent treatment from her father, a woman wrote:

> "Basically the silent treatment was a good thing for me. If my father was not talking to me I wouldn't be psychologically or emotionally abused in any way, I wouldn't have to listen to his ranting and raving about my mother and sister (the horrible names he called them/ how he was going to shoot them if I did anything wrong—in his eyes). I got to the stage where I said to myself if my father wants to act like a 2-year-old it was fine with me, at least it gave me a reprieve from listening to his abuse. It was heaven when he wouldn't talk to me and I made no attempt to try and break the silent treat-

ment. I wanted it to go on as long as possible. He was the one who started it every time and he was the one who cracked first. I was determined not to give him the satisfaction of talking first. Why should I talk first when I'm not the one who started the stupid situation in the first place? That I believed I didn't deserve anything I received."

In another instance, this wife gave her husband the silent treatment frequently. She explained that her husband preferred her to use the silent treatment because she was prone to talk too much:

"I think he [her husband] thinks it's nice to have some peace and quiet 'cause he always used to joke that he liked it when I gave him oral sex because I was quiet for 5 minutes!"

Perhaps for some the silent treatment offers a reprieve from other more aversive forms of interaction. Where people are in their search for a balance between having too much or too little silence may affect their reactions to being excluded and ignored. Those needing more attention and human connection may be particularly sensitive to ostracism; those seeking privacy and isolation may be somewhat immune to ostracism.

Variations in Long-Term Ostracism

We found that long-term ostracism meant different things to different people. Some people were ostracized by many individuals across the courses of their lives (provoking an attribution that perhaps they—the targets—brought it on). Others were ostracized by one person, either for a single event, in which case they endured one long continuous silent treatment (as did Lee), or for shorter bouts of the silent treatment given to them over and over again during the course of their relationship.

For example, this young girl experienced one long episode of ostracism by her schoolmates:

"In high school, the other students thought me weird and never spoke to me. I tell you in all honesty that at one stage they refused to speak to me for 153 days, not one word at all."

On the other hand, this woman experienced many episodes of the silent treatment from her father over the course of her life:

"The person who instigated the silent treatment was my father. It would happen very quickly and without any warning. The usual period of time was generally 2 weeks."

How might these two types of ostracism affect targets differently? For one thing, those who experienced one long continuous process of ostracism usually knew what had prompted it. One lady wrote:

"My husband of 45 years is giving me the silent treatment [still continuing after several months] due to the fact that someone told him I was meeting some man with whom I played bowls previously. This is quite untrue. I told him so and asked him, Who told him such lies? He wouldn't reveal his source of information but said he had also seen me meet this man. I explained he is punishing me for something I have never done. He gets up each morning, gets himself off to work, we sit at the same table and not a word is spoken and the same happens each night he eats his tea and adjourns to the lounge and watches TV and I am left to wash up, have my shower, and retire to my bed. Which I might add I've taken in the second bedroom since he accused me of this infidelity: I asked him why he didn't talk to me and why he was punishing me for something I didn't do, his reply was he had nothing to say and believes I did meet this man."

Those who experienced habitual shorter term episodes of ostracism usually indicated that they were not always aware of the reason for its use (as discussed previously). Both forms of ostracism are undoubtedly aversive, but perhaps for different reasons. Long-term continuous ostracism must be difficult simply because of its length of time and the likelihood that targets begin to see themselves as unworthy of any attention. Having to endure repeated episodes of short-term ostracism, while allowing targets brief respites of normalcy, are also mixed with higher levels of uncertainty (as to why it is occurring and when the next episode will occur).

Single or Multiple Sources

Many targets with whom we have had contact were subjected to ostracism by a single source, but some targets experienced ostracism by multiple sources. Often these multiple sources were other family members, but sometimes friends, coworkers, their church, and even the community at large ostracized targets.

"During my life from childhood to age 35 when I lived in my parent's home, my father could go up to 6 months without speaking to anyone or only one person in a family of five children. My sisters (two) and one brother (all older) used to apply the 'no speaks' to try to force me to do what they wanted and my other brother and self suffered. From age about 20 my mother applied the 'no speaks' for about 3 weeks whenever I changed employment—I worked as a secretary for many years and did not leave one position until I had another. During my marriage . . . my husband (after only 3 weeks) used the silent treatment regularly avoiding speaking to me for 3 or 4 weeks at a time although he did speak to our two daughters. The marriage ended after 21 years as I was ill and lost the energy involved in trying to provide some chat or, at least, a 'hello.' "

The woman introduced earlier who was ostracized by her high school classmates wrote:

"When I returned to school [after overdosing on Valium], the kids had heard the whole story and for a few days they were falling over themselves to be my friend. Sadly, it didn't last. They stopped talking to me again and I was devastated. I stopped talking myself then. I figured that it was useless to have a voice if no one listened."

A man wrote about his experience with ostracism from many sources when his schoolmates subjected him to it:

"I feel this descriptor is relevant to what occurred to myself at boarding school when I was in Year 7. For approximately 2 months I was excluded from any activities, social or academic, and apart from a very occasional jibe was not spoken to. I cannot remember the exact start of it but I remember they claimed to the housemaster who investigated it that I was a 'smartass' and full of myself. This may have been true as I had an elder brother at the school and was very cocky. There was also an incident where I was caught running down a dorm member to the identified best looking girl in the form. I was also newly integrated into the culture from a small rural town and my social skills were probably questionable. I remember attempting to integrate with other dormitories but was circumnavigated by my dorm members. I also remember attempting to gain their favor by acting out which resulted in my note being given to the teacher. Extra activities were occasionally conducted as I remember having to raise early to have a shower as they made sure they were kept full to prevent usage, and my journal being read to everyone when they stole it."

Another woman was ostracized by all the members of her family. She wrote:

"Too many times I realized I was always the last one to be involved in family plans (parties, family meals, outings, or picnics). Everything had always been discussed and decided upon when it got to me as though my opinions didn't matter. In 1990 I realized that phone calls and invitations from me were never returned. I wrote letters and they were not answered. Gradually everyone stopped talking to me. It was as though I ceased to exist. Family members actually turned their backs on me (at family funerals) and kept walking if I tried to catch up to talk. Even jumping in a car and racing off sooner than talk to me."

Being ostracized by one person, either continuously or frequently, is clearly painful, especially when the source of the ostracism is an important person in the life of the target. However, it may be even more painful for people who are ostracized by multiple sources. Attributions for a single source's behavior can plausibly rest on that source's cold shoulders. One can at least entertain the idea that it is something about him or her (the source) that makes him or her act so peculiar. When many people ostracize an individual, however, dispositional attributions to their characters become less plausible, and the target is left to bear more of the responsibility for their treatment.

Consequences of Long-Term Ostracism

How do targets of long-term ostracism think that it affects them? Clearly, these self-generated diagnoses must be considered at best possible and at worst inaccurate. Regardless of accuracy, such beliefs are worthy of examination. Targets report consequences ranging from self-destructive behaviors (indiscriminant bonding, suicidal thoughts and attempts, alcoholism) to aversive effects of ostracism on their physical and mental health. The woman ostracized by her high school classmates wrote:

"That was a very low point for me in my life and on the 153rd day [of being ostracized by her schoolmates], I swallowed 29 Valium pills. My brother found me and called an ambulance."

A woman whose mother and sister continue to give her and her daughter long episodes of the silent treatment wrote:

"I have and do suffer from deep depression and a feeling of worthlessness, and have contemplated suicide several times. Even though I consider myself a Christian, these thoughts still creep into my brain when I am at my most depressed. The only thing that is keeping me going is my daughter and what would happen to her should I die. I couldn't bear the thought of her suffering the same silent treatment though her life."

Other symptoms are less severe, but mentioned frequently, as is the case with this middle-aged woman:

"Why I am writing to you is that I can't take this treatment any longer—it's affecting my health. I suffer with severe headaches which all stem from tension."

In fact, almost all of our follow-up target interviewees (which will be examined more fully in Chapter 10) have volunteered that their physical and psychological health has suffered as a consequence of enduring ostracism. These include self-injurious behavioral patterns such as anorexia and bulimia, and most interesting, promiscuity, or what we refer to as "indiscriminate bonding." Our first indication of this consequence occurred in an interview with a woman in Toledo, Ohio, who said that, because of her father's constant silent treatment, she became promiscuous, seeking comfort and recognition of her worth by forming many brief sexual relationships with men. More recently, a woman wrote:

"[My husband's behavior] was affecting my physical and mental health. To compensate for the big freeze I had been submitted to I formed an inappropriate relationship which led to further complications in my life. I have lived a somewhat hermit-like existence since 1982 and restrict myself to a few loyal friends I can trust. I suffered loss of self-esteem, loss of control, loss of a sense of belonging, alienated and depressed. I still have a meaningful existence due to the cultural values passed on to me by my parents."

It may be that a lack of recognition and sense of belonging, coupled with an internalized feeling of low worth, motivate individuals to seek out others who will recognize their existence. Perhaps the standards that they apply to these others are substantially lower than otherwise would be the case, leading them to form ill-advised relationships with other individuals or groups.

Coping Strategies of Targets

Many targets have contacted us to ask how they should cope with their treatment. The words of this woman targeted by frequent episodes of the silent treatment in her life are common:

"I find *not speaking* a useless exercise and after all this practice, at
age 74, am still not able to cope so avoid anyone who tries it."

Perhaps not realizing it, she developed a behavioral strategy for coping
with people who use the silent treatment: she avoids them (another form
of ostracism?). A few targets, however, have described conscious strategies (cognitive or behavioral) that they claim have helped them cope
with the silent treatment. One woman, whose husband is prone to using
the silent treatment for 1 or 2 days for reasons of which she is unaware,
has accepted the periodic silence as nothing more than one of her husband's tendencies. She says she doesn't take it personally and she knows
it will end. Her strategy is to continue talking to her husband as though
he is talking back. She will say "What do you want for dinner?" and
then carry on a back-and-forth about various menu options. She even
grabs him by the arm and hauls him off to the movies. Eventually, he
wears down and begins to talk with her. Admittedly, this is the only person I know who has talked about using this technique, and it is not
likely that it would work for others. Even this woman describes the difficulty she and her husband have in returning to normal communications
after periods of the silent treatment:

"The most difficult aspect of this freezing out or directed venomous
silence is reestablishing a connection again. I read somewhere that
you should always be the first to start the peace process (women always are—nearly). Consequently, I'm the one who usually does 'the
bridge.' That's what we call extending ourselves to break the silence. That may come through touch, humor, or a few words that
have a bit of expression in them and are not purely information giving (e.g., so-and-so called)."

Most targets have not found a way to bring the source of ostracism
back into the fold of a normal communicative relationship. Instead, they
learn to cope internally. Here, on the surface, a woman claims she grew
to accept, enjoy, and even joke about her father's silent treatment. However, reading deeper into her statement, one gets the sense that her claims
are hollow:

"As I grew older the silent treatment didn't affect me at all, as I developed a mechanism/attitude to deal with the situation. Basically the
silent treatment was a good thing for me. . . . It even got to the stage
where I was joking about it to my mother, especially when the silent
treatment would go over the 2-week period. I would say, 'Wow he's
broken his record' etc. The last silent treatment I received was about
6 years ago when I went to work at an American summer camp

against my father's wishes. He thought the camp was going to be in Australia. One night at the local golf club I told him where I was going—the United States. During the course of the conversation he told me I wasn't allowed to go, and if I did that I wouldn't be welcomed in the house when I got back. At 23 years I rebelled against my father and went to the United States for 4 months. When I got back home he acted as if I didn't exist (in his eyes I was dead to him), that he no longer had a daughter. My father was an expert at this. I got home in August and until I moved to Sydney in February he didn't speak to me once. To this day he has never broken his record for the silent treatment. It will be 7 years in May next year since my biological father has spoken to me. I am better off this way. A relative once told me that I should go and talk to him, but my reply was 'Why should I?' At the present time my father is living by himself and has no contact with any of his so-called family. Apparently to him he has no family; we are all dead to him."

Like this Australian woman, many targets have indicated that the only way to cope with ostracism is to leave and rebuild their lives:

"When my third husband and I finally separated, for the fifth time in 9 years and after having him live in our garage for 12 months prior to this separation, I only felt relief and contentment when he was finally forced to leave. I broke up with my third husband in December, 1995, and this year met a kind, gentle man who treats me with dignity and respect and finds it extremely difficult to comprehend the lifestyle I've led up until the past few years. I have learnt to become assertive, confident, and like myself over the last 2 years and can no longer 'sit back' and allow anyone to treat me hardly nor react in a negative way."

Another woman wrote:

"My mother died when I was 30. It was quite difficult [for me]: she died during one of her silent periods and had not spoken to me for over 3 weeks. My father died a few years later; before he died he revealed that once my mother had gone 8 weeks without speaking to him. I grieved and missed my parents but with the death of my parents and the silent treatment a new freedom began, a time to be me and to fulfill my dreams."

When I talk about my research, the question I am most frequently asked is, "How does a person cope with ostracism, especially within the context of close personal relationships?" At present, this appears to be the question that will pose the most difficulty in my program of research.

SOURCES' PERSPECTIVES

Before we become so enmeshed in characterizing sources of ostracism as one-dimensional and evil, let us consider a story from Bill, the father of a teenaged son.

"Not so long ago, I had a row with my son, which was terminated by his use of extremely violent and foul language at me. I was so shocked and outraged by this incident that I instinctively, that is, without any thought about what should be my appropriate response, instigated a regimen of ostracism toward him. I did not speak to him, I did not acknowledge anything he said to me, or anyone else, in fact. I acted as if he were not even present. I did not set a place for him at the table nor did I provide for him in any meals that I prepared for the family.

"As I said, I slipped into this, although for me novel, paradigm without any premeditation and, hence, without any difficulty, and maintained it comfortably as if it were the natural way of family relationships. I was able to perpetuate it easily and without any discomfort for myself.

"After 2 weeks, I woke up one morning with a blinding flash of insight: 'What are you doing to your relationship with your son?' In that short period my son had already become intimidated by this treatment—he did exactly what his mother said at all times and whenever he spoke it was in a quiet whisper. I am ashamed to say that I was sort of pleased with the effect of my ostracism but, as I say, one day I suddenly realized that it was making him weak and submissive and that it was eroding the future quality of our relationship.

"To terminate the ostracism, however, was an extremely difficult process. I could only begin with grudging, monosyllabic responses to his indirect overtures. I was only able to expand on these responses with the passing of time and it is only now, about 6 weeks since the ostracism ceased that our relationship appears to be getting back to prerow normality. The pain and stress from a period of ostracism clearly impact on the principals for far longer than the actual period of ostracism.

"On your radio program last week, the case was mentioned of a husband who ostracized his wife for 40 years. I suspect that, in that particular case, the longer the ostracism persisted, the harder it became to stop, such that there came a point when, no matter how much that husband wanted to speak to his wife, it was just too difficult to do. This is what I felt after just 2 weeks of ostracism of my son—that if it had lasted much longer I might have not have been able to stop and that not only would our relationship have been de-

stroyed but also my son himself might have been permanently emotionally and physiologically disfigured. Further, as also suggested on
the radio program, it may even have led to illness and perhaps, ultimately, to his premature death.

"So the point of this letter is just to say that ostracism can be
like a whirlpool, or quicksand, if you, the user, don't extract yourself from it as soon as possible, it is likely to become impossible to
terminate regardless of the emergence of any subsequent will to do
so.

"The use of ostracism against one's immediate family might be
an instinctive reaction but its effects may be horrific. I have been
deeply shocked by the effect of its use in my family and will ensure
that it never happens again.

"I hope that this anecdote will help to add weight to any thesis
that you may be developing such that some good may come from
that harrowing experience."

Although similar in sentiment to many of the other source accounts,
this particular letter articulated best how ostracism can be perpetuated
for so long. It suggests that long-term ostracism may not be planned by
the source, but that there is something so addictive about the act of
maintaining silence and pretending that someone does not exist that it
becomes extremely difficult for sources to break with its use. In this father's letter, we can see hints about what causes this form of punishment
to become like "quicksand."

First, it is extremely effective, perhaps more effective than arguing,
yelling, or hitting. It was so effective that it both surprised and pleased
the father. Second, one can imagine what would have happened had the
father started to talk normally to his son after his demonstrative display
of silence. It would have been like an apology to admit that he had been
wrong to punish his son in the first place, and to acknowledge having
gone to such bizarre extremes such as not setting a place for his son at
the table. Finally, it seems as though the control and power that ostracism initially affords sources of ostracism suddenly comes back in full
force to control them. Let us briefly examine the letters from sources of
ostracism to see how they explain their behavior.

Reasons for Ostracizing

Unlike targets' claims that sources have no reasons or only trivial reasons to ostracize, sources give rational explanations for their behavior.
Consider the following letter from a woman who explains why she and
her coworkers are ostracizing their supervisor:

"My colleagues and I . . . work in the hospitality industry and our co-ordinator [manager] refuses to do any work—all she does is sit at her desk all day and read magazines. This has been going on for 9 months, so for the last three months we have given her the silent treatment. We felt that under the circumstances if she is not going to help us, then the best thing to do is completely ignore her. We now feel that it is all too much for her and life is a bit lonely at the top! It must be rather humiliating not to be spoken to day after day, and the lines of communication have completely broken down. The executive officer who is the boss above her has told us that we all have to work together as a team, but I'm afraid the damage is done and things won't right themselves as it's too far gone. The staff all work well together and the business has not deteriorated because of it, so we will just carry on as we are and continue the silent treatment. As for how she feels, I think deep down inside she is feeling the strain of it all, and she is losing control."

For this woman and her colleagues, the target basically asked for it. She wasn't a contributing group member, so they felt they needed to eliminate her from the group. From her description, her group is effective, and perhaps even more cohesive than before—the ostracism was justified.

As was the case with Bill, some explain that giving the silent treatment is their method of last resort. Only after other methods have failed do they consider using ostracism. Consider this young woman, who finds she is sometimes pushed into using the silent treatment:

"[I give the silent treatment only when] I can't match his quick-wittedness and retorts. I get too confused and too tongue-tied. I get tongue-tied and can't think straight so I just shut up because I don't want to put my foot in my mouth any further."

But for others the use of ostracism (i.e., the silent treatment) is clearly their first line of defense:

"I have often given the silent treatment to my husband, as I believed it was my best weapon. I believe it's . . . the most powerful weapon of the giver."

This next woman seems almost proud of the strategy of silence that she has discovered. In fact, she has perfected the technique down to specific details:

"I wipe them completely off the face of the earth. That means that I don't acknowledge them, I don't speak to them. Sometimes 'the glare' goes with the silence, but most of the time it's the silence and the stiff jaw. Stiff jaw, nose up . . . and give 'em the half-shut eye. Sort of dismissive glare, turn your head away. . . . "

Perhaps using the silent treatment as the last resort, seeing its effectiveness, feeling its power, leads some sources to using it as their first line of defense.

Short- and Long-Term Consequences of Habitually Using Ostracism

Most sources claim that the act of pretending that others do not exist is empowering. It gives them an enormous sense of control over their targets—control they may not otherwise experience. They observe that it brings their targets "to their knees," causing the targets to be overly compliant, even apologetic. Consider the thoughts of this young woman:

> "I am married with a 4-year-old daughter. I have often given the silent treatment to my husband, as I believed it *was my best weapon*. Before I got married 5 years ago I had no reason to use the silent treatment on anyone. Certain circumstances have changed all that. I don't use it as often as I once did, but I still resort to it when I have to. I believe it's . . . the most powerful weapon of the giver. It can make a grown man cry, without having to hit him over the head."

But there is an ironic twist to these feelings of control that some sources have noted. Like Bill, sources sense that at some point they themselves are controlled by the ostracism and find it difficult to stop using it. It is highly unlikely that Lee's husband (whose case began this chapter, in which he gave Lee the silent treatment for 40 years) would have imagined that his silent treatment would have lasted so long. Why does it? Bill suggested that the use of the silent treatment becomes self-perpetuating such that it becomes nearly impossible to break the cycle of using it.

Another explanation for sources' tendencies to use ostracism is that it has something to do with their personalities, particularly that they are stubborn or are well suited to holding grudges forever, as is the case with this middle-aged woman:

> "I'll hold a grudge till the day I die. I've still got a grudge against a 6-year-old boy who got me into trouble for playing 'I'll show you mine if you show me yours' behind the bike shed when we were in kindergarten."

Here, the self-described characteristic of stubbornness is used to account for its use, as this woman suggests in describing how both she and her husband use the silent treatment on each other:

> "We are both very, very stubborn. Sometimes we'll make the other really work to reestablish a communication zone. It's humiliating and degrading and childish and it makes me wonder about our relationship altogether."

Others, like the following woman, suggest that by using the silent treatment, they are able to offset the other person's power so that they might level the playing field:

> "I believe that it is a means of control and it empowers the person who is giving 'the silent treatment' and disempowers those upon whom it is being inflicted."

Still others suggest that their use of the silent treatment is more admirable (because it is more deniable?) than voicing their displeasure in other ways. This woman defends her use of the silent treatment to her former friend:

> "I recall feeling virtuous in that I did not raise my voice or become a nag but I also pretty well knew that the recipient would have preferred a chance at 'a verbal'—to talk/shout/clear the air."

Being exposed to the silent treatment within one's family while growing up is one of the most commonly voiced attributions for its habitual use as an adult. One target proclaimed:

> "It seems to be a learned behavior. And it affects every member of a family in which it is used."

This woman lamented her father's use of the silent treatment, claiming she vowed never to use it herself when she grew up:

> "I have given the silent treatment on occasions to people who have hurt me badly, but eventually start speaking to them again. However, I never forget and never forgive them. I too have stopped speaking to two people forever—that being my father and the boy who tried to rape me. My feeling toward them is I hope they both rot in hell for what they did to me. I can say my father taught me one thing at least—the silent treatment."

Another example of familial learning comes from this woman:

> "My partner and I have lived together for 10–11 years and we have tried to speak about and change our behaviors, but at this very moment I am giving him the silent treatment. This silence has lasted only about 24 hours. However, we have gone 1 whole week without speaking to one another. It is stressful, depressing, taxing, and painful. I also know it is very controlling. This behavior I learned from the best silent treatment giver in the world and that's my mother. She went for years with very little expression on her face, slamming things around, keeping her lips as thin as a dime."

And, in another example, a woman reports:

> "I was brought up in a family where my mother was the main exponent of inflicting the silent treatment on people—especially those close to her. She was raised by a mother who practiced the same methods. As a result, she and her two sisters also use silence as a means of expressing (or not expressing) their displeasure, My grandmother could go for months, even years, withholding communication. I am 35-years-old and I too have a tendency to use the silent treatment."

This woman admitted to having used the silent treatment in her family only to have learned of its destructiveness when her son used it on her.

> "I have been the recipient of the silent treatment for 2½ years by my now 17-year-old son. I have contacted lots of psychologists, counselors, privately and through the school, and have not been able to get any closer to solving this deadlock situation than I was at the beginning. My son decided to stop talking when I didn't accept his destructive behavior toward his brother. I pointed out to him that his brother's possessions, in that instance his plants, should be left alone in the garden and he had no right to kick them and damage them. It was culmination of sibling rivalry. I was told by a teacher friend of mine that this kind of ostracism must be learned behavior. I have to agree, since my father's response to anything unpalatable was always the silent treatment, or as my mother used to call it, '*das Scheigen im Walde*' (the silence in the forest). Analyzing myself in that respect, I have to concede that I responded that way too over the years, not over extended periods, but I did opt for 'not speaking' rather than confrontation, dialogue, or discussion. If anything, I have learned from my son how demoralizing, hurting, and bitter this treatment is and have stopped acting that way."

One woman noted how her use of the silent treatment seems to have been picked up already by her 4-year-old son:

"I'm probably passing it on to my 4-year-old because when he gets angry, he storms off. . . . He'll tell my youngest son 'Don't talk to Mum, I'm angry at her!' "

Finally, one woman sees her use of the silent treatment as involuntary, even physiological:

"Well, I wish I could just blow my top when people hurt me. But I can't, that's what it's all about. The left side of my chest closes off like a door shutting, and I can't talk. If it's a real bad hurt my whole chest closes off and its impossible to talk about it. And very often it doesn't seem to affect me, but goes straight to my chest and I have to stop and think what did that idiot say to affect me this way just as though there is some one greater than me taking offense at what's said. I really don't think I'm madder than anyone else. It just happens. It can take 3 days to a fortnight before I can get over it. Then it's gone. And I'll never bring the subject up again, especially to the ones I should."

The reasons that sources give for their long-term use of ostracism are varied. Some say they learned its power and technique early in their lives, but others suggest that they have come upon it only recently in their adult lives. Some, like Bill, seem to stumble upon it and watch themselves become enmeshed by it. Others see it as a response unique to their relationship (to level the playing field), while others simply reciprocate its use when it is used on them. Clearly, there is no single cause for its onset, but all agree that it is, at least in the short term, effective, empowering, and powerful.

What Do Sources Say Can Stop Them?

There appear to be two types of sources: the penitent and the proud. For the proud, there may be very little that can be done to stop them. Indeed, reading this chapter may make them more likely to use forms of ostracism because it will reinforce their view that it is powerful and effective. As one woman asserted:

"I'm gonna use the silent treatment till the day I die."

Likewise, a 65-year-old woman said:

"I use the silent treatment whenever there may be a fight or confrontation. The silent treatment accomplishes for me all the things that fighting does for other people: control, power, and punishment. It gives me pleasure, and I'm in control. I also think it is funny how people grovel. I never feel guilty or ashamed; because it's always justifiable. . . . The Rolling Stones talk about satisfaction. This is how I get mine."

The penitent, however, are a different story. They are sorry they used it, or that they still use it. They try not to use it, sometimes successfully, other times not. This woman's mother used the silent treatment on her from the time she was 14 years old. She wrote:

"I promised myself I would not repeat the pattern on my own children and was horrified when my eldest entered the teenage years and I found myself 'going silent' after one of our bouts. After a lot of hard work on my part I broke the cycle and am happy to say I have a great relationship with all my children."

Others have been more successful at suppressing their urge to use the silent treatment. One woman wrote:

"At times I have felt myself resorting to silent treatment of my children or husband but have been very aware of it and force myself to talk things out that same day, and not let things get how they were between my mother and me. I hated that."

Just as targets seem to have few answers on how to cope with the silent treatment, so sources have few suggestions as to how to get them to stop from using it. One source, however, offered a suggestion of what does not work:

"I get really mad when they go 'I don't know what I've done wrong.' Then I get even quieter. . . . I think that if they do something that bad and they don't know what they've done wrong, they are really stupid."

Do Sources Experience Any Negative Side Effects?

Despite gaining power and control over their targets, there is some indication that giving the silent treatment takes its toll on the sources as well. It is effortful, especially the "noisy" silent treatments that involve considerable thought, attention, and self-regulation. Take for instance this man (described earlier in the chapter), whose wife describes his silent treatment repertoire as consisting of:

(1) avoiding any bodily contact (i.e., would walk past you sideways so as not to touch you); (2) slept on the lounge or in the car until you begged him not to; (3) refused to eat any meals; (4) took away all financial support (i.e.,

had bank accounts transferred into his own name and allowed you no access to them); (5) refused to let you use the car.

Undoubtedly, having to attend carefully and constantly to one's own behavior in order to avoid the mistake of acknowledging another person's existence will deplete one's cognitive and emotional resources for other important activities. As one woman wrote:

"It is stressful, depressing, taxing, and painful."

Unlike targets, sources do not dwell on the psychological and physiological costs that they endure as a consequence of using ostracism on others. Whether there are such costs to them warrants further investigation.

CONCLUSIONS

I have presented several cases of real incidences of long-term ostracism. They reveal to us a remarkable breadth of experiences for targets and sources, and the variety of forms ostracism can take. They also inform us about the powerful effects that ostracism might have on its targets and even on its sources.

Our investigations into the causes and consequences of ostracism are aimed at determining the validity of the themes suggested in these cases. To do this, we take a variety of paths of inquiry. Some paths involve experiential simulations, others involve experimental laboratory manipulations, and still others rely on careful analysis of structured interviews. We look not only to social and situational causes of its use and impact, but on potential individual differences that lead some people to use ostracism habitually, and that make some people particularly susceptible to its impact. We hope that these paths lead us to some clearer understanding of this powerful and frequently used interpersonal behavior.

NOTE

1. See also Chapter 10, in the section, "Structured Interviews of Individuals with Long-Term Experience with Ostracism" for further discussion of the stories included in this chapter.

A Model of Ostracism

The preceding chapters described the broad varieties of ostracism, according to the personal accounts of those who used it on others and those on whom it was used. Personal accounts are valuable because they provide us with a richness of description and a depth of impact that is often missed in abstract theory and the responses to scaled questions used in experimental research. They are the first step in understanding the nature of the phenomenon. The next step is to formulate an integrated understanding of ostracism on which a program of research can be based. To this end, I present a model of ostracism in this chapter.

The development of a working model of ostracism is useful for a number of reasons. First, the phenomenon is sufficiently complex that it is imprecise to refer simply to "ostracism" and assume that (1) we are all envisioning the same sort of thing; and (2) the same causes and consequences hold true for all varieties of ostracism. Thus, one aim of the model is to offer taxonomic dimensions that allow us to pigeonhole specific types of ostracism. In this way, when I speak of one form of ostracism, others will know what I am talking about. While this may satisfy those who simply like to classify things, I did not undertake this task for that reason. Rather, it was my hunch that all forms of ostracism did not operate in the same way. Even though all forms of ostracism contain the common elements of ignoring and excluding, my observations led me to believe that various forms of ostracism were likely to have different causes, serve different purposes, produce different consequences, and have different interpretations.

Thus, I felt that it would oversimplify things to postulate that ostracism per se, no matter what its context, intention, or interpretation, always had the same effect. For example, would we imagine that an individual who was not acknowledged by a fellow elevator rider would feel the same as an individual who is not acknowledged by his or her friend? In both cases, an incident of ostracism has occurred, although some might not be inclined to label the elevator incident as ostracism. Why not? Imagine for a moment that we are interplanetary aliens visiting Earth for the first time. Imagine further that we understand the concept of ostracism to mean behavioral instances in which individuals (or groups) deliberately ignore and exclude other individuals (or groups). Given this definition, we would define the event that happened in the elevator as ostracism. But, because we are residents of Earth and understand the complex norms of our society, we may interpret the elevator incident to be normal, unremarkable, and inconsequential. Because of this, we may decide that it was not ostracism. But should its presumed effects define ostracism? If so, the definition and its effects become circular, preventing us from understanding why in some instances the same behavior is benign, whereas in other instances it can be devastating. This is precisely the reason that we need to have some sort of classification system, one that will indicate the incidences of ostracism that will have impact, and the sort of impact they might be likely to have. The primary reason for using this classification system is to suggest that an act of ostracism may or may not have particular consequences depending upon what form it takes and how it is understood. The taxonomic dimensions that I employ are incorporated into the theory so that my predictions take into account the type of ostracism about which we are talking.

The second reason for generating a model is that it allows the researcher to keep in mind the "big picture" during the course of the investigations. As each study progresses it becomes clearer how one set of findings may inform other aspects of the phenomenon—aspects that might otherwise be overlooked. Being mindful of the big picture also assists the researcher to undertake a systematic investigation of the phenomenon. It permits an accumulation of knowledge in such a way that each finding becomes a piece of a puzzle that ultimately will fit together. Without a model, knowledge would be uncovered haphazardly and relations between the findings would be less apparent. Instead, we may simply be left with a collection of factoids that do not enlighten us about the nature of ostracism. Previous work on ostracism was often characterized by a single experiment that had little or no big-picture context. It is not surprising, then, that the researchers themselves did not sustain an interest in conducting follow-up studies, and that their studies did not stimulate others to replicate and extend their findings, to determine limiting conditions, and to connect the findings to the broader social psychological literature.

The third reason for developing a model is that hypotheses can be derived from it that might not otherwise have been considered. Because the model presents an interrelated series of connections between types, causes, and consequences, testing one aspect of the model may inform another, and another, and so on. The results of one study testing one part of the model can trigger hypotheses that test other aspects of the model. The generation of new hypotheses can allow for tests of the model, such that it could be disconfirmed, qualified, or supported. This is perhaps the most useful aspect of working within the framework of a theoretical model.

There are, of course, disadvantages to generating a model to be used to guide an investigation, especially if it is done too early. A model can shroud the researcher with empirical blinders such that he or she rejects new findings or new ways of thinking because they do not fit the model. Without a model, a researcher might be more likely to follow his or her experimental findings wherever they may lead, resulting in potentially important serendipitous findings. Therefore, although the model guides me, I make a conscious attempt to remain curious about and fascinated by unexpected results. I have purposefully approached the phenomenon using a variety of methods, exploratory, descriptive, and observational, so that I would not be restricted by a single paradigm. Finally, I am constantly revising the model according to these unexpected findings. As such, this is truly a working model that informs, but is also informed by, the research.

THE MODEL

I present and refer to the model depicted in Figure 3.1 (see also Williams, 1997). I will describe the model presented in Figure 3.1 from top to bottom, although the model is not necessarily one that requires sequential investigations. That is, one can "jump around" in the model, searching the ostracism puzzle's border pieces as well as its middle pieces in no particular order.

I first discuss the classification of taxonomic dimensions (shown in the top left box of Figure 3.1). Then, I suggest possible antecedents of ostracism (top right box) and discuss potential moderators and/or mediators of its impact (the box one level down). The crux of the theoretical model is the postulate that four needs are affected by ostracism (the box two levels down). I propose that there is a temporal component to individuals' reactions to threatened needs. As a simplification to a temporal continuum, I consider three different time periods: immediate, short-term, and long-term reactions to ostracism (bottom box).

The primary purpose of the model is to delineate the consequences of ostracism on the person or groups who are being ostracized. The model is concerned with how individuals (1) perceive that they may be

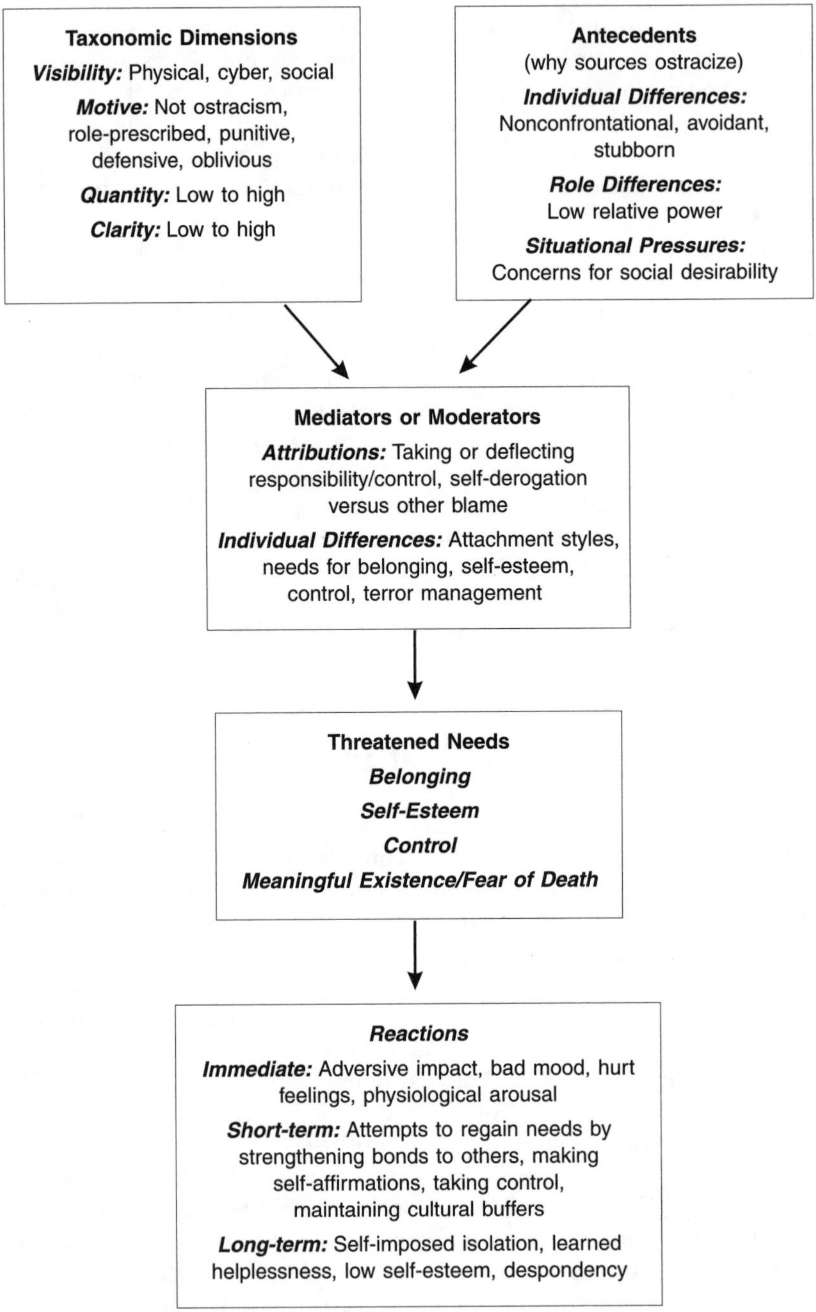

Taxonomic Dimensions

Visibility: Physical, cyber, social

Motive: Not ostracism, role-prescribed, punitive, defensive, oblivious

Quantity: Low to high

Clarity: Low to high

Antecedents
(why sources ostracize)

Individual Differences: Nonconfrontational, avoidant, stubborn

Role Differences: Low relative power

Situational Pressures: Concerns for social desirability

Mediators or Moderators

Attributions: Taking or deflecting responsibility/control, self-derogation versus other blame

Individual Differences: Attachment styles, needs for belonging, self-esteem, control, terror management

Threatened Needs

Belonging

Self-Esteem

Control

Meaningful Existence/Fear of Death

Reactions

Immediate: Adversive impact, bad mood, hurt feelings, physiological arousal

Short-term: Attempts to regain needs by strengthening bonds to others, making self-affirmations, taking control, maintaining cultural buffers

Long-term: Self-imposed isolation, learned helplessness, low self-esteem, despondency

FIGURE 3.1. Williams's (1997) model of ostracism.

targets of ostracism, (2) attempt to construct explanations for the ostracism, (3) vary in terms of their susceptibility to ostracism, and (4) react (physiologically, emotionally, cognitively, and behaviorally) to the threat to any or all four fundamental needs. Finally, their reactions are hypothesized to depend upon (5) how long they were exposed to the ostracism. Because the emphasis is on the targets' phenomenology, ostracism is hypothesized to have effects only when it is interpreted by the target him- or herself as ostracism, irrespective of whether the source intended the act to be ostracism. As long as targets think they are being ostracized, they will be affected by it.

Nevertheless, parts of the model are applicable to sources, and other parts may provide us with some direction when trying to understand how and why sources ostracize and what effects it has on them. For instance, when examining antecedents of ostracism, we consider the factors that lead sources to ostracize others. These factors may be emanating from characteristics of the targets, from the sources themselves, or from the situation. The classification of ostracism into different types may also apply to sources. On the one hand, a source may intentionally ostracize another person for purposes of punishment, or preemptively to defend against being harmed in some way by the person he or she chooses to ostracize. On the other hand, a source's act of ignoring may be completely unintentional, or may reflect a remotely conscious decision that the target simply did not matter enough to him or her to bother acknowledging. The sources' motives may influence how they behaviorally act out the ostracism. Finally, I propose that the same fundamental needs that ostracism can threaten in targets may be similarly threatened (or perhaps fortified) in the individuals who employ the ostracism. Whereas the model was not intentionally designed to predict specific effects on sources, it may nevertheless provide a beginning framework with which to explore the behaviors of ostracizers and the reactions they experience. I end the chapter by putting forth specific model-driven hypotheses regarding sources' intentions and behaviors and the consequences of ostracizing.

TAXONOMIC DIMENSIONS

The model describes the complexity of ostracism by classifying episodes of ostracism along four dimensions: *visibility, motive, quantity,* and *causal clarity.* I consider these dimensions theoretically independent and orthogonal to each other, but I concede that in certain cells of this large matrix real-life instances of ostracism might be virtually empty or substantially overrepresented.

Ambiguity

A recurrent theme in the four dimensions is the underlying ambiguity that seems peculiarly linked with episodes of ostracism. Unlike other forms of explicit rejection or derogation, such as verbal or physical aggression, ostracism could be considered a nonbehavior (or the absence of behavior), and as such is less tangible. Often ostracism occurs without explanation, making it difficult for the target of the ostracism to know whether it is really occurring. Sometimes it is perceived by targets even when it is not intended; other times it could be intended by the source, but not perceived by the target. Because ostracism can be employed in total or partial forms, as when the target of ostracism is still acknowledged but to a lesser degree than usual, targets may again have difficulty knowing for sure if they are truly being subjected to an ostracism episode.

The ambiguity that may be inextricably tied to ostracism can make the ostracism more powerful, or it may provide sources and targets a safe haven of suspended belief. For instance, if someone is suddenly on the receiving end of a possible episode of the silent treatment that is not set off by something obvious or announced by the source, then the inherent ambiguity of his or her situation may cause the target to generate a multitude of plausible reasons for deserving such treatment. Being forced to consider multiple reasons may result in higher levels of self-derogation than would likely have been the case if the precipitating cause of the silent treatment was clear, thereby making the ostracism more powerful. On the other hand, both targets and sources of ambiguous ostracism may be able to pretend that nothing is happening. By not forcing the issue by seeking clarification, both sides can convince themselves that nothing is wrong. In either case, the ambiguity of the specific episode needs to be considered, and may be related systematically to subcategories within each dimension.

Visibility

Imagine three instances that may occur in a prototypical situation. In the first, a married couple has a heated argument. After several rounds of mutual verbal assault, the wife leaves the room and locks herself in the bathroom. In the second, after the initial verbal argument, both partners remain in the room but stop talking, acting as though the other partner no longer exists. In the third, the argument develops over the course of e-mail messages. Suddenly, one partner no longer replies to the other's messages. These three instances are examples of the three levels in the visibility dimension: physical ostracism, social ostracism, and cyberostracism.

Physical ostracism involves withdrawing from or leaving the situation (e.g., leaving a room during an argument, being put in solitary confinement, being exiled). Physical ostracism describes the loss of visibility inherent in physical separation, which includes expulsion, banishment, exile, solitary confinement, time-out in a separate room, "being sent to Coventry," or, at an interpersonal level, spending less or no time with an individual, or removing oneself from his or her presence.

Social ostracism involves an emotional withdrawal that occurs in the physical presence of the target (e.g., removal of eye contact, not talking, and not listening). The source and the target, in social ostracism, remain visible to each other. Common terms such as "silent treatment," "cold shoulder," and "freezing out" are likely to refer to social ostracism. Ironically, even though victims are visible during social ostracism, it is with this type of ostracism that targets may actually feel invisible; victims of physical ostracism who are in fact not seen probably do not feel invisible.

Cyberostracism encompasses all forms of being ignored or left out in interactions other than those that are face to face, such as not receiving mail (whether e-mail or posted letters), phone calls, or other forms of communication (e.g., memos), or being ignored in chat rooms, MUDs (multiuser domains), or other forms of interpersonal communication or participation on the Internet.

Physical versus Social Ostracism

Separating ostracism into three levels of visibility is important only insofar as the levels produce different effects on targets. At present, my thinking has focused more on the difference between physical and social ostracism, so allow me to compare these two first. I offer some thoughts about cyberostracism at the end of this section. I propose that, to some degree, the power of ostracism lies within what it may symbolize to the target in its most extreme form. Physical ostracism symbolizes permanent exit, meaning that no further contact will occur. The targeted individual can nevertheless surmise that he or she is capable of being acknowledged, so much so that the source must physically leave in order to eliminate the target's influence over him or her. Social ostracism, however, symbolizes something quite different. Because the source has not removed him- or herself physically from the target, the source is communicating the message that the target's presence is inconsequential to him or her. Instead of symbolizing exit, social ostracism symbolizes death. This assertion is often met with considerable skepticism, but stay with me for a moment. The source is in effect saying, "This is what I would be doing if you did not even exist." Targets of social ostracism cannot make the assumption that their existence is acknowledged and influential, which they can do when they are physically ostracized. Instead, they are left to consider the symbolic message that they are invisible to the source, they have no influence, and they are not there. Obviously, I am not saying that targets consciously consider this possibility every time they are socially ostracized. What I am saying is that this notion of their invisibility and inconsequentiality is subconsciously primed and has devastating potential. In this regard, I view social ostracism to be far more insidious than physical ostracism.

If we consider not the symbolic but the more concrete message communicated by the three levels of visibility, we are also left to surmise that physical ostracism has the lowest potential for harm. Physical ostracism signals disapproval and an unwillingness to engage in bilateral conflict resolution. But it also permits thoughtful reflection regarding behaviors that caused the ostracism in the first place and a chance for the individuals involved to "cool down" or to prevent the escalation of regrettable words or actions. In this sense, physical ostracism, which may in some ways seem the most extreme form, may be easiest to cope with. Thoughtful introspection and deescalation of anger may be more difficult to accomplish while being socially ostracized. During social ostracism, one is continuously reminded about being ignored. As Boehm (1986) states, "To inflict such exclusionary treatment on a living person who has nowhere else to go is an ultimate punishment—in some ways worse than solitary confinement or death, since the person is reminded continually of the active and total rejection that is taking place" (pp. 313–314). Instead of allowing the individual to reflect upon whatever instigated the conflict, social ostracism might result in increasing anger or hurt, persistent attempts to recapture the attention of the ostracizer (e.g., by insincere apology, or by escalating verbal or physical abuse), or retaliation in kind.

Is ambiguity systematically linked to subcategories of ostracism? If so, in which subcategory of visibility is the ostracism least ambiguous? It could be argued that physical ostracism is the least ambiguous. Except for not knowing how long the physical ostracism will last (which, admittedly, could be a very important type of ambiguity), the target has clear evidence that the source is no longer in his or her presence. Exclusion and ignoring have occurred. In social ostracism, the source is still present; all bonds have not been severed—there is still a visual bond—and a clear decipherable act of separation has not taken place. The point here is that each level of visibility may be more or less likely to be ambiguous, which may have implications for interpreting and coping with ostracism down the line.

Cyberostracism

Should cyberostracism produce different outcomes from social or physical ostracism? In one respect, it is similar to physical ostracism: the target cannot see the source. However, with cyberostracism the mode of communication (e-mail or regular mail) is the expected form of connection. That is, one would probably only feel cyberostracized to the extent that some form of nonvisual communication was expected. If one participated in a routine mail exchange and suddenly one stopped receiving replies to one's letters, then one might feel cyberostracized. But if an exchange of letters was not expected, then it is unlikely that an individual would feel ignored or excluded by not getting a letter in reply. Thus, the fact that visibility is not broken off or removed makes cyberostracism different from physical ostracism. If, however, the routine mail (or e-mail) messages cease to arrive, then there is a similarity to physical ostracism in that the source is no longer in the electronic (or communicative) presence of the target. As such, I would expect the effects to be largely similar to physical ostracism.

There can also be similarities between cyberostracism and social ostracism, in that with certain types of nonvisual (mostly electronic) communication there is still an implied presence of the other person. For instance, if messages are being sent back and forth among a group within a chat room, but no messages are being directed to one specific individual, then that individual is likely to feel ostracized while still in the electronic presence of the others. The same thing applies to those interminable silences that occur occasionally during a telephone conversation that is going awry. Thus, cyberostracism itself may communicate the same symbolic and concrete messages as physical or social ostracism, depending upon whether targets feel as though they are in the communicative presence of others.

What about the ambiguity that is attached to cyberostracism? In this respect, cyberostracism presents the greatest potential for ambiguity. The target will ask him- or herself, Am I being ostracized, or did X [the source] not receive my last message? Did X reply, but for some technological reason the reply went astray? Is X away from the computer or out of town? Or am I actually being ostracized? This additional ambiguity may makes things worse for targets because it causes them to ruminate about all the possible reasons they are being ostracized, many of which may be self-deprecating. Moreover, targets might well take advantage of this ambiguity and engage in plausible denial that anything bad is happening or was intended. We shall see in Chapter 8 how targets of cyberostracism deal with the additional layer of ambiguity.

Motive

The model postulates five potential motives that targets could attribute to sources for their apparent act of ostracism. The possibility that up to five potentially plausible reasons could explain being ignored and excluded adds yet another layer of interpretive ambiguity for targets. In fact, it may be the exception rather than the rule that targets can convince themselves absolutely that only one motive explains an act of ostracism. I hypothesize that the motives presented below vary in their power to threaten the fundamental needs. I begin with the most innocuous motive, and work through to the motive I believe can be most harmful.

Not Ostracism

This describes instances in which targets notice a behavior that could be interpreted as ostracism, but then rationalize that the behavior was something else. They may convince themselves that the source did not see or hear them, or was otherwise distracted. They (the targets) may decide that they are being overly sensitive (perhaps paranoid) to inattentive behaviors. The source's behaviors may well be indicative of ostracism (such as when a source provides little eye contact, does not speak to the target, or does not react to what the target is saying or doing), yet may plausibly be interpreted as not intended to be an act of ostracism. It is quite likely that this particular motive is considered with the highest frequency. Except for exceptionally clear instances of ostracism in which its use is explicitly announced, this motive may always linger as a possibility. As a result, the motive of *not ostracism* fuels the ambiguity of any ostracism situation because there is always the possibility that targets are not intentionally being ignored. We may anguish over why our friend, spouse, or coworker did not look at us or speak to us this morning, but we will almost certainly consider the possibility that it was not intentional, that his or her mind was on other issues, and that we are blowing things out of proportion. Whether this type of ambiguity is harmful or protective is not clear. If an individual is not sure that he or she is being ostracized, its very possibility may cause intrusive consternation and rumination such that ongoing activities or thoughts are disrupted. Furthermore, individuals may entertain (or be influenced to entertain) notions that they are being paranoid, which undoubtedly reduces their self-confidence and reliance upon their own intuition, feelings, and thoughts. On the other hand, the possibility that one is not being ostracized may provide individuals a safe mirage to deny ostracism when it is actually happening that may keep the individual from experiencing its most harmful effects.

Role-Prescribed

This motive is inferred when acts of ostracism are noticed in a context in which such behavior is socially endorsed, occurring in situations in which individuals are not expected to acknowledge the presence of others. For example, elevator riders; passengers on trains, planes, or buses; passersby on the street; or even people waiting tables in a restaurant may experience being ignored by others but discount its importance because it is normatively or culturally commonplace. The *role-prescribed* motive is similar to *not ostracism* in that if individuals contemplate this as the explanation for being ignored, then they may be able to safely deflect the potentially negative impact of being ostracized. However, there may be a fine line between what is tolerated as being role-prescribed ostracism and what might be attributed to a manifestation of power, indifference, or rudeness. Once again there is the possibility of ambiguity. If, for instance, persons who wait tables in a restaurant attribute the fact that the customers are not acknowledging them to the customers feeling superior to them and deeming them unworthy of their attention, then the impact of such behavior could be quite harmful. I refer to this type of perceived motive as "oblivious ostracism" and will discuss it shortly.

Defensive

This motive refers to instances in which the target believes that the source is ignoring or excluding him or her in order to avoid being hurt or ostracized him- or herself. For example, if John believes that Jane is going to be angry with him because she saw him flirting with a coworker at his office party, John may try to avoid the accusation and a scene with Jane by avoiding Jane. If Jane correctly interpreted John's avoidance as his attempt to protect himself from her scorn and derision, then she would be taking into account the possibility that John's motive for ostracizing her is defensive. Another example is the individual who appears to ostracize him- or herself from the larger group to avoid being ridiculed for looking or acting different. If the target interprets the ostracism to be motivated by defensiveness, then the prospect that the source is trying to intentionally hurt the target is replaced by a consideration that the source is merely trying to protect him- or herself against something that the target may do or say. In this regard, the target knows several things. The target knows that the source is aware of his or her existence and the target also knows that the source is concerned about the target's evaluation of him or her and fears confrontation. As negative as this motive may be, the target must also feel a certain degree of control over the source. Nevertheless, the issue of ambiguity still arises. It may be quite difficult to distinguish between defensive ostracism and ostracism that is intended to be harmful or punishing.

Punitive

Targets inferring this motive assume that they are being ostracized as a form of punishment. The perceived goal of the punishment may be to correct the target's undesirable behavior (rehabilitative), to eject the target from the other individual or group (rejection), or simply to inflict hurt on the target (retributional). *Punitive* ostracism refers to acts of ignoring that are perceived to be deliberate and aversive. Exile, banishment, shunning, and the silent treatment are examples of this. Clearly, it would be unpleasant for targets to assume that this is the motive for the ostracism. It would suggest to the target that he or she was bad or had done bad things to deserve such treatment. It would also, however, suggest to the target certain things that would not be so debilitating. First, as the "object of inattention," the target of punitive social ostracism may become highly self-aware, a psychological state often experienced by people who are the object of attention. Although this in itself may be aversive, because it may draw attention to one's own inadequacies, it also makes salient one's existence. As bad as negative thoughts about the self are, they at least serve the purpose of acknowledging the existence of the self. It is this message that is communicated in the last motive—that the self does not exist or is not worthy of existence.

Oblivious

This is the motive for which targets infer that their own existence is unnoticed or inconsequential to the source. It is not regarded as punishment; punishment would imply intentional and effortful behavior on the part of the source; it would also imply that the targets were worthy of punishment. Instead, targets feel that sources are oblivious to their presence and that their own existence is unworthy of the sources' attention. When individuals infer that others do not acknowledge them because of their status, stigma, race, or religion, then they consider the motive of oblivious ostracism.

Some of the best examples of oblivious ostracism can be found in literature and film. In Ralph Ellison's (1952) *Invisible Man*, the unnamed black protagonist claims, "I am invisible, understand, simply because people refuse to see me" (p. 3). Rather than being the object of inattention, the obliviously ostracized person feels invisible and unworthy of attention. Ellison's invisible man goes on to say, "You often doubt if you really exist" (p. 3). In Ayn Rand's (1957/1992) *Atlas Shrugged*, she describes Dagney Taggert's perception of being ignored by her lover: "He acted, not as if she wasn't present, but as if it did not matter that she was" (p. 237). Lina Wertmüller's film *Swept Away* (Cardarelli & Wertmüller, 1975), the lower-class protagonist (played by Giancarlo Giannini) finds himself swabbing the deck of a luxurious yacht while the beautiful blonde wife (played by Mariangela Melato) of the yacht's owner suns herself in the nude. Privy to his thoughts, the audience hears him complain about how he believes that her lack of modesty reflects her belief that he is no more important to her than a dog—that in fact she might even be more likely to acknowledge the existence of a dog than of himself. Again, we see the difference between oblivious ostracism and any other intentional form of ostracism. This woman was not trying to punish him; she simply did not care enough about him to acknowledge his existence.

Another example comes from Muzafer Sherif and his colleague's (1961) book on his Robber's Cave field experiment, in which two teams of boys were first driven to competition and hostility, then to interdependence and friendship. Where was Sherif during his investigation? How was he, an adult authority figure, able to observe the boys' behaviors without inhibiting them or causing them to behave in a socially desirable manner? A little known fact is that he accomplished his goal of being an unobtrusive observer by becoming the maintenance man—his own version of being invisible (I'd like to thank Lee Ross for bringing this to my attention). The children probably noted his presence at some level of their awareness, but were sufficiently unconcerned with his evaluation or reactions to let it bother them. In this respect, the children obliviously ostracized Muzafer Sherif. Note that one status differentiation, age, was overridden by another status measure, wealth or occupation. Note also that he, like the protagonist in Ellison's *Invisible Man*, exploited his invisibility. So, on the one hand, being a target of oblivious ostracism could be the most debilitating experience imaginable. On the other hand, at least occasionally, a wily individual may recognize his or her condition of invisibility as a potential opportunity to act without fear of evaluation or capture.

Quantity

Ostracism varies in terms of the quantity of behaviors used to signal the ostracism, varying from low levels of *partial* ostracism to the highest level of *complete* ostracism. For example, targets of ostracism may perceive that sources will only answer questions put to them directly, but will not elaborate or initiate conversation on their own. Targets may notice reduced levels of eye contact, briefer utterances, and loss of inflected affect. Partial ostracism could be signaled by short, barely sufficient replies to queries, or could include a minimum concession to social norms (e.g., saying "Excuse me" when passing by, or answering "Nothing" to the question, "What's wrong?"). Similarly, in Boehm's (1986) hierarchy of ostracism, the lowest degrees of ostracism include coolness in tone of voice and denial of eye contact. All these behaviors may signal partial ostracism, but, of course, they may also signal any number of other things. Perhaps the source is deep in thought, upset about something unrelated to the target, drowsy, or even intoxicated. Here is yet another opportunity for ambiguity to rear its ugly head. Partial ostracism makes it more difficult for the target to make clear interpretations and react appropriately, but it may also allow the target to pretend that ostracism is not occurring.

Complete ostracism is certainly more extreme in its performance. The source makes no replies to the target's questions, initiates no conversation, withdraws all eye contact. The target gets the feeling that he or she is being looked *through* rather than looked *at*. In sum, for complete ostracism, all forms of social intercourse and acknowledgment are cut off. There appears to be a trade-off between the extremity of the form of ostracism and its inherent ambiguity. The more complete the ostracism, the less ambiguous it becomes. However, to the extent that ambiguity can provide a safe haven of denial for the target, no such protection is offered by complete ostracism. When completely ostracized, targets are left with no other option but to surmise that they are being ignored and excluded. Whereas complete ostracism could be experienced more negatively (compared with partial ostracism), it may also be easier to detect, evaluate, and cope with.

Causal Clarity

The last dimension is causal clarity, on which ostracism may also vary along a continuum. In some situations, the cause of ostracism may be clear in that the source explicitly announces his or her intention to ostracize the target (e.g., situations where ostracism is imposed by law). The Amish use high causal clarity when ostracizing individual members who violate their rules. For the Amish, everyone is aware that the punishment for disobeying the elders is *Meidung* (shunning). Low causal clarity would occur in situations where there is no explicit announcement of ostracism and instead the target merely notices behaviors that could suggest that he or she is being ostracized. In Franz Kafka's sketch "Gemeinschaft," he writes of five men excluding a sixth for no reason (even to themselves) other than he is not one of the five (reprinted in Rehbinder, 1986). Undoubtedly, the sixth man must have devoted considerable thought as to why the others were excluding him, just as we all would when confronted with unexplained ostracism. Although Kafka's story is purposely absurd, there are similar occasions when we find ourselves ostracized by friends, coworkers, or family without any accompanying explanation.

In certain circumstances, causal clarity may be closely linked to motives. If ostracism is explicitly announced, the reason for the ostracism may be fairly apparent or easily derived. When causally unclear, however, the motive for ostracism will not be readily surmised, and attributional ambiguity will prevail.

Once again, the importance of this dimension lies in the plausibility that variations in it are likely to be associated with its impact and the means with which we cope with it. And, as before, one reason for this difference is because of concomitant variations in ambiguity. Low causal clarity is, by definition, ambiguous, whereas high causal clarity is not. With low causal clarity, not only are targets left to wonder if they are being ostracized, but even if they decide that they are, they are left to ponder sources' motives. All this thinking, which undoubtedly includes considerations of being needlessly paranoid along with myriad legitimate reasons why such treatment is deserved, can be potentially damaging and obstructive in and of itself. It may even trigger doubts of one's existence if one considers the ostracism's motive to be oblivious (e.g., "Am I here?," "Is my existence meaningful?"). If the ostracism is causally clear, and the motives are obvious, then targets will at least be able to understand the treatment, and to narrow their range of reactions to the specific issues at hand.

ANTECEDENTS

What instigates ostracism? Why ostracize a person rather than verbally or physically confront him or her? When is one type of ostracism more likely to be used than another? These are the issues that are considered under the heading of *antecedents*. Antecedents to ostracism can be broken down into three broad categories: characteristics of the *source*, characteristics of the *target*, and characteristics of the *situation*.

Source characteristics acknowledge that there may be important individual differences that separate people who are likely to use ostracism from those who are not likely to use it. Some people may be more inclined to use ostracism tactics as opposed to verbally expressing their emotions or resorting to violence. Some sources may rely on using ostracism to maintain control over the interaction, or to prevent verbal or physical abuse. For instance, people with lower levels of self-esteem may be more inclined to preempt anticipated derogation by "cutting dead" the person(s) they think will derogate them. This may allow these individuals who are less adept at managing other forms of interpersonal conflict to have substantial influence. Source characteristics may also dictate the type of ostracism that is preferred. Certain types of ostracism may be preferred by some sources over other types. Some may prefer to use partial ostracism so as to be able to deny that they are ignoring the target. After all, if a source answers a target's question (albeit without affect or interest, and with a monosyllabic response), then the source can rightly maintain that he or she was not ignoring the target.

Target characteristics may also predict the occurrence of ostracism. Some individuals may simply possess certain undesirable characteristics or behave in ways that cause others to ostracize them. These characteristics may include insensitivity to others, obnoxiousness, chronic complaining, loudness, perceived dangerousness, or other unpleasant characteristics. Although even suggesting this possibility may be perceived to be "politically incorrect" in that it blames victims, it would be foolish to ignore the possibility that some people elicit ostracism because of what they do or say, or how they look or smell (see Goffman, 1963). Target characteristics may also include aspects about themselves for which they have little or no control. People with certain stigmas or who belong to certain classes within society may be more likely to be ignored and excluded by others. Ralph Ellison's *Invisible Man* presented this case most eloquently. Being a black man in a society in which black men were considered less than human resulted in the feeling that one was invisible to society at large.

Finally, social/situational forces may act to facilitate or inhibit the use of ostracism. For instance, an individual may choose to give his or her partner the silent treatment at a party, for not only is it a socially acceptable means of "fighting" with the partner in public, but it also can be denied if confronted ("No, I'm not angry with John, I'm just tired"). The "unobservable" and deniable nature of ostracism would also allow it to be used quite easily in the workplace by employees without fear of the recriminations that would accompany verbal abuse or violence.

MODERATORS AND MEDIATORS

In the model, I propose several moderators or mediators of ostracism. At this point, I am not prepared to predict the factors that are merely moderators versus the factors that actually mediate the effects. So I will approach this issue cautiously at this point and refer only to moderators. For example, attributions of responsibility for the ostracism by the target should moderate its effects. Specifically, targets who attribute responsibility *externally*, that is, who view ostracism to be the fault of others or as arising from the situation, should be less affected than those who attribute the responsibility for the ostracism *internally*, that is, to themselves. Likewise, targets who attribute the cause of the ostracism to the fact that they are members of groups (e.g., "I am black and they don't like blacks") may cope more easily with ostracism than those who attribute the ostracism to unique personal characteristics that they possess.

Another class of moderators is personality and the individual differences of targets. Although I suspect that ostracism is not particularly pleasant for the majority of people, it is also likely that not everyone reacts to ostracism in the same way. Various personality differences may account for different levels of perceiving ostracism, being susceptible to ostracism, or characteristic patterns of response to ostracism. For instance, extroverts may respond more strongly to ostracism than introverts, because extroverts are more dependent on the opinions of and bonds with other people.

Another individual difference that should be related psychologically to targets' reactions to ostracism is their variation in attachment styles. Bowlby (1977) investigated attachment behavior by examining the way in which infants forged emotional bonds with their caregivers. Ainsworth (1989) created a paradigm, "the strange situation," to examine attachment patterns based on responses to the child's separation from his or her parent. In this paradigm, parents returned to a room after a brief absence, but were instructed to ignore their children. Three attachment styles were observed: secure, avoidant, and anxious/ambivalent (or resistant). Secure children made contact with their mothers and then freely explored their environments. Anxious/ambivalent children were more likely to cling to their mothers, apparently afraid to leave their sides. Avoidant children tended to ignore their mothers, almost as if they were reciprocating ostracism with ostracism. These infant attachment patterns have been hypothesized to generalize to adult attachment styles in romantic relationships (Hazan & Shaver, 1987). Given that the original paradigm used to determine attachment styles stemmed from an ostracism episode, it seems quite likely that attachment styles may predict targets' reactions to being ostracized. Specifically, secure individuals should be least affected by ostracism (or should cope with it in healthier ways), anxious individuals should be more vigilant for episodes of ostracism and react more negatively, and avoidant individuals should be more likely to disengage from those who ostracize them, possibly by using ostracism in retaliation.

OSTRACISM THREATENS FOUR FUNDAMENTAL HUMAN NEEDS

The core theory of the model is that ostracism, in comparison to other aversive interpersonal behaviors, has the unique potential to threaten up to four fundamental human needs. These needs are the need to *belong*, the need for *self-esteem*, the need for *control*, and the need for *meaningful existence*. A great deal of research and theory supports the importance of each of these needs for human motivation and survival. Human beings need and seek to increase their sense of belonging (Baumeister & Leary, 1995), self-esteem (Steele, 1988; Tesser, 1988), control (e.g., Burger, 1992; Peterson, Maier, & Seligman, 1993; Seligman, 1975), and meaningful existence (Greenberg, Pyszczynski, & Solomon, 1986; Greenberg et al., 1990; Greenberg et al., 1992). Although proponents for each need claim that their need subsumes the others, the model assumes each need to be uniquely important to the individual.

I will use the word "needs," rather than "desires" or "wants" or "drives," because there is substantial evidence that when any of them are lacking, people "exhibit pathological consequences beyond mere temporary distress"—which is a critical defining element of needs (Baumeister & Leary, 1995, p. 498). These needs are not exclusively threatened by ostracism; in fact, they represent a synthesis of fundamental motivational needs assumed to underlie most human social behavior (see, e.g., Smith & Mackie's [1995] thematic encapsulation of the field of social psychology). I believe, however, that these needs are peculiarly and almost immediately triggered by even short-term exposure to ostracism. I am also not arguing that these needs are necessarily mutually exclusive; indeed, the authors who champion each need often indicate that the other needs are subordinate to, and serve in the maintenance of, their particular need (Greenberg et al., 1992). I will leave to others the task of debating which of these needs envelop the others. It is sufficient for my purposes to merely recognize the importance of these needs, particularly as they relate to ostracism.

In this section, I present arguments for why ostracism, compared to other interpersonally aversive behaviors (such as argument and verbal or physical confrontation), threatens these four needs. Presenting the voluminous research that supports the proposition that each need is fundamental is beyond the scope of this book, but I do provide readers with reference citations if they would like to explore the evidence for these propositions on their own.

Belonging

Ostracism is hypothesized to deprive targets of their sense of belonging. Baumeister and Leary (1995) put forth a compelling argument that the need to belong is the most fundamental of all human needs. They argued that this need is not only emotionally desirable, but also evolutionarily adaptive (Baumeister & Tice, 1990; Buss, 1990). The need to belong "involves two criteria: First, there is a need for frequent, affectively pleasant interactions with a few other people, and second, these interactions must take place in the context of a temporarily stable and enduring framework of affective concern for each other's welfare" (Baumeister & Leary, 1995, p. 497). They reviewed many studies that showed that the absence of affiliation and intimacy with others produces a host of negative psychological consequences, including depression, anxiety, stress, and physical and mental illness. Being ostracized may be one of the clearest methods of attacking a sense of belonging.

People can be criticized or chastised for any number of behaviors, and can feel badly about themselves with respect to those behaviors, but as long as the disagreement does not lead to ignoring or expulsion, the targeted individual can still feel attached to the individual or group who is punishing him or her—belonging and connectedness remain despite disapproval. Yet, when the silent treatment or some other form of ostracism is meted out, then the explicit or symbolic message is that the offending person risks losing his or her attachment to the other individual or group. Whereas Baumeister and Leary (1995) argue that all forms of disapproval may trigger fears of rejection, ostracism would seem to be the clearest and most direct method of evoking such a fear.

Self-Esteem

It is argued that "people are guided by a strong, fundamental desire for self-esteem" (Baumeister, 1994, p. 84) and that there is "consensus that self-esteem is a vital human need" (Greenberg et al., 1992, p. 913). Many theorists argue that the need for maintaining high self-esteem is pervasive and adaptive (e.g., Greenwald, 1980; Steele, 1988; Tesser, 1988). Self-esteem is central to many theories as a primary determinant of self-efficacy and mental health (e.g., Bandura, 1997; Barnett & Gotlib, 1988; Leary, Tambor, Terdal, & Downs, 1995). Ostracism threatens targets' self-esteem because it is associated with punishment; it carries with it the implicit accusation that the target has done something wrong (of course, the feeling of threatened self-esteem may simply be an indicator of threatened belonging—see the sociometer hypothesis developed by Leary et al. [1995]).

As I discussed in Chapter 1, ostracism is most commonly regarded as a response to deviant or inappropriate behavior, or, in some instances, to one or more physical characteristics of the individual that sets him or her apart from the rest (e.g., physical handicap, different color, carrier of a disease, etc.). As such, it carries with it the message that something about the individual is bad or unwanted. This message directly threatens an individual's sense of self-esteem and may lead to an internalized belief in one's undesirable nature and shortcomings. In the short run, individuals are rather resilient to attacks on their self-esteem: they either use defense mechanisms, or redeem themselves in the specific domain of attack, or affirm their goodness in other domains (e.g., after failing a driving test, individuals can bolster their self-esteem by thinking about how good they are at parenting) (Steele, 1988). In the long run, however, continued diminution of their self-esteem can lead to negative expectations and self-fulfilling prophecies resulting in a downward spiral toward lower self-esteem and undesirable behaviors.

Control

There is considerable evidence that without feelings of control, individuals (indeed, many organisms) exhibit learned helplessness and become depressed (Seligman, 1975). As with belonging, maintaining control is considered by some to be "a fundamental human motivation" (Friedland, Keinan, & Regev, 1992, p. 929; see also Bruneau, 1973; Taylor & Brown, 1988; Taylor et al., 1992). Furthermore, researchers claim that the belief that one has control in situations (i.e., self-efficacy) allows the individual to persist in the face of failure and to succeed (Bandura, 1997). I propose that ostracism threatens targets' perceived control over their interactions with the source(s). Exchanging verbal accusations or punches with sources, though unpleasant, can still provide targets with a sense of control or influence over the interaction. A sense of control is greatly diminished, however, when sources give no reactions to targets' queries or provocations. Unlike most other forms of aversive behavior, ostracism involves a unilateral stance by one person (or group) over another. There is no give-and-take. In a verbal argument, regardless of the intensity and insulting nature of the verbal barbs, it is still the case that each person is responsive to the other. Despite its negativity, participation in such give-and-take continues to provide a sense of control. What one person says affects (has control over) what the other person says. The same thing can be said for physical aggression. Although unpleasant and potentially dangerous, there is still the opportunity for a responsive exchange. A person who is physically threatened can escape, or cover him- or herself in an attempt to ward off further blows, or can attack back—all these actions involve control. But someone who is ostracized is deprived of the bilateral nature of conflict. No matter what is said or done, the other person appears unaffected, as though the victim of ostracism did not exist.

Control is further diminished when the ostracism is low in causal clarity or when multiple motives are plausible. This sort of control is called "interpretive control" by Rothbaum, Weisz, and Snyder (1982), who contend that the ability to understand an aversive or traumatic event is an important step in the coping process. Even in the absence of direct or primary control, interpretive control provides a certain element of order and meaning to life (Janoff-Bulman & Wortman, 1977).

Meaningful Existence

Ostracism, perhaps more than any other form of aversive control, is a poignant metaphor for what life would be like if the target did not exist. Because ostracism involves a withdrawal of attention or recognition by others, individuals exposed to it may be reminded of their fragile and temporary existence, and its lack of meaning and worth. They may even be reminded of their own death. Theory and research indicates we have a need to maintain our beliefs in a *meaningful existence* (e.g., Cooley, 1902; James, 1890; Mead, 1934) and to avoid thoughts of our own death (Solomon, Greenberg, & Pyszczynski, 1991). In fact, it could be argued that ostracism symbolizes death. While we are being ostracized, it could occur to us that this is what it would be like if we were dead, the sort of realization Charles Dickens evoked in Scrooge in *A Christmas Carol*. In terror management theory, Greenberg et al. (1986; Solomon et al., 1992) argue that a fundamental human anxiety that drives social behavior is our fear of our own mortality and meaningless existence. Individuals are motivated to constantly manage the terror of death and the prospect of having a meaningless existence. The terror management position claims that "people need self-esteem because it is the central psychological mechanism for protecting individuals from the anxiety that awareness of their vulnerability and mortality would otherwise create" (Greenberg et al., 1992, p. 913).

Other authors also allude metaphorically or literally to the similarity between ostracism and death. As I mentioned before, William James (1890) likened the phenomenological horror of being socially ostracized to feeling as though "every person we met cut us dead" (p. 294). Mahdi (1986) argued that the most severe form of ostracism is the "termination of life" (p. 295). Service (1975) wrote that the usual punishment by any society is some amount of disapproval or withdrawal, the most extreme being ostracism, which he describes as "in primitive society a fate practically equivalent to death" (p. 54). In writing about the ostracism used by primates, Lancaster (1986) states, "the 'cold shoulder' is only a step along the way to execution" (p. 216). In Gruter's (1986) account of Amish shunning, she writes, "Meidung [shunning in this rural community] means slow death" (p. 274). As a final example, Boehm (1986) considered the connection between death by execution and social ostracism and concluded: "The act of execution is not much more than the strongest manifestation of the 'silent treatment' itself when this [treatment] persists for a long time. Either involves what amounts to the social death of the individual" (pp. 313–314). Based on these accounts of ostracism, it does not seem such an enormous leap to suggest that ostracism (perhaps particularly social oblivious ostracism) threatens an individual's sense of meaningful existence and offers a terrifying glimpse of what things would be like if one were dead. Both of these reactions ought to bring us closer to the terror that Greenberg, Solomon, and Pyszczynski believe we fight so diligently to buffer.

REACTIONS TO OSTRACISM: TEMPORAL STAGES

I suggest three distinct stages that characterize reactions to ostracism; these stages correspond to the length of time targets have to endure the ostracism. *Immediate* reactions to being ostracized include hurt feelings, anger, damaged mood, and physiological arousal. These effects are relatively cognition-free, but give way soon after to short-term effects, which do involve cognition and interpretation.

Because ostracism may threaten all four needs, the *short-term* effects of ostracism are predicted to drive individuals (behaviorally, emotionally, and cognitively) to regain these lost or threatened needs. For instance, threats to belonging can be remedied by establishing new bonds with others. Self-esteem may be regained by increasing one's self-importance or by remembering past achievements. Control may be reestablished by taking a leadership role in a situation or exerting control over the lives of others. And threats to meaningful existence may be remedied by reasserting life goals and sense of purpose. This notion of a direct causal link between needs deprivation and needs fulfillment has been suggested or demonstrated for belonging (Baumeister & Leary, 1995), self-esteem (Steele, 1988), control (e.g., Friedland et al., 1992; Pittman & D'Agostino, 1989; Pittman & Pittman, 1980; Wortman & Brehm, 1975), and meaningful existence (Greenberg et al., 1990).

If, however, an individual endures *long-term* ostracism, his or her attempts to regain these needs may give way to despair and helplessness. This is consistent with research and theory on long-term loss of control (Peterson et al., 1993; Seligman, 1975; Wortman & Brehm, 1975) and rejection (Leary, 1990). I hypothesize that lengthy exposure to continuous or repeated episodes of ostracism will lead to detrimental psychological and health-related consequences. Instead of making deliberate attempts to regain his or her lost or threatened needs, the target will succumb to the lost needs and internalize the meaning that their loss represents.

For loss of a sense of belonging, there would be a prolonged lack of connection with others that may lead to feelings that one does not belong anywhere. The constant threat to self-esteem is likely to feed a downward spiral of self-belief and affect, resulting in chronic low self-esteem. Prolonged loss of control over the environment and other people is likely to lead to learned helplessness. The sense of no acknowledgment or feelings of invisibility may then force people to question the purpose and the worth of their existence and be a constant reminder of their death.

APPLICATION OF THE MODEL TO SOURCES

As I discussed at the outset of this chapter, my initial intention was to formulate a working model that would provide a useful framework within which to explore the phenomenon of ostracism in its effects on targets. Since developing this model, I could not help but notice that in many respects the model could be quite useful as a preliminary framework within which to understand the causes of the source's behavior and the effects that employing ostracism might have on them too. Let us briefly consider the aspects of the model that seem most relevant to this application.

Motives

Just as targets can perceive and interpret the motives of sources, so can sources' intentions be related to the same motives. Sources may have no intention of ostracizing an individual, but because they are distracted, or lost in thought, they may ignore someone. For sources, this would be *not ostracism*. Likewise, sources may not intend to hurt targets' feelings or in any way project a feeling of superiority in instances where it is socially and culturally appropriate to not acknowledge other people. One may choose to ignore people in the elevator or a seatmate on a bus simply because it is thought to be the polite or proper thing to do. In this case, the intention is *role-prescribed*. Ostracism arising from either of these motives should impose little or no depletion of cognitive and emotional resources in sources.

Defensive ostracism is preemptive in nature, and may be used in anticipation of negative, threatening feedback from another, or even to expected ostracism by others; it is meant more as ego protection or as a means to suspend vanishing control over the situation, rather than as an offensive weapon. Baumeister and Leary (1995) suggest that when people do not believe that they will be regarded in ways that will lead to acceptance, they might avoid absolute rejection by disaffiliating. By doing this, they "reduce the risk of saying or doing something that others might regard negatively . . . giving others few reasons to reject" (p. 520). In Basso's (1972) examination of a Western Apache tribe, he noted several occasions in which community and family members traditionally ostracized individuals. These occasions included not talking to recently widowed women or to adolescents who had recently returned from their initial exposure to modern society. The underlying pattern in all these occasions was that the sources of ostracism anticipated that the targeted individual would either be dangerous or crazy, or would derogate them. Widows were feared to be possessed and returning adolescents were feared to hold condemning attitudes of their tribe and family. So, to preempt the derogation, other tribal members chose to ostracize first and wait for the target to come to them and speak (in a civil manner).

Sources' motives to ostracize may be *punitive*, arising from a desire to condemn or correct the target. This motive for ostracism is the one most widely referred to in the anthropological, ethological, and sociological accounts discussed in Chapter 1. In these perspectives, ostracism is assumed to be punitive, with the primary function to either temporarily or permanently exclude an offending individual. If temporary, the punishment is intended to modify the behavior of the offending party by making it more appropriate. It is also a means to resolidify the remaining members of the group, apparently by reminding them of what behaviors define the group and by giving them an out-group member to whom they can compare themselves.

Unlike not-ostracism and role-prescribed motives, punitive or defensive motives should be characterized as more deliberate and effortful, especially if the acts of ignoring and unresponsivity are unusual within the given context. Of course, interactions with the visibility dimension would also determine the extent to which effort was required. If physical ostracism is employed, then sources need not be under constant surveillance of their own behavioral reactions to the target. For social ostracism, however, defensive and punitive ostracizing sources must be vigilant regarding their own behavior and constantly remind themselves of their task in order to maintain it consistently. Clearly, within social ostracism, either defensive or punitive ostracism should deplete cognitive (and emotional) resources in the sources who use it more than would be the case for the other motives.

Oblivious ostracism may be similar to not ostracism in terms of sources' awareness of their own behavior or intentions. If an individual consciously and deliberately decides to ignore a person because of class, race, or other differences between themselves and the targets, then it could be argued that the employment of such a strategy was punitive or scornful in nature. True oblivious ostracism, implied by the word "oblivious," suggests that ignoring is so automatic and routine that sources employing it are unaware of their behavior. It is unlikely that a source who is engaging in oblivious ostracism would be able to acknowledge his or her own behavior, unless, perhaps, it was pointed out to them. From the source's perspective, oblivious ostracism occurs when the presence of the target simply is of no consequence to them. There should be little or no effort exerted in oblivious ostracism, unlike the mindful premeditation and continuous maintenance required with punitive or defensive ostracism. Instead, all that is needed is the smallest amount of awareness that, for the source, the target individual is unimportant and unworthy of further attention.

Quantity

From the source's perspective, the choice to employ partial ostracism may reflect upon strategic considerations. The source may desire to avoid escalation of conflict or retaliation, or may resort to an opportunistic exploitation of ostracism's ambiguity. A clever source can maintain deniability ("I wasn't ignoring you, I said 'Excuse me'!") in order to avoid being held accountable for using ostracism. Choosing complete ostracism would probably reflect intense anger and a lack of concern for disguising it. Because it would be more difficult to deny having used complete ostracism, regard for future consequences of the act would be relatively low. For face-saving purposes, it would be easier for sources to cease using partial ostracism and reestablish communication than it would be for sources who use complete ostracism. Partial ostracism and social intercourse differ only in matters of degree, whereas there is a qualitative and noticeable break between complete ostracism and open (even unpleasant) communication.

Effects on Fundamental Needs

Are sources' fundamental needs affected when they use ostracism? It is plausible that they are affected, although probably not in the same way as targets are. Employing ostracism should reduce a source's feeling of belongingness, at least to the target. If a group uses ostracism, then belongingness might actually be strengthened within the ostracizing group (as suggested by anthropologists and animal behaviorists). If ostracism is used as a corrective measure, rather than for purposes of permanent exclusion, then feelings of belonging may be relatively unchanged. The effects of ostracizing on self-esteem are open to debate. One could feel justified and vindicated by its use, and suffer little damage to self-esteem. One's self-esteem may even be bolstered to the extent that the consequences of ostracism on the targets are pleasing to the source. Still, the damage done to a target for whom the source cares may make the source feel bad for using it. Finally, there is no reason to suspect that sources' feelings of meaningful existence should be threatened. Sources should still feel acknowledged and influential. Perhaps noting one's influence can even inflate one's sense of meaningful existence.

Probably the clearest effect of using ostracism on any of the fundamental needs is associated with control. Whereas targets' need for control is threatened, it is reasonable to assume that sources' need for control is fortified. The control is shifted from the target to the source, because the source enjoys unilateral power within the relationship. The source can control when communication and recognition is resumed, whereas the target cannot. So, at least in the short term, the source should feel empowered with heightened control.

Temporal-Related Consequences

For control, there is some reason to believe that there may be a similar temporal aspect to the consequences of using ostracism on sources as that proposed for the effects of ostracism on targets. The short-term benefit of ostracizing may well be to feel empowered, gaining control in a situation in which one may not have had control otherwise. But once ostracism is employed, how does one end it without essentially becoming accountable for having used it, or worse, having to apologize for its use? The end of an argument can be signaled by silence, but what signals the end of silence? Anything involving speech, eye contact, or acknowledgment can potentially suggest that the source is "giving in." In order not to appear apologetic or even accountable for using ostracism, the source may feel compelled to continue with ignoring, with exclusion, with silence. In this regard, the initial empowerment gives way to being under the control, not of the target, but of the ostracism itself. In Chapter 2, I presented instances of sources who ostracized their partners for years. It is doubtful any of them anticipated such long-term ostracism when they began it. Rather, in order to save or maintain "face," they fell under the control of the commitment to maintain the ostracism, even to the point that they forgot the original reason for having employed it initially. In this sense, then, there may be an important qualitative temporal shift in sources of ostracism from feeling control to feeling controlled.

CONCLUSIONS

This model provides a framework in which to examine the causes and consequences of ostracism. With continued research, certain aspects of the model will undoubtedly be modified. It may be necessary to add, within the taxonomic dimensions, a temporal category. Exposure to single short-term episodes of ostracism may be quantitatively, and more importantly, qualitatively different than exposure to repeated or long-term continuously running episodes of ostracism. Another motive that may be conceptually distinct from the five presented is true disengagement. That is, a person may desire to disengage temporarily or permanently from another and use ostracism to achieve this goal. I have to date considered this desire to be enveloped within the defensive motive, because the source was preemptively defending against desired bonds by the target, but this way of thinking may require too much of a stretch in logic. Similarly, I have also considered an example of the defensive motive sources wishing to "cool down" so as not to say or do something they would eventually regret (or to "cool down" a volatile target or situation). Perhaps, this too is really a separate motive that deserves to be distinguished from defensively ostracizing a target to protect one's feelings and self-esteem.

Further research will be required to assess whether these possibly different motives do indeed have distinctly different manifestations and consequences. If so, they need to be considered as separate motives. For the time being, I will use the model presented here to direct and provide a framework for the research I have undertaken, presented in the upcoming chapters.

Forty Minutes of Silence

Narratives of Short-Term Episodes of the Silent Treatment

In Chapter 2, I presented a number of interviews and letters from people who had experienced various forms of ostracism in their lives. These accounts often depicted a dyadic form of ostracism between individuals who were in close personal relationships. The common term for this particular sort of dyadic ostracism is "the silent treatment." It is not clear from where the term originated, but Ferguson (1944) noted that merchant sailors used the term to describe social punishment of men at sea. Certainly, however, the phenomena occurred long before the term was coined. Other terms or phrases mean roughly the same thing, including "the cold shoulder," "freezing out," and being "sent to Coventry" (a town where, during World War II, English soldiers were ignored by the countryfolk, especially the women, because the women feared their reputations would be sullied).

In this chapter, I present two lines of investigation into the silent treatment. The first was done in collaboration with Wendy Shore and Jon Grahe (Williams, Shore, & Grahe, 1998). In two studies, we examined how individuals understood the behaviors that comprised the silent treatment and the feelings that were associated with those behaviors. The theoretical model presented in the preceding chapter was used as a framework within which to understand the participants' responses. The behaviors were coded to determine where in the model's taxonomy the silent treatment was located. The feelings were then coded to test the central theoretical predictions of the model: Do people feel that the behaviors associated with ostracism threaten targets' needs for belonging, self-esteem, control, and meaningful existence? Additionally, we looked for evidence that these needs could be actually fortified in the sources who use the silent treatment.

The second set of studies was conducted by Kristin Sommer, myself, Nancy Ciarocco, and Roy Baumeister (Sommer, Williams, Ciarocco, & Baumeister, in press). In this research, we asked individuals to provide us with written narratives in which they recounted the last time they gave someone the silent treatment and the last time someone gave it to them. Once again, we tested aspects of the model dealing with needs threat in targets and fortification in sources.

Both lines of research offer a first detailed analysis into the common, but until now, overlooked interpersonal phenomenon of the silent treatment. Most of the episodes in these accounts were of relatively short duration—hence the reason for this chapter's title. The temporal shift in reactions to ostracism discussed in the preceding chapter suggests that we should expect reactions to short-term and long-term ostracism to be substantially different. In essence, desires and actions to regain senses of belonging, self-esteem, control, and meaningful existence should characterize short-term reactions to the threatened needs. Individuals facing continuous or long-term episodes of ostracism, however, will eventually exhibit helplessness, resulting in enveloping feelings of alienation, low self-worth, and despair. I will return to analyses of long-term episodes of the silent treatment (and other forms of ostracism) in Chapter 10.

SOME BACKGROUND INTO THE SILENT TREATMENT

The silent treatment is a widespread form of social rejection. But it is less than rejection in some ways and more than rejection in other ways. The silent treatment is not verbal or physical abuse. The target is not insulted or punched. As such, it is less than other forms of rejection. On the other hand, the silent treatment involves the playing out of a role, a pretending that the target does not exist. In that sense, the silent treatment is more than rejection—it is a dramaturgical metaphor for separateness, meaningless, and even death.

Recall the classic Uncle Remus story of the "Tar Baby" (Harris, 1948). Brer Fox, exploiting Brer Rabbit's gregarious nature, devised an ingenious plot to capture Brer Rabbit, by dressing up a baby made of tar and sitting it along a path that Brer Rabbit frequently traveled. When he came upon the stranger, Brer Rabbit attempted to engage the tar baby in polite conversation. The tar baby did not respond. After repeated attempts to communicate, Brer Rabbit became angrier and more frustrated with the tar baby's unwillingness to give him the civility and recognition he thought he deserved. To get a response from the tar baby, Brer Rabbit punched and kicked him, eventually getting both fists and both feet stuck in the tar. His sticky predicament allowed a gleeful Brer Fox to capture Brer Rabbit without resistance (of course, Brer Rabbit later "out-foxes" Brer Fox by using reverse psychology—"Please don't throw me into the brier patch"—but that's another story!).

Evidence of the use of the silent treatment or behaviors similar to it has been documented in the work on power tactics within close relationships (Kipnis et al., 1980). Falbo (1977) referred to explicit announcements that verbal interaction will be withdrawn as "threats." From this literature, it appears that the silent treatment would be regarded as an "indirect or weak," "nonrational," and "unilateral" tactic. It is indirect because it is not confrontational, it is nonrational because it does not involve logic or reasoned persuasion, and it is unilateral in that it can be used without approval, consent, or contribution by the target. Buss (1990, 1992) regarded the silent treatment as a behavioral option for interpersonal manipulation in his cross-cultural research. Additionally, Rosenfeld (1979) suggested that males avoid self-disclosure (a form of silence) in order to increase their control over their relationships.

Understanding the silent treatment within the existing power tactic labels, however, is problematic because the silent treatment can be classified under competing categories. The silent treatment is often subsumed under a more general category, such as "disengagement" or "withdrawal," which includes leaving the premises temporarily or permanently, pouting, locking oneself in one's room, or truly disengaging. The more demonstrative type of silent treatment that may include active nonverbal displays of anger, heavy sighs, and stomping about do not appear to qualify as "weak," and may not reflect the same concept as withdrawal. After all, if we take the term literally, it is a "treatment," something applied to someone who needs something corrected. In this sense, it is active, effortful, and involving.

The silent treatment (or something similar to it) has been documented as being used by young children, particularly girls (Asher & Coie, 1990; Barner-Barry, 1986; Cairns & Cairns, 1991), and with adults, by employers and coworkers on whistleblowers (Faulkner & Williams, 1999; Miceli & Near, 1992). The silent treatment could fall under Gottman's (1979, 1980) general category of disengagement behaviors, which he believed to be symptomatic of relationship distress. It is especially destructive when combined with contempt.

How common is the silent treatment? Nearly 70% of U.S. citizens have admitted to receiving the silent treatment from their romantic partners, and only slightly less have admitted using it on their partners (Faulkner et al., 1997). Although a similar poll has not yet been undertaken in Australia, audience reactions to interviews I have given there suggest that the incidence rate may be just as high. In fact, when I describe the silent treatment at various gatherings, most people indicate that they have either used it or received it. For something so common, there is surprisingly little knowledge about what it is, how it works, and how it makes people feel.

William James (1890) suggested that to be "cut dead" and to go "unnoticed" by others would be worse than the "most fiendish punishment." The silent treatment may well be the most frequently used method of cutting people dead. What is it about the silent treatment that is so bad? To begin answering this question we must first understand what behaviors comprise the silent treatment. Then we need to examine how these behaviors make us feel. Finally, most interest in the effects of ostracism has focused on those who are targets of such treatment; little is known about what effects it has on those who use it. That the silent treatment is so common suggests that it must provide certain benefits for those who use it, so we examined the impact that the silent treatment had on its perpetrators as well.

Our investigation began with two studies in which we assessed individuals' perceptions of the silent treatment. This provided us with a richer descriptive foundation for what the silent treatment entails. We then asked the same individuals to indicate how either giving or receiving each particular behavior would make them feel. After doing this, we began to understand the consequences of the silent treatment. Finally, we looked for themes that emerged in these descriptions that inform the theoretical model of ostracism discussed in the preceding chapter.

STUDY 1. THE SILENT TREATMENT: PERCEPTIONS OF ITS BEHAVIORS AND ASSOCIATED FEELINGS

Twenty-three undergraduate males and 25 undergraduate females from the University of Toledo participated in Study 1. Upon arrival at the laboratory, they were each issued a packet divided into two parts, the order of which was counterbalanced. One part pertained to *giving* the silent treatment, the other to *receiving* the silent treatment.

In the section providing instructions for *giving* the silent treatment, participants were asked to imagine giving the silent treatment to their best friend. They were instructed to consider what specific behaviors they engaged in, particularly any behaviors they did that they normally would not do and any behaviors they did not do that they normally would. They were instructed to list only outward behaviors and to avoid listing feelings. They were encouraged to provide detailed descriptions, including details they might consider minor or unimportant. After they had listed their behaviors, they were told to report specific feelings they had when giving the silent treatment that were associated with the behaviors they listed on the previous pages. For each behavior they listed, they were asked to describe the emotions, moods, and feelings they associated with that behavior.

For the section associated with *receiving* the silent treatment, participants were instructed to imagine that their best friends were giving them the silent treatment. Again, they were asked to list the specific behaviors that their best friends engaged in, especially the behaviors that their best friends did that they normally would not have done and the behaviors their best friends did not do that they normally would have done. After completing this section, participants were asked to list a feeling they would have when they experienced each of these behaviors.

The participants took about 40 minutes to complete the study. They listed an average of just under eight behaviors when giving the silent treatment and just over seven behaviors when receiving it. In all, 528 behaviors were listed. Screening for overlap, we arrived at 152 unique behaviors. The five most frequently listed behaviors were not making eye contact (listed by 73% of the respondents), not talking (54%), making a definite effort to ignore (42%), trying to avoid all contact (40%), and not responding to any questions or comments (40%). It is rather ironic that the most frequently listed behavior for the *silent* treatment involved the visual rather than the auditory sense.

We coded the behaviors in order to locate the silent treatment in reference to other forms of ostracism, according to the taxonomy presented in the model. The vast majority of the behaviors (94%) were coded as social ostracism: being ignored and excluded by others in one's presence. Almost as many (87%) were coded as having a punitive motive: to punish the target. Half the behaviors were coded as partial ostracism, and over half of the behaviors listed by participants were coded as having an unclear cause—that is, the behavior itself was not attached to a declaration of intent.

Because participants' responses were coded overwhelmingly as social, punitive ostracism (83% of all participants indicated this joint classification), subsequent analyses were restricted to those feelings that were associated with behaviors coded as social, punitive ostracism. Analyses were not limited by the quantity and causal clarity dimensions because of the greater range of responses along those dimensions.

Pattern of Needs Threat and Needs Fortification

We were interested in determining whether the silent treatment actually affected the four needs postulated by the ostracism model. To the extent that the silent treatment affected a particular need, we sought to determine whether that impact was best described as fortification or threat. To do this, we trained two judges whose agreements were generally good to code each feeling response associated with each behavior. For simplicity's sake, we chose the ratings of a single judge for the analyses. The judge rated each feeling as suggesting a fortification (e.g., "makes me feel powerful"), a threat (e.g., "makes me feel that I'm a bad person"), or as having no impact (e.g., "nothing in particular") on each of the needs of belonging, self-esteem, control, and meaningful existence. We also included ratings of anger (e.g., "makes me mad") because after an initial examination of participants' responses, we discovered that feelings of anger were evident.

We felt that having an independent judge rate the feelings was a particularly stringent test of our hypotheses. The judge had to determine whether the feeling represented a fortification or threat to each need. We trained the judge not to project or infer beyond what was actually written. Whereas the participants may have had more access to what they meant when they listed the feeling, the judge did not. Therefore, we expected generally low scores for each need, but we felt that even low scores would be encouraging at this step.

Because each participant listed a different number of behaviors (hence, a different number of feelings), proportions rather than raw frequencies were used as the dependent variable. Proportions were computed by dividing the frequency of fortification, threat, and no impact responses for each need and feeling by the total number of behaviors listed for giving, and then for receiving, for each participant. For each participant, their proportions did not necessarily reach 1.0 because, overall, 28% of participants' feelings responses could not be coded.

Despite the stringency of relying on the ratings of an objective judge, 10% of the feelings could be coded as reflecting an impact (either fortification or threat) on belonging (e.g., "alone," "alienated," "lonely"), 34% on self-esteem (e.g., "dumb," "I feel good," "guilt"), 20% on control (e.g., "frustrated," "helpless," "in control"), 8% on meaningful existence (e.g., "useless," "invisible," "worthless"), and 31% on anger (e.g., "pissed off," "angry").

Direction of Impact of the Silent Treatment

Analyses were then performed to determine whether the silent treatment either threatened or fortified each need. Twice as many feelings were coded as indicating needs threat over needs fortification. A difference was detected for needs as well, such that the silent treatment was coded as having the greatest impact on self-esteem, followed by control, then belonging, and finally meaningful existence. The impact on anger was just as high as that on self-esteem.

Effects on Each Need

Further analyses resulted in different patterns of threat and fortification for each need. Let us examine each need separately.

- *Belonging.* When the silent treatment was perceived as impacting on belonging, that impact was more likely to be coded as threatening than fortifying. In addition, an impact on belonging was more likely to be perceived when participants described *receiving* the silent treatment rather than *giving* it. However, participants' responses were never perceived by the objective rater as indicating a fortification of belonging, regardless of whether they were describing giving or receiving the silent treatment. Threats to belonging were perceived as more frequent when participants described receiving as opposed to giving the silent treatment.

- *Self-esteem.* When the response could be coded as impacting on self-esteem, that impact was more likely to be threatening than fortifying. Both *receiving* and *giving* the silent treatment resulted in greater threat than fortification of self-esteem; however, this difference was greater for receiving than for giving the silent treatment.

- *Control.* As predicted, the need for control was threatened more than fortified when *receiving* the silent treatment, but there was no difference between the proportion of control threat to control fortification when *giving* the silent treatment. This slight reversal was the first sign that giving the silent treatment may to some extent fortify more than threaten the need for control.

- *Meaningful existence.* When the silent treatment is perceived as impacting on the need for meaningful existence, that impact is a threatening one. In fact, like belonging, participants' responses were never perceived as indicating a fortification of this need.

- *Anger.* Use of the silent treatment, whether being given or received, resulted in feelings coded as increasing rather than decreasing feelings of anger.

Summary of Findings for Study 1

Several interesting findings emerged from Study 1. First, participants listed a surprisingly large number (152 to be exact) of unique behaviors that exemplified what they meant by the silent treatment. From this alone it appears that the silent treatment is multidimensional, complex, and ambiguous. It is ambiguous because not only might so many different behaviors be exhibited during the silent treatment, the same behaviors might mean something altogether different. Avoiding eye contact, folding one's arms, and listening to loud music might mean that one's attention is directed elsewhere, that one's arms are tired, or that one preferred loud noise. Because many of these behaviors might be indicative of other things, determining whether or not the behaviors at any particular point in time indicate the silent treatment may be quite puzzling for targets. Likewise, the inherent ambiguity that accompanies the behaviors associated with the silent treatment affords sources the ability to deny using it.

Second, despite the reference to silence in the term, the most frequently mentioned silent treatment behavior involved a visual component: "to avoid eye contact." Still, silence was implicated in many of the responses ("not talking," "avoiding all contact"), although some behaviors were difficult to define according to exactly what specific responses constituted them (e.g., "making a definite effort to ignore").

Third, the trained rater, using a conservative system in which subjective guesses were minimized, regarded most of the listed behaviors as fitting into the social and punitive types of ostracism. Apparently, leaving the room—an instance of physical ostracism—is not commonly incorporated into peoples' understanding of the term "the silent treatment."

Fourth, there were a reasonable percentage of responses that could be coded as affecting each of the four hypothesized needs: belonging, self-esteem, control, and meaningful existence. This emerged despite the fact that the objective rater typically coded short descriptions of participants' feelings in the absence of any contextual information that could be used to make inferences about the participants' intended meaning. Additionally, participants' responses were also rated as affecting feelings of anger.

More compelling were the interesting relations we observed between giving and receiving the silent treatment and the direction that the impact had on the hypothesized needs. Initially, we speculated that giving the silent treatment might fortify the needs in the source that it deprives in the target. We were postulating that perhaps the target's belonging, control, self-esteem, and meaningful existence was sucked out of him or her and absorbed by the source. Overall, however, the silent treatment was more often associated with threatening rather than fortifying needs, particularly for belonging, self-esteem, and meaningful existence. Regardless of whether individuals were associating feelings for behaviors of giving or receiving the silent treatment, feelings of belonging, self-esteem, and meaningful existence were coded as being threatened. A different pattern emerged for control, however, such that when giving the silent treatment, control was just as likely to be coded as threatened as fortified. When receiving the silent treatment, however, control was more likely to be rated as threatened. This provided us with initial evidence that giving the silent treatment offers its sources a certain degree of perceived control.

We recognize that having objective raters to code responses was, on the one hand, a conservative approach, but on the other, one that is perhaps misleading. It is possible that if people judged their own reported behaviors and feelings in relation to the model, a different pattern may emerge. Individuals would presumably know what they meant by the feeling they listed, and therefore could more appropriately code feelings according to the tenets of the model.

In Study 2 we asked participants to judge their own behaviors and feelings, after first explaining the taxonomy of the model to them and then explaining the concepts of needs threat and fortification. If subjective and objective judgments are similar, then a similar pattern of results should emerge to that of Study 1. We note here that we also had the trained rater code the responses. This indeed replicated the pattern as before, so any differences that emerged with the participants' ratings can be attributable to differences in their inferential perspectives.

STUDY 2. PERCEPTIONS AND SELF-RATINGS OF THE SILENT TREATMENT

Twenty-two men and 41 women from the University of Toledo participated in this study. The task was essentially the same as in Study 1, except now, after having listed the behaviors and feelings, participants listened to a brief tutorial on the model given by the experimenter (see Chapter 3), while following along in their Study 2 packets. After receiving the tutorial, participants were told to code their behaviors on the four taxonomic dimensions and then code each feeling associated with those behaviors on each of the four needs (plus anger). This time we added apology as a category because we have noted in our interviews that people who give the silent treatment often do not feel the need to apologize, and people who get the silent treatment often feel compelled to apologize in order to end the silence. For each feeling, participants were asked to judge whether that feeling represented a threat, a fortification, or no impact for each of the four needs, plus anger and apology.

Participants listed an average of about 12 behaviors each when giving and when receiving the silent treatment. A total of 1,087 behaviors were listed. As in Study 1, a trained judge did a conservative "literal" screening for overlap, resulting in 224 unique behaviors. The five most frequently reported behaviors were not making eye contact, not talking, not calling as usual, making a definite effort to ignore, and trying to avoid all contact.

The participants' perceptions of their own behaviors in relation to the taxonomic dimensions of the model revealed a pattern similar to yet more variable than that of the trained judge in Study 1. Participants coded about three-quarters of their behaviors as social ostracism. For motive, they coded over half of their behaviors as punitive, with the other four motives represented approximately equally. Participants coded a quarter of their responses as partial ostracism, and almost half as complete ostracism (30% were coded as normal interaction). Finally, when asked to code for the causal clarity dimension, participants regarded almost half of their behaviors as causally unclear, and a little less as being causally clear. Because the highest joint classification of visibility and motive was social and punitive (42%), we again restricted our subsequent analyses to responses given only to those social, punitive behaviors.

We first addressed the extent to which each listed feeling was perceived to affect each hypothesized need (plus anger and apology). We suspected that the blind rater's judgments in Study 1 underrepresented the extent to which the needs and feelings were being affected because the judge's decisions were based solely on a literal, and not subjective, interpretation. Because participants were judging feelings that they themselves generated, we expected an increased proportion of responses to be coded as having an impact on the need or feeling in question. This was indeed the case for belonging, control, meaningful existence, and apology. Participants coded about a third of their feelings as having an effect on belonging, self-esteem, control, anger, and apology, with slightly less effect on meaningful existence.

We then analyzed the responses to determine whether the impact was needs fortification or needs threat. As in Study 1, participants coded more feelings as indicating needs threat than needs fortification. And, once again, the patterns of threat and fortification were different depending upon the specific need.

- *Belonging.* Regardless of whether the silent treatment was being given or received, belonging was much more likely to be perceived as being threatened than fortified.
- *Self-esteem.* A similar pattern was observed for self-esteem: participants coded their feelings as self-esteem threat more than self-esteem

fortification. Unlike in Study 1, in Study 2 this pattern was particularly true of receiving the silent treatment, but not of giving it.

• *Control.* When receiving the silent treatment, participants perceived more threat to control than to fortification; however, when giving the silent treatment, participants perceived that their need for control was more likely to be fortified than threatened.

• *Meaningful existence.* Similar to the pattern of results for self-esteem, when the silent treatment impacted on the need for meaningful existence, that impact was perceived to be more threatening than fortifying. In addition, receiving the silent treatment resulted in more perceived threat than fortification in meaningful existence, whereas giving the silent treatment resulted in no differences between threat and fortification.

• *Anger and apology.* Participants perceived the silent treatment as increasing anger rather than decreasing it. Receiving the silent treatment did not affect reported needs to apologize, but giving the silent treatment resulted in a lower net obligation to apologize.

Summary of Findings for Study 2

The results of Study 2 mostly replicated and strengthened the patterns observed in Study 1. Over 200 unique behaviors indicative of the silent treatment were listed. Afterward, the participants were given a brief training session on the ostracism model and were asked to go over their listed behaviors and rate each according to the model's taxonomy. Not only were they able to do this without apparent difficulties, but they appeared to make finer and more varied distinctions than did the objectively trained rater of Study 1. Then they were asked to rate their corresponding feelings according to the needs-threat aspect of the model. Again, they completed this task without any requests for clarification or help.

Once again, our participants understood the silent treatment to be generally social, but they were also more inclined to view their behaviors as instances of cyber- and physical ostracism than the objective judge did in Study 1. Consistent with Study 1, they rated the motive behind the behaviors as primarily punitive, but they also more frequently referred to the other four motives. As was the case in Study 1, they viewed the silent treatment as varying substantially with respect to quantity and causal clarity.

The four hypothesized needs—belonging, self-esteem, control, and meaningful existence—were largely viewed as being threatened by the silent treatment, but the only evidence for fortification was for control. The person who employs the silent treatment gains control, despite losing a sense of belonging. In Study 2, the net effect of ostracizing someone was less clear for self-esteem and meaningful existence; for both needs, there was just as much fortification as threat.

Clearly, anger is a prominent emotion fueled by both using and receiving the silent treatment. The fact that anger plays such an important role may provide us with some ideas about why the silent treatment may be self-sustaining, at least at first. Because it makes both sides angry, there may be less willingness to talk things out initially, and pressures to "save face" may be high. Apology, which was not detected sufficiently by the trained judge in Study 1 to be included in the analysis, was detected by the participants themselves, and displayed an interesting pattern. When receiving the silent treatment, participants' feelings indicated ambivalent pressures: just as strong to apologize as to not apologize. When giving the silent treatment, however, the net effect was for the source to feel less of a need to apologize.

SUMMARY OF STUDIES 1 AND 2

The typical dictionary definition of the silent treatment is relatively simple. *Merriam-Webster's Collegiate Dictionary,* 10th edition, defines the silent treatment as "an act of completely ignoring a person or thing by resort to silence especially as a means of expressing contempt or disapproval." Yet the participants in our studies described the silent treatment as 224 unique behaviors, many of which involve acts other than silence. This suggests that the silent treatment is complex and multidimensional. The large list of behaviors also may speak to our extensive experience with it. Presumably, our language and depth of understanding for an object, concept, or phenomenon is enriched by experience. That there are so many possible behaviors that might indicate the presence of the silent treatment suggests that the participants had a thorough understanding of what the silent treatment was and how it was manifested. This is consistent with the Faulkner et al. (1997) survey that indicated that between two-thirds and three-quarters of the U.S. population admit to receiving the silent treatment from and giving it to a loved one.

No sex differences emerged in the analyses, nor did the sex of the participant interact with any of the other variables. Previous research suggests that sex differences might have been expected. Cairns and Cairns (1991) reported that girls were more likely than boys to use forms of ostracism like the silent treatment. The Faulkner et al. survey mentioned above revealed that women reported using the silent treatment slightly more than did men, which is also consistent with the power tactics literature (Buss, 1992; Falbo & Peplau, 1980; Kipnis, 1984). Apparently, even if the frequency of giving the silent treatment is different for males and females, it is not described differently by members of the two sexes.

WHERE IS THE SILENT TREATMENT
IN THE TAXONOMY?

Using the taxonomy put forth in the model of ostracism discussed in Chapter 3, the silent treatment is by and large regarded as social and punitive. By "social," we mean that it is used most often in the presence of its targets, rather than through physical expulsion or avoidance. By "punitive," we mean that it is used as a form of aversive control over others. That it is regarded as primarily social is interesting in that it would seem that the clearest and easiest indication of ignoring someone might be to physically leave that person's company. Nevertheless, the silent treatment was understood generally to be something one did while in the presence of the treatment's target. The punitive motive ascribed to the silent treatment is consistent with the notion that the silent treatment is considered to be an intentional act (hence, a "treatment"), and of the five motives, punitive is probably the most clearly intentional.

The quantity of ostracism appears to vary in people's perception of the silent treatment, as does its clarity. That is, the quantity of ostracism used in the silent treatment may be partial, mixed with normal interactions, or it may be complete, such that no "normal" interaction occurs. Additionally, the causal clarity behind the reason for its use (as in "I'm not going to talk with you") may or may not be present.

The data support the proposition put forth in the theoretical model that the silent treatment influences feelings of belonging, self-esteem, control, and meaningful existence. We would argue that it is a powerful weapon that offers its sources a large array of behavioral options and that simultaneously threatens four fundamental human needs.

How the silent treatment behaviors affect these needs depends to some extent upon whether the silent treatment is being given or received. In general, all needs were threatened when receiving the silent treatment. Individuals who give the silent treatment risk loss of belonging, but gain feelings of control. Self-esteem and meaningful existence are equally fortified and threatened when individuals give the silent treatment.

If giving the silent treatment threatens users' needs for belonging, self-esteem, and meaningful existence, then why use it? Perhaps the answer lies in the immediate control that it apparently offers individuals who use it. Although the act of giving the silent treatment may be aversive and threatening to the source, the purpose of using the silent treatment may be to correct an undesirable behavior of the target. Thus, the temporary threat to the source's other needs may be an acceptable price to pay for other longer term benefits.

The addition of anger and apology to associated feelings may require refinement in the model. The data suggest that people give the silent treatment because they are angry, and that when they receive the silent treatment it makes them angry. Obviously, because of the nature of this study, the direction of these causal links is only assumed to work in this fashion. Anger, however, is an emotional reaction (and possibly an instigation for action) rather than a need. Still, its role in understanding the antecedents and consequences of the silent treatment cannot be underestimated. Also, the silent treatment appears to impact a desire to apologize, but again it impacts differently on receivers and givers. Receivers' feelings were rated as reflecting about an equal amount of pressure to apologize as to not apologize, but givers were rated as feeling fewer obligations to apologize. I believe an unusual feature of ostracism is that because it can be regarded as a nonbehavior, it is easy for someone using it to deny that he or she is employing such a tactic. This, in turn, relieves the source of having to apologize for using it. Such relief would not be available for other, more obvious forms of aversive behavior, such as verbal insult or physical violence. It is also interesting to note that, compared to those who are insulted or hit, targets of the silent treatment feel some compulsion to apologize to the person who was using the silent treatment on them. Again, this points to the unusual power of the silent treatment. It is essentially a "stealth" tactic that affords users incredible power over their targets, while allowing them to deny using it and in some cases obligating the target to apologize.

The silent treatment is used by children, teachers, family members, coworkers, and relationship partners. The results of Studies 1 and 2 suggest there are many behaviors that might imply the presence of the silent treatment, and that these behaviors impact fundamental human needs. Further, except for control, either receiving or giving the silent treatment threatens most needs.

In the next set of studies, we look at narrative accounts of actual instances of both giving and receiving the silent treatment. Will the results suggested in the first two studies that were devoid of any particular context generalize to actual silent treatment events, as interpreted by the actors in the silent treatment episode?

NARRATIVES OF THE SILENT TREATMENT

The purpose of this research was to explore in a broader sense how people recall their experiences of the silent treatment (Sommer et al., in press). We asked participants to write a narrative account of the last time that they gave the silent treatment and the last time they received the silent treatment. The previous two studies simply analyzed how people interpreted the term *silent treatment*: What behaviors constituted the silent treatment and what feelings were associated with those behaviors? In the next two studies, we went beyond this context-free and somewhat limited approach by asking respondents to provide accounts of their own experiences with the silent treatment. By using the autobiographical narrative method, we hoped to obtain evidence to complement that found in Studies 1 and 2, and to further test various predictions of the model.

The Narrative Method

In the next two studies, we developed a detailed coding scheme to test several hypotheses derived from the model. The predictions were tested using the narrative method. University students wrote one story about a time they were exposed to the silent treatment and one story about a time they used the silent treatment on someone else.

The analysis of narratives has several advantages and is complementary to experimental methods. Narratives are rich in detail, not constrained by the expectations of the researcher, and possess higher levels of external validity. There are, however, potential concerns about the use of narratives. For instance, there is debate about how participants go about choosing their anecdotes: should they select the most memorable, the most recent, or perhaps, the most representative anecdote? We chose to ask respondents for their most recent experience in order to increase the generalizability and representativeness of the episodes.

Autobiographical narratives often yield evidence for perspective biases (Baumeister & Catanese, 2001). Perpetrators (or sources) will often de-emphasize the long-term negative consequences of their behaviors and maintain that any problems they caused have long been solved. By justifying their objectionable behaviors and also denying the long-term impact of these behaviors, perpetrators are able to avoid feelings of guilt or shame. Victims (or targets), conversely, emphasize their own suffering and maintain that the transgression continues to have implications for their lives (Baumeister, Stillwell, & Wotman, 1990). Continued suffering entitles victims to further compensation from the perpetrator and provides a means of eliciting concern and support from others (Baumeister & Catanese, 2001; Baumeister et al., 1990; Baumeister, Wotman, & Stillwell, 1993).

We expected that sources and targets would present different interpretations of their experiences. Sources should downplay the negative consequences of their behavior by maintaining that the problem was eventually resolved. Targets, conversely, should be less likely to portray the situation as resolved and instead would emphasize the negative consequences of being ignored. We also expected that sources would emphasize the utility of having used ostracism on their partners, whereas targets would deny such utility and denigrate its use.

Predictions Derived from the Model

First, we predicted that targets would report greater negative impact when they were unaware of the cause for the silent treatment (causally unclear) than when they were aware of it (causally clear). This prediction is based on the idea that simply knowing about the cause of an event, rather than being able to exact change, can provide sufficient control (called integrative control) to individuals that can help them cope with traumatic or aversive events (Rothbaum et al., 1982). Thus, knowing the cause of something can provide a certain degree of order and meaning to one's life (Janoff-Bulman & Wortman, 1977). Furthermore, in the absence of causal clarity, targets may search for plausible reasons for being subjected to the silent treatment. These reasons might include their possible misdeeds, offensive statements, or transgressions, causing them to generate a host of self-deprecating attributions for their treatment. Finally, causally unclear ostracism may be more likely to jeopardize the perceived stability of the interpersonal bond. Knowledge of a specific cause may provide clues as to if and when the silent treatment will likely end. People who do not know the reason may be more fearful as to when (or if) the silent treatment will end, and whether or not it signals the end of the relationship.

Second, we expected targets to report greater negative impact when they interpreted the motive for the silent treatment to be oblivious rather than punitive. The results from Studies 1 and 2 suggested that the silent treatment is primarily an interpersonal strategy with a punitive motive. However, one important way in which the silent treatment deviates from other forms of social rejection is in its capacity to affect targets even when it is not intended to punish. Oblivious ostracism is defined from the target's perspective and refers to situations in which a person feels so unimportant as to escape the attention of others. We predicted that oblivious ostracism would be especially devastating to targets because they may interpret the silence as a sign that they simply do not matter. When the ostracism is perceived as punitive, targets can at least be comforted in the knowledge that they mattered enough to evoke a negative emotional reaction. When sources are regarded as being oblivious to the target, then this may represent a much stronger attack on targets' feelings of belongingness, self-worth, and meaningful existence.

Third, we coded sources' reasons for giving the silent treatment in order to determine if, as suggested in Studies 1 and 2, they perceived increased control when they employed it. Because the silent treatment is unilateral, allowing no give-and-take with the target, and often deprives the target of the relevant information with which to explain it, sources enjoy an increase in power and control over the targets.

STUDY 3. NARRATIVES OF YOUNGER UNIVERSITY STUDENTS

Participants were 167 (90 female and 77 male) undergraduates recruited from introductory psychology classes at the University of Toledo. They wrote two personal stories about their prior experiences with the silent treatment. Of the 334 possible responses, 53 were either absent or too short to code. The remaining 131 source stories and 150 target stories comprised the data for Study 3 ($N = 281$).

Participants first wrote a story about an occasion they were the target of the silent treatment. Instructions for the target condition were as follows:

> We are interested in the use and effects of ostracism in interpersonal relationships. By *ostracism*, we mean the purposeful ignoring or shunning of an individual by others. Perhaps you know it as "the silent treatment." In any case, we would like you to remember the last time you were subjected to the silent treatment. Write down the circumstances that led to you being ignored and how you it made you feel, think, and behave. What were the ultimate consequences of being ignored?

Participants then wrote a story about a time in which they had used the silent treatment. Their instructions read:

> Now, think back to the time you last used the silent treatment on someone else. What led to you using this treatment? Why did you choose silence rather than some other way to deal with the situation (like direct confrontation, arguing, etc.)? What were the outcomes of using the silent treatment on this person?

Coding

• *Causal clarity.* Causal clarity referred to whether the target understood the reason for the silent treatment. The narratives were coded as either causally unclear (the reason for the silent treatment was not known or understood), causally clear (it was known or understood), or that causal clarity could not be determined from the information provided.

• *Needs threatened.* The target narratives were coded for the mention of each of the four needs that I propose are threatened by ostracism: belongingness, control, self-esteem, and meaningful existence. They were also coded for two reactions that could repair or defend against a threat to belongingness and self-esteem: seeking external relationships and self-affirmation, respectively.

• *Outcomes and interpretations of silent treatment.* Several outcome variables were coded in order to examine the different ways in which sources and targets recalled and described their experiences. These included: ostracism was effective in securing desired outcome (e.g., "He stops harassing me right away"), the problem was discussed or resolved (e.g., "We finally talked it out"), the source gained power or control (e.g., "I chose this method so I would not say something I'd later regret,"), the target reciprocated the silent treatment (e.g., "I decided to remain firm in my resolve and ignore his behavior"), the target withdrew (e.g., "I spoke only when spoken to"), and the target resented being manipulated (e.g., "I didn't appreciate having to grovel for forgiveness").

• *Emotional outcomes.* Possible emotional outcomes included anger, frustration, hurt feelings, guilt, loss of pride, feeling scared, experiencing loss of trust and feeling upset, lonely, rejected, uncomfortable, confused, bad, and stupid.

• *Reasons for ostracism.* The list of reasons for ostracism was partially drawn from the five motives I propose in my ostracism model, and we added a few others that might be interpreted as falling outside those motives. These included punitive, defensive, oblivious, and role-prescribed, as well as time out (to calm down), confrontation avoidance (to avoid a full-blown argument), to communicate a problem (to communicate one's anger or disappointment in the other's behavior), that the silent treatment was easier (because the treatment was easier than fighting), as a last resort (when confrontation proved ineffective), and to terminate the relationship (to end or sever one's ties with the target).

For the purposes of testing the prediction that the oblivious motive was more likely to increase negative consequences for targets, we combined all motives other than oblivious (no responses were coded as "not ostracism") and labeled them as *intentional*. The reason for this prediction was that regardless of the differences, targets who thought the silent treatment was intentional all perceived that the sources were taking the effort to attend to them and recognize their existence.

Results of Study 3

• *Narrative length.* On average, target narratives were 81 words and source narratives were 68 words. For each variable, coders recorded a "Yes" or "No" indicating whether that variable was present versus absent, respectively.

• *Causal clarity.* We compared causally unclear and causally clear target narratives to determine whether unclear ostracism resulted in greater threat. Silent treatment episodes that were causally unclear predicted stronger threats to belongingness and self-esteem than did causally clear episodes. Contrary to expectations, causally unclear episodes were not associated with greater perceived loss of control.

• *Oblivious ostracism.* Silent treatment episodes coded as having an oblivious motive predicted greater threats to belongingness than the combined intentional motives and were associated with higher levels of seeking affiliation with others. These findings suggest that the failure to be noticed by others may deprive individuals of the basic need for belongingness and meaningful existence, and that such deprivation surpasses that created by ostracism that is perceived as punitive or intentional.

• *Perspective differences.* Source and target narratives were compared to determine whether individuals' interpretations of silent treatment episodes depended on the role or perspective they took. Sources were more likely than targets to indicate that the source got what he or she wanted, and that the issue had been discussed or resolved. Consistent with the findings from Studies 1 and 2, the analyses also showed that the sources were more likely to say they gained control. Targets' narratives, conversely, were more likely to portray the target as reciprocating the ostracism, withdrawing, and resenting the manipulation.

These perspective differences indicated that sources and targets of the silent treatment characterized their experiences differently. Whereas sources emphasized the utility of the silent treatment as a means of achieving power and control, targets focused more on their own withdrawal and resentment. Sources were also more likely than targets to consider the episode as resolved. The present findings suggest that attitudes about the silent treatment depend largely on perspective. The silent treatment is viewed as effective and appropriate by those giving it but not by those receiving it.

• *Emotional outcomes.* We recorded the adjectives used for the type of emotion(s) experienced prior to, during, or following the silent treatment. Because most of the silent treatment episodes occurred within the context of interpersonal conflicts, we expected high levels of anger among both sources and targets. Yet targets were expected to experience a disproportionately higher number of additional negative emotions stemming from the sources' response to conflict. As expected, anger was a prevalent emotion in both target and source narratives. However, compared to source narratives, target narratives yielded a greater percentage of several other negative emotion categories, and targets reported a greater total number of negative emotions than sources. The results suggest that the silent treatment resulted in a broader array of negative experiences for targets than for sources.

Reasons for Ostracism

Sources and targets generated many reasons for the silent treatment. Targets generated consistently fewer reasons than sources, with the exception of the oblivious ostracism category (which is defined primarily from the target's perspective). As occurred in Studies 1 and 2, punitive emerged as the most frequent reason for ostracism in both source and target narratives. Another reason frequently mentioned by sources was the desire to avoid a confrontation, which may fit conceptually within the category of defensive motives.

There were certain limitations with Study 3 that we wanted to correct in Study 4. We did not counterbalance the order in which source and target narratives were completed; all participants completed the target narratives first. In Study 4, the perspectives were counterbalanced. Moreover, in Study 3, we relied solely on the experiences of university freshmen and sophomores who were predominantly in their late teens and early 20s. In Study 4, we attempted to replicate the findings of Study 3 with an older, professional sample.

Besides testing the same set of hypotheses, another aim of Study 4 was to investigate the effects of trait self-esteem on the use of, and reactions to, the silent treatment. Nearly all the experimental work examining individual differences in social rejection has been done outside the domain of the silent treatment per se (e.g., Fenigstein, 1979; Nezlek et al., 1997). Thus, our investigation into the ways in which self-esteem may moderate the causes or consequences of the silent treatment was largely exploratory, but we generated a few predictions based on previous theory and research.

Predictions of the Effects of Trait Self-Esteem

Self-Esteem and Perceptions of Being Ostracized

Our first prediction was based on our observation that theories often link self-esteem with perceptions of inclusion or acceptance (e.g., Abrams & Hogg, 1990; Cooley, 1902; Rogers, 1959; Tajfel & Turner, 1986), and recent studies demonstrate that people low in self-esteem are more likely to perceive and react negatively to exclusion by others

(Harter, 1993; Leary et al., 1995; Nezlek et al., 1997). Therefore, we hypothesized that people with lower self-esteem would be more likely to report receiving the silent treatment by others.

Self-Esteem and Reactions to Receiving the Silent Treatment

Our second prediction dealt with the relationship of targets' self-esteem to their reactions to the silent treatment. We expected that individuals with higher self-esteem would be less likely to suffer partners who gave them the silent treatment, and would be more likely to sever themselves from such relationships. This is because individuals higher in self-esteem are more likely to assume they have the ability to attract alternative partners, and thus may feel less invested in their relationships (Rusbult, 1993; Rusbult, Morrow, & Johnson, 1987). According to interdependence theory (Kelley & Thibaut, 1978; Rusbult, 1993) people will exhibit constructive rather than destructive responses to interpersonal conflict when they are more invested in their relationships (Rusbult et al., 1991). Indeed, several studies have shown that highly committed (i.e., more invested) individuals exhibit more loyalty and attempts at problem solving than less committed individuals (Rusbult, 1993; Rusbult et al, 1991). Additionally, individuals who are higher in self-esteem may be less likely to assume blame or responsibility for problems in collaborative relationships (Greenwald, 1980). This, in turn, may make higher self-esteem individuals react with even less tolerance to their partners' use of the silent treatment: they may be more inclined to assume its use reflects the dispositions of their partners rather than due to something they did wrong. Therefore, low self-esteem targets of the silent treatment, who are more motivated to maintain their relationships and who are more likely to assume blame, will make greater efforts to conform to the source's desires.

People high in self-esteem, then, would be less committed to their current relationship partners and less willing to respond constructively to their partners' anger. In fact, Rusbult et al. (1987) found that self-esteem correlated negatively with one's willingness to accommodate angry partners and correlated positively with the tendency to exit the relationship during periods of marital distress.

Self-Esteem and the Use of the Silent Treatment

We also examined whether self-esteem predicted people's likelihood of using the silent treatment. Our prediction pertained to when individuals used the silent treatment motivated by defensiveness. Based upon research by Murray, Holmes, MacDonald, and Ellsworth (1998), individuals with lower levels of self-esteem who were led to feel bad about themselves responded by withdrawing from their partners in a defensive, self-protective manner. Given this proclivity, we expect that individuals with lower levels of self-esteem may, when they perceive imminent rejection, be more likely to use the silent treatment as a preemptive strike. Therefore, we expected that defensive ostracism would be more common among people with lower as opposed to higher levels of self-esteem.

Another reason that individuals who are lower in self-esteem may be more likely to use the silent treatment is that they may feel that they cannot express themselves effectively during a conflict. People with low self-esteem have lower feelings of efficacy (Burger, 1995; Deci & Ryan, 1995) and are more socially anxious (Leary & Kowalski, 1995). If attempts to justify their anger or behaviors to their partners fail, people who are lower in self-esteem may, therefore, resort to silence.

STUDY 4. NARRATIVES OF OLDER UNIVERSITY STUDENTS

Participants were 130 individuals enrolled in a continuing education seminar. Most were female (91%) medical professionals (mostly dental hygienists and nurses). The procedure was the same as in Study 3, with three exceptions. First, the order in which respondents completed the narratives was counterbalanced. Second, all respondents were asked to complete a trait self-esteem scale prior to completing the narratives. Third, all participants were asked to report how frequently the silent treatment was used on them and how often they used the treatment on others. These last two items were assessed in order to examine the relationships between self-esteem and experiences with social ostracism in everyday life. Coding categories were identical to those used in Study 3.

Of the 260 possible narratives, 45 were either absent or too short to code. Final analyses were based on 111 source stories and 104 target stories (N = 215 stories).

After they completed both target and source narratives, respondents answered the following two 100-point questions:

1. Some of us have had the silent treatment used on us a lot, some occasionally, some rarely, and some never. How would you rate yourself on the frequency with which the silent treatment has been used on you?
2. Some of us use the silent treatment a lot, some occasionally, some rarely, and some never. How would you rate yourself on the frequency with which you use the silent treatment on others?

Results of Study 4

Target and source narratives averaged nearly 100 words in length. Once again, interrater agreement was moderate to high for all coding dimensions. The order of the narratives had no effect.

- *Causal clarity.* As in Study 3, causally unclear silent treatment episodes were associated with greater threats to self-esteem than those coded as being causally clear. However, against predictions (and unlike the null finding in Study 3), causally clear ostracism was associated with stronger threats to control than causally unclear ostracism.
- *Oblivious ostracism.* The effects of oblivious ostracism on feelings of belongingness and other basic needs were similar to those found in Study 3, though low statistical power prevented most of these comparisons from reaching significance. Significance was achieved only for threats to self-esteem, with oblivious ostracism causing greater threats to self-esteem than other motives for ostracism.
- *Perspective differences.* As in Study 3, sources were more likely than targets to report that ostracism was effective. Consistent with the previous three studies, sources were more likely than targets to report increased control. Targets, conversely, were significantly more likely than sources to report their own withdrawal, reciprocation of the silent treatment, and resentment of its use.
- *Emotional outcomes.* Emotional outcomes were very similar to those in Study 3, except that sources reported levels of frustration comparable to those of targets. Targets reported a greater overall number of negative emotions than did sources, suggesting that fatigue or order effects cannot explain the perspective differences in emotional outcomes obtained in Study 3.
- *Reasons for ostracism.* As in Study 3, targets most often thought the silent treatment was being used to punish them. Targets generated very low frequencies for the other motive categories. Sources were equally likely to report using ostracism for punitive reasons, to avoid confrontation, to achieve a time-out, or as a last resort. For exploratory purposes, we coded the real (source's perspective) or perceived (target's perspective) reasons for the silent treatment. Sources were specifically queried for their reasons for choosing silence over other responses to conflict. Thus one would expect a higher frequency of reason categories in source compared to target narratives. Yet, if targets' perceived reasons for the ostracism roughly matched sources' actual motives, then source and target narratives should evidence approximately equal proportions of each reason category. However, in both Studies 1 and 2, targets gener-

ated a lower frequency of nonpunitive reasons. This suggests that targets may have overestimated the frequency with which sources meant to hurt them. Perceptual or motivational biases may lead targets to underestimate the role of nonpunitive motives in sources' behaviors (e.g., "The argument was too aversive for him" or "She needed to cool off"). Instead, targets may have focused on their own negative outcomes and assumed that the source meant to inflict hurt or suffering (Baumeister et al., 1990). Research shows that empathy does reduce such biases (Chen, Froehle, & Morran, 1997), but targets may have had difficulty empathizing with sources who said nothing.

COMBINING THE COMMON RESULTS
OF STUDIES 3 AND 4

One purpose of Study 4 was to replicate the findings of Study 3 in an older, professional (and primarily female) sample. For the most part, this was successful. There were some inconsistencies, however, and therefore we conducted a meta-analysis on both studies to see which effects were reliable.

• *Causal clarity.* The results indicated that targets of causally unclear ostracism suffered significantly greater threats to belongingness and self-esteem than did targets of causally clear ostracism. Causally clear ostracism was associated with greater threats to control than causally unclear ostracism. I will return to this anomalous finding in a moment.

• *Oblivious versus intentional motives.* Oblivious ostracism was marked by stronger threats to belongingness, self-esteem, and meaningful existence. It was also associated with increased affiliation following the silent treatment. This set of findings is consistent with the predictions of the model. Whereas punitive and other intentional forms of ostracism are unpleasant and can have substantial impact in their own right, oblivious ostracism is even worse. These findings lend credence to William James's (1890) assertion that failure to be noticed by others exerts a more detrimental impact on one's sense of self than negative attention by others. Most instances of ostracism described by targets in both samples were viewed as punitive, and yet targets were consistently more threatened by instances in which others were not trying to ignore them but rather were oblivious to their presence.

The hypothesis that people prefer negative attention to indifference has received support from studies in developmental psychology. Based upon their research with elementary schoolaged children, Gallimore, Tharp, and Kemp (1969) concluded that negative attention reinforced undesirable or incorrect behavior in children who had a high need for social approval. Others studies have revealed significant positive correlations between perceived parental rejection and negative attention-seeking behavior (Peretti, Clark, & Johnson, 1984; Saxena, 1992). These lines of research help to explain why the negative attention characterizing intentional ostracism may be less threatening than the indifference suggested by oblivious ostracism. People would rather receive negative attention than no attention at all.

• *Perspective differences.* Compared to target narratives, source narratives were more likely to characterize the silent treatment as effective and as a means of gaining control. Sources were also more likely than targets to claim that the problem was eventually resolved or talked out. Conversely, targets were more likely than sources to focus on target withdrawal, resentment toward the source, and reciprocation of the ostracism. Finally, targets reported a higher number of negative emotions than sources. These findings are consistent with previous research revealing strong perspective biases inherent in various forms of interpersonal transgressions (Baumeister & Catanese, 2001).

EXAMINING THE ROLE OF SELF-ESTEEM IN THE USE OF AND REACTIONS TO THE SILENT TREATMENT

Self-Esteem and Frequency of Giving/Getting the Silent Treatment

As predicted, low self-esteem individuals reported being ostracized more frequently than did high self-esteem individuals. Low self-esteem was also associated with an increased use of silence on others. This is consistent with Leary et al.'s (1995) proposition that there is a link between chronic rejection and trait self-esteem such that low self-esteem participants (lows) reported feeling rejected more frequently than did high self-esteem participants (highs). Low self-esteem was also associated with an increased use of silence on others. This finding sheds light on the social worlds of people with low self-worth. Intuitive reasoning would lead one to hypothesize that lows (who perceive higher levels of ostracism) would be less likely than highs to engage willingly in behaviors that threaten the interpersonal bond. The finding that lows were more likely to give others the silent treatment suggests that the link between self-esteem and interpersonal rejection is more complicated than previously recognized.

Self-Esteem and Reactions to the Silent Treatment

Also as predicted, low self-esteem was associated with increased use of defensive ostracism, whereas high self-esteem predicted the use of ostracism as a means of terminating the relationship. This set of findings indicates that, though people with low self-esteem may use the silent treatment more in general, they use it in a defensive way, not as a deliberate means of severing the relationship. This finding for low self-esteem individuals is consistent with Murray et al.'s (1998) recent finding that low (but not high) self-esteem individuals who were made to focus on their own faults or shortcomings subsequently devalued their partners and expressed reduced needs for their relationships. Murray et al. speculated that lows were rejecting their partners before their partners had the opportunity to reject them. Low self-esteem may thus have a self-fulfilling aspect to it: perceptions of impending rejection or criticism from others leads to the rejection of others, which in turn disrupts belongingness and lowers self-esteem (Leary et al., 1995). Partners of low (but not high) self-esteem individuals rate their partners and their relationships more negatively over time (Murray, Holmes, & Griffin, 1996).

Support was also attained for the hypothesis that targets' level of self-esteem would predict their decisions to leave their ostracizing partners. Individuals with higher levels of self-esteem were more likely to report that they terminated their relationships with their ostracizing partners. This finding supports Rusbult et al.'s (1987) research showing that high self-esteem individuals, who generally possess greater relationship alternatives, are more likely to exit the relationship when dissatisfied with their partners. A partner's excessive use of the silent treatment may indeed cause such dissatisfaction.

WHY DO TARGETS EXPERIENCE MORE CONTROL WHEN THE CAUSE IS UNCLEAR?

We predicted that the consequences for targets would be worse if they were unclear as to the cause of the silent treatment. This prediction found support when we examined reports of belonging, but not for control. In fact, loss of control was more often associated with causally clear instances of the silent treatment than with instances that were unclear. Why? Perhaps this unanticipated finding was because we operationally defined control threat as "a reduced ability to control one's own or others' behaviors or outcomes." This operationalization was probably insensitive to changes in interpretive control, which refers to the ability to make sense of one's environment. Perhaps this definition precluded the control gained with causal clarity of simply *knowing* what the cause was, even if action could not necessarily be taken to exact change on one's self or others. Unfortunately, the content of the narratives revealed that respondents did not focus on this type of control.

The findings for causal clarity suggest that sources may choose to withhold an explanation for the silent treatment when the primary reason is to punish the target. By withholding an explanation, sources will maximize the loss of sense of belongingness and self-esteem experienced by targets. From the source's perspective, then, punishment is probably best accomplished by keeping the reasons for one's silence secret. However, refusing to offer an explanation may also reduce the likelihood that one will receive reparation. That is, targets will likely find it difficult to appease or compensate the source when they have no knowledge of what they have done to bring about the silent treatment.

A final intriguing possibility is that in some circumstances targets may take advantage of the ambiguity of causally unclear ostracism by choosing to deny that the source is actually giving them the silent treatment. In this sense, targets gain a certain degree of control by cognitively reframing the situation. In Chapter 10, we will examine this possibility further. Not only can sources benefit by pretending that they are not giving the silent treatment, but apparently targets can also benefit by pretending that they are not getting it.

CONCLUSIONS

We investigated the silent treatment using two paradigms. The first paradigm involved two studies that examined peoples' understanding of the silent treatment. Specifically, what behaviors comprised it, and how did those behaviors make them feel? The second paradigm used narrative analysis to examine peoples' accounts of the last time they gave and received the silent treatment. The results of both paradigms produced a fairly clear picture. Targets of social ostracism suffer some damage to mental well-being. They lose a sense of belonging, self-esteem, control, and—to a lesser extent—meaningful existence. Sources gain a sense of control, despite losing a sense of belonging.

The second paradigm also supported predictions from the model that causally unclear ostracism is more threatening to belonging than causally clear ostracism, and that oblivious ostracism is more damaging to targets than other intentional forms of ostracism.

Finally, some interesting individual differences emerged from the narrative analyses. Low self-esteem individuals were more likely to use the silent treatment, and they perceived that they received it more often too. They used it, however, more as a defensive tactic than as a means to end a relationship. Unfortunately, if their partners have high levels of self-esteem, it appears that their strategy will backfire. High self-esteem individuals are more likely to end a relationship when they are given the silent treatment. Likewise, when high self-esteem individuals use the silent treatment, it is more likely to signal their desire to end the relationship.

Although we have been able to shed a great deal of light on a heretofore overlooked phenomenon, more research is clearly needed into the causes and consequences of the silent treatment. Do sources of the silent treatment incur any intrapsychic costs? Preliminary evidence suggests that there may be important, self-regulatory costs associated with ignoring others. In one study (Sommer, Ciarocco, & Baumeister, 1999), participants were asked to ignore or speak freely with another person. Results revealed that participants who ignored another person persisted for a significantly shorter period of time on the anagram task than those who spoke freely. For sources of ostracism, short-term gains in control may be offset by a reduction in their larger capacities for self-control.

The use of controlled experiments that directly manipulate factors such as causal clarity and the perceived reasons for ostracism are also needed to provide converging evidence for the present findings. These approaches are discussed in the forthcoming chapters.

Later in this book, I discuss our research using structured interviews with long-term sources and targets of ostracism, many of whom have been involved with the silent treatment continuously for several years (Williams & Zadro, 1999). Recall the woman discussed in Chapter 2 who was not spoken to or looked at by her husband for the last 40 years of his life. It is evident from these interviews that targets of long-term silent treatment undergo severe psychological distress, ranging from feelings of helplessness and alienation, to depression and suicide attempts. Almost all targets also report physical distress as a result of long-term exposure to the silent treatment, and many volunteer that they would rather be verbally abused or beaten than given the silent treatment. When asked to explain, targets say that beatings at least signify that the source recognizes their existence. Further, targets argue that a person could go to friends or the authorities with bruises from beatings, but there is nothing they can show others to prove that they have been victimized by silence. Perhaps the studies in this chapter found relatively weak support for the hypothesized impact of the silent treatment on meaningless existence because the episodes were of limited duration. Long-term exposure to the silent treatment may signal, at some point, the pointlessness of one's existence.

The silent treatment is powerful. I marvel at the unique power and qualities of the silent treatment, but I do not endorse its use. Although initial reactions to the silent treatment may be to regain senses of belonging, self-esteem, control, and meaningful existence, finding means to do so may be dysfunctional. To regain their sense of belonging and self-esteem, silent treatment victims may try to seek out anyone else with whom they can form a bond and get approval, thus exposing themselves to unscrupulous others who might exploit this desire. Increased attempts to regain control might take the form of more provocative and aggressive behaviors aimed at eliciting some sort of response out of the source (as was the case with Brer Rabbit). This may lead to verbal and physical violence. And desires to regain a sense of meaningful existence may motivate the individual to do something, anything, in order to be recognized. Clearly, many dysfunctional harmful acts can gain people such needed recognition.

The Scarlet Letter Study

Five Days of Ostracism

I feel like I am a ghost on the floor that everyone hears,
but no one can talk to. I want to be noticed!
—MR. BLUE, 1996

Imagine arriving at work and being greeted by your coworkers as though you possessed a contagious virus or, perhaps worse, like you were not even there? No matter what you did or said, your fellow workers steered clear of you and did not respond to you. Even when tasks required group effort, your contributions seemed to fall on deaf ears. Your coworkers did not ask for your input as they usually did, nor did they argue or disagree with you. How would you react? How would it make you feel? What thoughts would you generate to explain or make sense of their behaviors?

Now imagine being on the other side of this scenario: you and your colleagues are ignoring one particular coworker throughout the day and are pretending this person does not exist. Why are you doing this? Is it difficult and distracting to ignore your coworker, or is it a simple and effortless task? After all, not talking to or looking at someone else requires nothing of you. Or does it? How does actively ignoring your coworker affect your attitude toward him or her? How does it make you feel about yourself?

In this chapter, I describe an examination and analysis of such a situation in which my colleagues at the University of Toledo and I were the participants (Williams, Bernieri, Faulkner, Grahe, & Gada-Jain, 2000). To afford my colleagues and myself a thin veil of anonymity, I will refer to us as Dr. Black, Dr. Brown, Mr. Blue, Ms. Yellow, and Ms. Pink. For the record, I'd like to identify my colleagues by their real names before I provide the details of the study. They are (in no particular order) Frank Bernieri, Sonja Faulkner, Neha Gada-Jain, and Jon Grahe. The five of us planned to ostracize a different person in our group each day over a period of a week. We recorded our thoughts, feelings, and behaviors in an open-ended, event-contingent, self-report record. These records were later typed out verbatim, synchronized by time and day with each other so that reactions to specific episodes could be compared, and coded by two nonparticipating individuals.

We assessed the cumulative exposures to frequent episodes of ostracism that occurred in a normal work setting over a period of a day (for each target) and a week (for sources).

We used a role-playing method to study lengthy intervals of ostracism within a closed system. Shaftel and Shaftel (1976) stated that role play in its simplest sense involves assuming a role to practice the behavior required in various situations. Unlike acting, which uses predetermined words and actions to entertain others, role play involves experiencing a problem or situation that is governed by its own constraints in order to further one's understanding of the situation (Van Ments, 1983). Role play is used in various forms in schools, industrial training, the military, and counseling as a means of educating and demonstrating how the roles people play in day-to-day life potentially effect the outcome of a situation.

Role play also has a place in psychology as a research technique that allows psychologists to examine phenomena within ethical constraints and without undue expense or danger. One of the most notable instances of role play in psychology was the Stanford Prison Study conducted by Haney, Banks, and Zimbardo (1973; Haney & Zimbardo, 1998). Haney et al. randomly assigned mentally and physically healthy male college students the roles of either prisoners or prison guards in a 2-week prison simulation. Six days into the simulation, the study was halted due to the increasing brutality of the prison guards and the declining health and spirits of the prisoners. The study demonstrated the power of role play, indicating how easy it is to fill a particular role (even if the role is randomly allocated) to the point where reality and role play merge.

The role-play method we adopted may have more mundane and experimental realism than a typical role-play method because we were always "playing" ourselves in our natural roles. In effect, we took part in a real-life simulation because our experiences lasted an entire week and occurred completely within the context of our lives (we were not stuck in the basement of some psychology laboratory—just on the sixth floor!).

What was the best way to record our reactions, feelings, thoughts, and behaviors? A traditional method is the self-report questionnaire. At the end of the week, we might have given ourselves a questionnaire asking such things as "How many times during the last week have you felt rejected, ignored, or ostracized?" Such measures could be useful as descriptions of our global perceptions of our social activity, but they should probably not be viewed as descriptions of actual social behavior. Instead, they are best seen as personalized impressions of social activity that have been percolated, construed, and reframed through various perceptual, cognitive, and motivational processes (see Wheeler & Reis, 1991, for a discussion of the specific problems of selection, recall of content, and aggregation). Another commonly used method of studying ongoing events is behavioral observation. But we refrained from enlisting someone to come to our floor to observe us for a week, take copious notes, and perhaps videotape us, because that would have made us feel like we were animals in a zoo. As strange as this week was going to be, we didn't want to make things more artificial by having strangers following us around.

We decided to use an unstructured event-contingent self-recording (see Wheeler & Reis, 1991, who discuss the structured types) because it seemed the best way to collect detailed data about ongoing, spontaneous ostracism events. This method required making a report every time an event meeting a preestablished definition occurs. The best known example of this method is the Rochester Interaction Record (RIR— Pietromonaco & Barrett, 1997; Reis & Wheeler, 1991; Wheeler & Nezlek, 1977), but it has also been used successfully to examine other processes (e.g., the Rochester Social Comparison Record—Wheeler & Miyake, 1992; the Iowa Communication Record—Duck, Rutt, Hurst, & Strejc, 1991). The event, in short, can be anything. The key to success in using this method is the unambiguous definition of the event requiring a report and the timeliness of reporting following the event itself. Rather than using a checklist-style record (like the experiments noted above), we decided to use an open-ended, diary-style format that did not presuppose relevant categories or responses. As such, the present method is qualitative in nature, amenable to descriptive rather than quantitative analysis.

THE SCARLET LETTER STUDY

General Plan of the Study

The five members of the social psychology graduate program at the University of Toledo (two faculty, both male, and three graduate students, two females and one male) served as participants. Together we discussed and informed ourselves about the purpose and procedure of the study. We each had an office on the sixth floor of the northwest wing of a large university building. No other offices were housed on this wing, although undergraduate research assistants and participants in other studies were often present.

Five sealed envelopes were distributed among us at a preparatory meeting held the Friday afternoon prior to the Monday on which the study would begin. Inside each sealed envelope was a different colleague's name. The outside of the envelope was obfuscated such that, even if held to the light, the name inside could not be read. In open discussion, each person chose a different day of the week (Monday through Friday) and wrote it on the outside of their envelope. The envelopes were handed to the first author, who would be in charge of them during the study. We agreed that at the beginning of the study (the following Monday before 8:00 A.M.), I would take the envelope marked "Monday," open it, and then place a scarlet letter "O" above the office door of the person whose name was contained within it (as shown in Figure 5.1). The same procedure would be followed for the remaining 4 days. This meant that four of the participants would not know if it was his or her day until he or she came to work on that particular day, but Friday's person would know that he or she was the last target by process of elimination. There was one exception to this rule. Because Ms. Pink was scheduled to present her research at a weekly discussion meeting on Friday, we

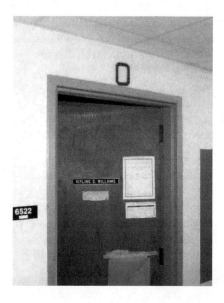

FIGURE 5.1. The scarlet letter "O" above the author's door on his day to be the target.

agreed that if she was not assigned to the target role by Wednesday, she would take her turn as target on Thursday.

We agreed that, for each day, all four participants would ostracize the individual who had the scarlet letter "O" above his or her door. The definition of ostracism stemmed from a discussion of the taxonomy outlined in my model (see Chapter 3), but generally included any act that was intended or perceived to involve ignoring, exclusion, or rejection. We did not place restrictions on the precise method of ostracism to be employed, but left it up to our own devices. If something had to be said to a target because of academic-related issues, the target could be spoken to, but in the manner of one who was otherwise not talking to that person. Targets could do whatever they wished: they could keep to themselves, attempt to talk with the others, leave the sixth floor, invite others up to their office, or anything else.

We agreed to make open-ended, event-contingent, self-recordings whenever an *episode* occurred that made us think of ostracism. We also allowed ourselves to make entries whenever we found ourselves ruminating about ostracism. Because of this, many of us wrote entries just prior to the study's commencement, in anticipation of what lay ahead. We were encouraged to record affective, cognitive, and behavioral entries and to write our entries as temporally close to the episode as possible. We were to make entries throughout the week whether we were ostracizing (sources), observing the ostracism, or enduring the ostracism (targets).

Typically, in role-play studies, debriefing is unnecessary. The participants are not deceived, and they are well aware that they are simply playing a role, so they are unlikely to have their feelings hurt. Nevertheless, despite the fact that we were fully aware of the study and its purpose, we agreed that a poststudy debriefing session would be helpful to air any hard feelings and to reestablish group harmony. On the Monday following the Scarlet Letter Week, we met over lunch for a 2-hour debriefing session.

Overview and Highlights of the Week

A chronological summary of the week's events follows in an attempt to capture the psychological climate and phenomenological experiences of the participants.

Entries Prior to Monday

Several participants chose to make entries prior to the first day of the experiment. Dr. Black noted that he tried to clear up any lingering disagreements among group members prior to Monday so that there could be no confusion as to the reasons for the ostracism. He was worried that participants could misinterpret the motives behind their ostracism and respond in anger. He expressed concerns about already feeling paranoid.

Ms. Pink wrote that she was not worried at all, and feared most of all that she wouldn't take the week seriously. In fact, she thought she might start giggling. She thought the week would be a bust, not likely to reveal anything interesting because it was premeditated and explicit. On the other hand, she believed that if this sort of role play would ever affect her, it would be during this time period when she was feeling particularly vulnerable.

Ms. Yellow discussed the study with her friend and said that it could be quite valuable phenomenologically, but that she doubted that it would affect her. She did, however, wonder if it would adversely affect her productivity.

Dr. Brown indicated he was "sort of" planning a strategy, but gave no details. He wondered how he would communicate effectively during the week. He hoped to be the first target and was especially fearful that his day might be Friday, the day of his departmental colloquium.

Mr. Blue also wanted to be the "O" first—to get it out of the way. He wrote that he felt apprehensive, aroused, and ambivalent toward the coming week. He thought he might feel negative affect when being the target of ostracism, but might actually enjoy being a source.

Monday

Dr. Brown's name was drawn first. Dr. Brown wrote, "I was filled with anticipation as I walked up the fifth flight of stairs. As I walked down the sixth-floor hall I slowly realized I might have the 'O.' " He considered how to react: "Maybe I'll engage in anticipatory retaliation. I saw Dr. White [another colleague] on the fifth floor and I went out of my way to tell her that I got the 'O' and that she needn't participate." Later that day, Dr. White invited Dr. Brown to join the group at a bar to watch *Monday Night Football*. He thanked her, but declined, and asked her not to invite the rest of the group until after he had left the office for the day.

Social comparison processes among the sources were evident on the first day. Dr. Black wrote, "I've talked with Ms. Pink and now Mr. Blue about how they are dealing with ignoring Dr. Brown, whether he's tested them, and just how it's going."

Normal activity appeared to be obstructed for everyone. Dr. Brown wrote, "My interaction with Mr. Blue and Ms. Yellow was extremely awkward. I found myself speaking faster than usual, almost as if to rush through. Motivationally, I want to withdraw. Contact is effortful and there's a growing sense of dread associated with having to deal with the ostracizers." Examples of paranoia also seeped in: "I have wondered about the contiguousness of this manipulation. I don't think any of the practicum students are in on it but I did find myself wondering about this at times throughout the day."

Being a source of ostracism also proved to be difficult, but in different ways than being a target. Dr. Brown remarked on how Dr. Black accidentally looked up at him and then quickly retracted his gaze, uttering a sound that suggested regret for reacting when he should not have. "I think I caught him off guard. He didn't turn around like he normally does. I found myself smiling and laughing like a Milgram teacher [this is a reference to Milgram's famous obedience studies, in which his naïve teachers sometimes laughed nervously when they were shocking the learner]. This must be very arousing. I think there is less stress on me than on the ostracizers. I noticed Dr. Black holding his hands to his face." Regarding Ms. Yellow as source, Dr. Brown said, "She cracked (or wilted, or rebelled, whatever). I think I learned something. O is fragile." Ms. Pink (a source) wrote, "The silent treatment takes control away from the user, too, when you think about it. It requires a huge amount of effort to remember how you're supposed to act—it's like the ostracism takes over you!" Finally, Mr. Blue remarked how distracting it was to ostracize Dr. Brown: "I also noted that the ostracism took so much mental effort that I have little memory of the purpose or content of the interaction. This is troublesome because he [Dr. Brown] told me something he would like me to do, and I can't even go ask him what it was."

The sources, who felt badly for Dr. Brown, experienced noticeable anxiety. "So far all day I've felt really sorry for Dr. Brown. This may not be affecting him at all, but I feel this is déjà-vu—do you remember how certain kids were always either picked on or left out at school? That's what I'm reminded of—I always used to feel sorry for those kids. . . . I don't like not being able to engage in the behaviors that I normally engage in." Although the clarity of the ostracism was high in that we all knew why we were doing it, thoughts of ambiguous causality nevertheless percolated. Dr. Brown wrote about being a source, "In retrospect, I felt a bit punitive. In other words, there might have been a tendency to indulge in some tit-for-tat behavior."

Finally, there was the feeling that the first day was exceptional, that what was experienced could be chalked up to first-day jitters and that the rest of the week would be easier and less interesting. Dr. Brown wrote, "Getting the hang of this thing. I've got a sense that with practice we'd settle into some sort of efficient communication."

Tuesday

This was Ms. Yellow's day. As the newest member of our group, Ms. Yellow considered herself lowest on the totem pole and generally spoken to less often than the rest of us under normal circumstances. She made interesting attributions about her situation: "It'll be easier for me to take ostracism since this is not my country, people don't acknowledge my existence all the time. I don't think they even realize that I may feel ignored at times because I'm the youngest and junior-most on the floor. So, who cares. . . . " After having washed her lab coat the night before, she wore it proudly during the day. But, of course, no one paid attention. "I wish they had looked . . . but even if they did they wouldn't know why I'm walking around with it . . . they're not very sensitive." By the time she came out of her office at the end of the workday, everyone had already left. "Wanted to catch the 6 P.M. shuttle and all the labs and computers were to be shut down! Ran like a mad woman to shut all computers . . . almost reflexively saying aloud 'Why the hell did they not tell me they're leaving???' Was really mad at everyone for a few minutes. But then I simultaneously was telling myself that they weren't suppose to, this is not on purpose, blah blah. . . . "

Ms. Pink did not always remember to play her role as source. Ms. Yellow seemed quite appreciative when Ms. Pink actually spoke to her: "Felt good that she spoke to me and was polite. It was her usual response but felt better than usual. Everything seems to have so much meaning."

Dr. Brown wrote some interesting reflections upon his return from exile. When he walked in that morning he wrote of his first contact, a greeting to Mr. Blue and Ms. Pink, "Apparently, a need developed which was satisfied by that greeting. Can't help but wonder what would happen with prolonged exposure . . . very satisfying." He also noticed that some of the sources were now trying to make up for the ostracism. "Ms. Pink made a peace offering. An interesting one: unpalatable raisins."

As Dr. Brown was the first to compare being a target to a source, he revealed, "I found it to be much easier [being a source] and the act carried no amount of excitement or anxiety." Dr. Brown also noted what may have been a status difference in being a source with high status relative to a lower status target: "It seems more natural to me to overlook or ignore students than my colleagues or closest friends."

Nevertheless, Dr. Brown was looking forward to getting back to normal with Ms. Yellow: "Tomorrow I'm looking forward to greeting Ms. Yellow. I'm curious as to whether the greeting will be as rewarding to her as the one I received from Mr. Blue and Ms. Pink this morning."

Wednesday

Mr. Blue was the target, one day before his birthday. He began by writing in a humorous tone, "For some reason no one is talking to me today, and there is a scarlet 'O' in front of my door. I decided earlier this week that when it was my day, I would make it difficult for everyone else and keep talking to them." But, in his first attempt, he noted, "I just needed to tell him something and he ran way. I was quite amused actually."

The sources noticed Mr. Blue's strategy. Wrote Ms. Pink, "The little shit is trying to talk to me about everything under the sun. I'm pretty proud of myself though—I'm pursing my lips and not looking at him."

Later that day Mr. Blue's amusement seems to have dissipated some. "I am going to give the paper to Jude [an undergraduate research assistant] and ask him to give it to Dr. Brown, because I really don't want to be ignored by him again."

Mr. Blue believed being a source was particularly difficult for Ms. Pink. He wrote, "I think it was very difficult for her not to engage me, because we always interact and discuss personal issues. It was hard for me too, because I keep getting confusing attributions. I feel like I am a ghost on the floor that everyone hears, but no one can talk to." Later, when Ms. Pink broke role and talked to him, Mr. Blue echoed Ms. Yellow's reaction: "I saw Ms. Pink in the hall, she forgot that she was ignoring me and we maintained eye contact for about 5 sec. which felt wonderful. I actually got a full interaction."

Mr. Blue's strategy turned to evoking any sort of response as the day progressed: "It is funny that I have begun using tactics to force them to acknowledge me. I don't care if I anger them, I just want someone to notice me."

Once Mr. Blue returned home that evening, he continued his quest to be recognized. He said he wanted to "find out what ostracism was like over the phone," so he called Dr. Brown, Dr. Black, and Ms. Yellow. Dr. Brown and Dr. Black upheld their source role even on the phone, but Ms. Yellow talked to Mr. Blue until he reminded her.

Thursday

Because of the exception clause, on Wednesday we knew Thursday would be Ms. Pink's day. She appeared prepared. "Today is my day to be ostracized and I think I'm going to enjoy it. I know that sounds crazy, but I'm looking at it as a game, a challenge. It's a battle of wills, a contest: I bet I can do a better job counterostracizing them, if that's the expression." She was quite effective in her strategy. She remarked, "I walked right past them, didn't look at them—they didn't even exist."

Most sources admitted she did a better job ostracizing them on the day she was "O" than on the days she was a source. Dr. Black wrote, "Seems like Ms. Pink is using defensive ostracism, not trying to talk to me since she knows I won't talk with her."

Nevertheless, the day was beginning to take its toll on her as it neared its end. "This is absolutely no big deal today, but it does demonstrate one important point: I certainly would not want to work in an environment like this on a daily basis."

Because of Ms. Pink's tactic of "counterostracizing," as she put it, being a source apparently felt different. "I didn't really feel that guilty today because, as I said, it was as though she was ostracizing me, so, in a way, it was sort of annoying. Another feeling I had was that her presence today was like the presence of a stranger, whom we don't feel compelled to introduce ourselves to, and who doesn't seem interested in us."

Friday

This was Dr. Black's day, and it was unusual for several reasons. Because Ms. Pink was presenting some preliminary dissertation data in a social area practicum, it was the first time that all members of the social area were required to be in each other's presence. Typically, these practica were noted for enthusiasm, arousal (coffee was served), interruption, and peripatetic discussion. It should be noted that Dr. Black usually drank the most coffee and interrupted the most.

Second, Dr. Brown was scheduled to present a colloquium to the entire Psychology Department at noon, yet another opportunity for all social area members to be present, although in the company of others.

Finally, it was the final day of the Scarlet Letter Study, which made it unique as well. There would be no convenient opportunities for making up with the target on the following day and no chance for Dr. Black to use his experience as target to affect his behavior toward the next target.

Apparently, anticipating that Friday was his day affected his sleep Thursday night: "I woke up this morning thinking how odd it was that I actually dreamt about this; that it must be affecting me more than I thought." He dreamt that not only were his colleagues ostracizing him, but so was his wife. He told her she didn't have to do that because she wasn't part of the study, but she continued ignoring him anyway. This dream, in fact, came true on Friday night when Dr. Black joined his wife and her coworkers, whom he had not met before, at a bar. No one looked at him or signaled for him to come to their table, and when he did sit at their table, no one looked at him or talked to him for several minutes. Finally, they broke down and laughed.

Upon arrival at the office, he encountered two colleagues in the hallway who talked among themselves and didn't make eye contact with him. His first response was, "Sort of humored, but in a defensive sort of way."

Unlike Mr. Blue, Dr. Black had not initially planned a strategy. But after a few ostracism episodes, he found himself reacting much the way Mr. Blue had. Dr. Black's primary motive was to be acknowledged, to cause the others to break role. Before attending the morning's practicum session, he cut himself a small scarlet "O" and put two-sided adhesive tape on its back. Soon after Ms. Pink began her presentation, Dr. Black stuck the "O" on his forehead. Several of the students noticed and smirked or openly laughed. Dr. Black wrote, "I felt victorious . . . I got them to acknowledge me." But Dr. Brown did not notice the "O" for almost 30 minutes. When he did, he was visibly angered and annoyed, saying, "How long has that been on your head?" Ms. Pink and Mr. Blue replied, "The whole time." Dr. Brown said, "Take that off. It isn't necessary!" Dr. Black wrote, "I got a rise out of him—Good!" But Dr. Black's feelings of success were mixed with regret: "He chastised me, he's mad at me—I feel like I want to get into his good graces. I also wonder if you guys want to find more to criticize about my comments than you usually would." Thereafter, provoking a response became paramount for Dr. Black: "I beep at Dr. Brown as I pass him (I'm driving back to school, Dr. Brown's walking). He waves. I laugh . . . I got him again! Oh, to be recognized." Finally, Dr. Black writes, "I'm seeing my goal today as trying to get people to recognize my existence, with good or bad evaluation—it doesn't matter."

Dr. Brown's ostracism during the practicum was perhaps his most extreme of the week. "At one point toward the end I attempted an active ostracism act by speaking over Dr. Black as he was finishing a point and switched the topic of discussion. So, as he was finishing a sentence (before he did finish) I blurted over him, 'Let's move on. . . .' This was perhaps the most active, hostile, deliberate, 'O' I achieved during the whole week."

Later that day, Dr. Brown gave a departmental colloquium in front of some 50 people. Despite the fact that he was being evaluated by his peers and students in a very public forum, the ostracism intruded into his thoughts while on the podium. He wrote, "I start my talk and notice Dr. Black in the classroom. I catch him nodding occasionally (acknowledging a point or two). This was extremely painful for me. Perhaps in some sense it was the most difficult aspect of the entire week." After the talk, Dr. Black wrote, "I said 'Very good talk, Dr. Brown.' He looked up, said, in sort of a begrudging, unaffective, below-his-breath mutter, 'Uh, thanks.' I realized how much worse that was than if he'd acted like I didn't talk at all (at least I think so). It was like he really didn't like me, but knew he had to say thanks."

Other paranoid attributions (Kramer, 1994) continued to surface for Dr. Black. He wrote, "No matter how much I know why they're doing that, there's a part of me that wonders if it isn't something else. This is so weird."

Content Analysis

The diaries ranged in length from 2,259 to 5,186 words. The number of separate entries (comprised of words devoted to a single event) ranged from 29 to 44. There were 119 unshared entries (singular entries for an event that was not recorded by anyone else), 21 entries shared by two participants, five shared by three, three shared by four, and one shared by all five participants. In contrast, there were only 45 events that, as written, involved no interactions (mostly musings about the week), 60 events that involved two interactants, 32 involving three, four involving four, and eight in which all five participants were involved.

Targets used almost twice as many words per day as sources. Targets also used more emotional terms than sources. The valence of these affective terms was predominantly negative. The only exception to this pattern was when targets were describing a source who broke role; when this happened, there was a higher proportion of positive affective entries than negative.

Nonverbal Behaviors

Sources and targets both averaged 2.8 entries per day to describe their own nonverbal behaviors. But targets made considerably more entries relating to sources' nonverbal behaviors (7.8 per day) than sources made of other sources' nonverbal behaviors (0.4 per day). Moreover, sources made only 1.9 entries per day regarding targets' nonverbal behaviors. This difference between perceptions is similar to the findings of several investigators (DePaulo, 1992; Ekman & Friesen, 1969) who have noted that expressive behavior is difficult to control and to monitor for the actor (i.e., the source). This is exacerbated when under high cognitive load, such as when one is speaking or planning to speak. In our case, of course, the source was preparing not to speak. For an observer (i.e., the target), however, the speaker's nonverbal expressive behavior is quite salient and easily available for scrutiny.

Another intriguing possibility is that this divergence regarding non-verbal entries between targets and sources reflects a form of compensating interpersonal modalities. This argument would be analogous to the notion that a blind person's acute hearing compensates for his or her loss of sight: targets, who are not spoken to, may be more sensitive to the nonverbal behaviors of sources.

Themes

Ease of Ostracism

Dr. Brown observed that "each ostracizer is unique. It does not feel like the same phenomenon with each person." Although there was considerable variation in the way in which sources ostracized the target, the ease of ostracizing a target was most consistently affected by the nature of the relationship between the target and the source. In general, ostracism was perceived as difficult to do and difficult to take. Several sources indicated their difficulty with ostracizing. Dr. Black wrote, "Whoa . . . that was really difficult." Ms. Yellow wrote, "It was so difficult!" Dr. Brown observed, "It was extremely difficult to act that way." For sources, two aspects of the relationship between themselves and the target seemed particularly important: the preexisting bond and the status differential.

The closer the preexisting bond between the target and the source, the more likely the experience of ostracism was documented as aversive. For example, on ostracizing Ms. Yellow, Dr. Black wrote, "I didn't have as much of a reaction to this as I did to yesterday's discovery, and I don't know if that's because I probably interact less with Ms. Yellow on a daily basis, anyway, or because Dr. Brown's collegial status with me is more important." Similarly, Dr. Brown wrote about having to ignore Dr. Black during Dr. Brown's departmental colloquium, "It really killed me to attempt to ignore him during the talk. This was the one instance where I felt I was paying a supreme price for being an ostracizer." Mr. Blue wrote of ostracizing Ms. Pink, "I don't look forward to this because I typically interact with Ms. Pink on a personal level. By ostracizing her, I am eliminating an important source of social interaction. . . . I felt more guilty all day, because of all the group, I desired to ostracize her the least. I felt like she didn't exist and that we were treating her so badly."

The ease associated with ostracizing a target was also affected by the status differential between target and source. In general, sources found ostracizing a target of higher status to be extremely difficult. Mr. Blue wrote, "I think it was more difficult to ostracize higher status individuals." Similarly, Dr. Brown reported, "Quite easy to do, actually, in the high-status role." Yet, when ostracizing a higher status target, it seemed to give the source feelings of greater power and control. Mr. Blue wrote, "I also felt more powerful being able to ostracize an individual of higher status." Even Dr. Brown made a similar comment about when he ostracized Dr. Black: "The act of 'O'ing him certainly changed that [Dr. Black's higher status] during the meeting. For me, I felt a very clear and strong status differential where he was on the low end." On the other hand, sources who held higher positions of authority experienced little difficulty in ostracizing lower status targets. Commented Dr. Brown when he ostracized Ms. Yellow, "Quite easy to do, actually, in the high-status role. Didn't even seem that rude. It seems more natural for me to overlook or ignore students than my colleagues or closest friends." Similarly, Dr. Black wrote of ostracizing Mr. Blue, "Ostracizing Mr. Blue was somewhat difficult although not as difficult as Dr. Brown. This is either because (a) Dr. Brown was our first victim and I've become habituated, and/or (b) Dr. Brown's status as my colleague made it more difficult, and/or (c) Dr. Brown seemed more hurt by my response than Mr. Blue."

The difficulty in carrying out the ostracism also appeared to take its toll on the participants' cognitive capacity. Mr. Blue noted, "The ostracism took so much mental effort that I have little memory of the purpose or content of the interaction. This is troublesome because [Dr. Brown, the target] told me something he would like me to do, and I can't even go ask him what it was."

Of the same occasion, Ms. Yellow observed, "Talked to Mr. Blue [a cosource] about the lab meeting . . . strangely, both of us heard and remembered the wrong schedule. Both of us forgot what Dr. Brown said. . . . It is so effortful to pay attention to what he's saying."

Apparently, this effect did not solely affect those ostracizing someone higher in status, as Dr. Brown observed when he was ostracizing Mr. Blue: "He gave me some information. In my effort to 'O' him [Mr. Blue] I think I might have tuned out the message. I don't trust the information processing or transfer from an 'O' victim."

Signs of relief, either after an ostracism episode or at the conclusion of the week, were another indication that ostracism was effortful. After one episode in which Ms. Yellow was a target, she wrote, "Was a relief to see them go. It's exhausting to play this act." Then, after the week was over, Ms. Yellow wrote more generally, "Relief. Thank God this is over. I did it for this week but even another day or few more hours would have been so exhausting!"

Strategies Used to Ostracize

Sources often expressed the intention to use a particular strategy to ostracize. Dr. Brown wrote, "A dilemma: How do I play it?" Often, these strategies were expressed prior to the day's events. Sources primarily expressed the intention to use avoidance strategies. Dr. Brown wrote, "My plan today is simply to avoid contact. I might choose to go down different stairwells today. So the ostracism will be more noncontact than awkward, nonspeaking contact. If any business can wait until tomorrow it can wait." Dr. Black noted, however, "I feel like I'm looking for him to ignore him; like I've got to be supervigilant. Weird, seeking out someone to ignore." A bit of method acting also crept into the strategies. Of another target, Dr. Black wrote, "In anticipation of ostracizing him, I was already imagining or feeling angry with him."

New strategies also emerged for sources after initially unpleasant confrontations with targets. Dr. Black wrote, "It seems like I've taken the easy way out, and basically avoided Dr. Brown at all costs." Mr. Blue lamented, "I am basically physically ostracizing him. However, since he doesn't know that I wanted to interact with him, and since he has probably been busy all day, my physical ostracism of him isn't really impactful." Dr. Brown too found a less unpleasant way to ostracize: "So, passive neglect is what is happening so far. I'm fairly comfortable with this strategy."

Strategies Used to Cope with Ostracism

Like sources, targets also planned a strategy for how they would cope with being ostracized. Prior to the day's events, targets expressed the intention to either defensively ostracize or, conversely, to seek recognition from sources. Ms. Pink exemplified the former strategy: "I'm determined not to look at them, talk to them—basically pretend that none of them exist." Mr. Blue, on the other hand, wrote, "I decided this week when it was my day, I would make it difficult for everyone else and keep talking to them." Both strategies appeared to be aimed at taking the initiative to forestall the effects of being ostracized.

After a confrontation with a source, targets expressed more instances of countering the ostracism by seeking recognition. Dr. Black wrote, "I'm seeing my goal today as trying to get people to recognize my existence, with good or bad evaluation—it doesn't matter." Mr. Blue wrote, "I just decided to call everyone tonight, just to see what happens and how it makes me feel. It is funny that I have begun using tactics to force them to acknowledge me. I don't care if I anger them, I just want someone to notice me." Even Ms. Pink, who tried to use "counter-ostracism," forced recognition at one point: "I have to be in Dr. Black's office at some point today because I need to use the computer. That's okay, and if he wants me to leave, he's going to *have* to talk to me. . . . He will have to be verbally explicit if he wants me out of sight."

Compensation

Compensation is the term we used to characterize sources who were motivated primarily by the desire to make amends to former targets for any discomfort the target may have experienced while being ostracized. Three forms of compensation were observed: anticipated compensation, actual compensation, and acts interpreted as compensation. It should be noted that only Dr. Brown made entries related to compensation.

Anticipated compensation included instances in which sources stated their intention to make amends for their behavior. Dr. Brown wrote, "I'm looking forward to seeing Ms. Yellow. I feel a strong need to give her a hearty 'good morning' with a warm smile. I think I need to compensate a bit for yesterday." Actual compensation included acts performed by sources to make amends for the ostracism. One such instance involved verbal greetings and interactions. For instance, Dr. Brown wrote, "Talked to Mr. Blue. Good/satisfying interaction. I feel we made nice-nice." During the ostracism of Dr. Black (in which Dr. Black had e-mailed Dr. Brown positive feedback about Dr. Brown's colloquium), Dr. Brown wrote, "I made a promise to myself that I would reply to his message at 12:01 A.M. that night." Finally, acts interpreted as compensation included instances that were perceived by former targets to be compensation acts, such as those unpalatable raisins offered to Dr. Brown by Ms. Pink mentioned earlier.

Ambiguous Motives

It was perhaps most surprising that instances of motive confusion were reported. This was not expected. Indeed, it was anticipated that no motive confusion would be a shortcoming of our role-play study. Whereas motives (inferred by targets, intended by source) are likely to play an important role in determining the consequences of the ostracism, by agreeing ahead of time to ostracize each other for the purpose of the study we thought we had essentially restricted the motive alternatives. Nevertheless, many entries recorded some form of motive confusion. For instance, here Dr. Brown (as a source) reported an episode that suggested that what appeared to be ostracism was, after all, not ostracism. He wrote, "I noticed a paper from Ms. Yellow [target] on my door. She placed it there sometime late this morning. I noticed I hadn't retrieved it yet. I'm wondering if she noticed it was 'not retrieved' and if she would interpret this as an 'O' act. This would be unintentional on my part. I simply wasn't ready to read it, and I've been so busy I didn't know exactly what to do with it (where to place it so it wouldn't be lost or forgotten, as I am apt to do). I'm retrieving it now." Similarly, Ms. Pink, as a source, wrote, "I think he [Dr. Black, the target] was frustrated that he didn't have the floor, but it really had nothing to do with the ostracism. That's just the way practicum is, and why practicum on any given week can become frustrating."

We also reported defensive motives, that is, in some cases we speculated that someone was ostracizing as a self-protective strategy. Dr. Brown (as a target) wrote, "How do I play it? My first reflex is to 'ostracize first in anticipatory retaliation.' Not meant to be offensive, however. I think it's a defense. If I ignore everybody then I won't notice or care if they are ignoring me." Ms. Pink, who epitomized defensive ostracism on her "O" day, wrote, "I bet I can do a better job counterostracizing them, if that's the expression. I'm determined not to look at any of them, talk to any of them—basically pretend that none of them exist. This may or may not make it easy for them—they may be relieved, or they may be bummed out that I'm taking away their fun. This is a perfect example of Dr. Black's point that ostracism begets ostracism. I have the attitude, 'Anything you can do I can do better.' " Others perceived Ms. Pink's defensive motive. For example, Dr. Black (as source) observed, "Seems like Ms. Pink is using defensive ostracism, not trying to talk to me since she knows I won't talk with her."

Targets also inferred punitive motives, and some sources feared that their behaviors would be interpreted punitively. In one example, as Dr. Brown observed his behavior as an ostracism source, he wrote, "In retrospect, I felt a bit punitive. In other words, there might have been a tendency to indulge in some tit-for-tat type behavior. It wasn't a very salient motivation but in retrospect I think it existed, even though the cause for the 'O' was well understood."

There were also instances of what could be considered oblivious ostracism—that is, the ostracism was perceived to be occurring not as punishment, but as a reflection of the lack of apparent importance the target had in the source's eyes. For instance, Dr. Brown (as a source) made this observation: "It seems more natural to me to overlook or ignore students than my colleagues or closest friends."

Variations on the Completeness of the Ostracism

Although we had agreed to ignore the target totally, in fact, sometimes ostracism was quite complete, whereas other times there was simply a reduction in the usual amount of communication and other characteristics of social intercourse. For example, Mr. Blue (as a source) wrote, "Dr. Brown [the target] stopped me in the hall to set up our meeting, and I had to leave. This was a situation when we had to communicate, so I responded to his questions, but did not make eye contact." On the other hand, Dr. Brown (as a source) writes of his complete ostracism, "Avoided acknowledging all of her [Ms. Yellow, the target] contributions. Oriented my body and face towards Mr. Blue the entire time."

Ambiguous Acts of Ostracism

The degree to which the ostracism was clearly being given and why also varied throughout the week. Sometimes the acts of ostracism were highly ambiguous, as when Dr. Brown (as a target) made this rather conspiratorial attribution: "My first thought was that the act was deliberate. They [Dr. Black and Mr. Blue] deliberately chose to walk past my door talking to let me know they were ostracizing me. I'm questioning this attribution but it occurred reflexively. I'm guessing now that I'll probably attribute *every* behavior I see or 'don't see' today in this context." Dr. Brown (as a target) makes a similar observation about Ms. Yellow's (a source) behavior: "I just heard Ms. Yellow unlock her door and get something from inside her office and I immediately thought 'She's ignoring me.' It's pretty much becoming an obsession." Then there were entries that contained no ambiguity, as when Mr. Blue (as a source) wrote, "There was no ambiguity to the cause of the ostracism . . . the interaction was much less stressful this time because I noticed him smiling so I was sure that he was making the correct attribution." And Dr. Brown writes of his ostracism of Dr. Black, "I'm sure, however, that if I attempted such a maneuver on him [Dr. Black, the target] and he did not attribute my action to an 'O' or a role play that he would never have let it slide." These last two examples also support the idea that as clarity increases (or conversely, as ambiguity decreases), ostracism appears to have less negative impact.

Evidence of Coping with Different Threatened Needs

As I discussed in Chapter 3, ostracism appears to have the unique capability to undermine four fundamental human needs in its targets. Meanwhile, some of these needs may actually be fortified in the sources. Let's briefly focus on entries that could be considered to reflect upon these four needs: belongingness, control, self-esteem, and meaningful existence.

Belonging

It was expected that being ostracized directly threatens targets' feelings of having a bond, a sense of connectedness, a feeling of belonging to others. Ms. Yellow (as a target) wrote, "When they [the sources, Mr. Blue and Dr. Brown] did not incorporate my suggestion it did feel like they are one." Ms. Pink (as a source) made sympathetic belonging-related observations concerning two targets, first Mr. Blue, then Dr. Black. Of Mr. Blue she wrote, "I know that he has a higher need for affiliation than the rest of us, so maybe this really is affecting him." Of Dr. Black, she wrote, "I know Dr. Black probably would have liked to have joined in, because he likes to talk about Thursday night television (*Friends*, *Seinfeld*, etc.)."

It was hypothesized that a consequence of threatened belonging is to try to regain that sense of belonging in some other way. This could be by joining other groups, talking with others, trying to please others more, and so on. For example, Mr. Blue (as a target) observed, "I also noticed today that I wasted most of the day talking to practicum students about non-school-related issues. This may be an anomaly or maybe I just was overcompensating for being shut out of my normal social interactions." Dr. Brown (as a target) wrote, "Talking to Jude [an undergraduate student] more than usual." And, in one of the more surprising self-disclosures, Dr. Black (as a target) wrote, "I feel like I need to hug someone."

An examination of sources' entries related to belonging fortification also seems to suggest that ostracism threatens belonging for both targets and sources. Mr. Blue (as a source) wrote, "I don't look forward to doing this because I typically interact with Ms. Pink on a personal level. By ostracizing her, I am eliminating an important source of social interaction."

Control

Ostracism is hypothesized to deprive targets of a sense of control, causing them to experience feelings of frustration. With other types of interpersonal conflict, such as verbal or even physical arguments, the interchange can be and often is bidirectional. However, because others are ignoring the target during ostracism, targets' counterattacks fall on deaf ears and blind eyes. When Dr. Black was a target, he observed, "It was very frustrating!!! I almost gave up and didn't make the comment. It was like the *Twilight Zone*." Both Dr. Brown and Ms. Pink made diary entries at the same time, and they concurred with Dr. Black's feelings. Dr. Brown wrote, "He [Dr. Black, a target] yielded and did not object nor attempt to regain control of the conversation." Ms. Pink commented, "One time he [Dr. Black, a target] was trying to talk and everyone else was talking too. I think he was frustrated that he didn't have the floor."

As a consequence of threatened control, targets are likely to try to regain control through provocative behaviors that demand responses in the sources. When Mr. Blue was the target, he frequently attempted to regain control. Sometimes, he simply thought about how to get control. He wrote, "Well, Ms. Yellow left for the day and didn't say good-bye, even though she passed right by me. I wanted to shoot her with a rubber band or smack her on the head to get her attention." Later Mr. Blue acted on his desires. After work, he wrote, "I just decided to call everyone tonight, just to see what happens and how it makes me feel." Dr. Black also acted in ways to regain control when he was a target. After he was the target of ostracism in the practicum meeting, he made this entry: "Then, after about 5 minutes where no one looked at me, I stuck a red 'O' on my forehead." About an hour later, Dr. Black found another opportunity to provoke a response, this time by beeping his car horn at Dr. Brown, as mentioned earlier. These attempts did not go by unnoticed. Dr. Black wrote of Mr. Blue's provocative behavior, "Mr. Blue's [the target] testing us." Dr. Brown wrote of Dr. Black's attempts, "The guy 'tricked' me into completing a social exchange. I was a bit angry at myself, as if someone scored a point on me during some kind of competition because of my carelessness. I thought 'I've got to be more on guard.' "

In sources, we saw indications that ostracism increased their sense of control. For example, Ms. Yellow, as a source, wrote, "It felt powerful to do what everyone was doing—ostracizing and specially since I'm the junior-most." Mr. Blue (a source) wrote, "I didn't really feel anything about him [Dr. Black, as a target] other than [having] greater control over the interaction." Sources often reported feeling empowered as a result of ostracizing. Mr. Blue (a source) wrote, "I felt uncomfortable ostracizing him [Dr. Brown, the target], but I also felt more powerful being able to ostracize an individual of higher status." Mr. Blue made an observation that suggests the power shifts away from the target, when he wrote of Dr. Black (the target), "I felt like he lost a couple notches in status." And Dr. Brown made this insightful observation of the relative status between him and Dr. Black after he ostracized Dr. Black: "One last thing. Dr. Black [the target] has a bit more status than me here for a number of reasons. However, the act of 'O'ing him certainly changed that during the meeting. For me, I felt a very clear and strong status differential where he was on the low end. This was partly due to his unusually passive behavior but partly also to my willingness to assume, accept, or assert a higher status position. It wasn't a conscious thing nor was there any intention behind it but it was there and kind of occurred naturally."

However, Ms. Pink, as a source, made an intriguing observation: "I don't like not being able to engage in the behaviors that I normally engage in! The silent treatment takes control away from the user too, when you think about it. It requires a huge amount of effort to remember how you're supposed to act—it's like the ostracism takes over you!" This observation is consistent with those made by long-term users of the silent treatment in structured interviews (Williams & Zadro, 1999). Perhaps control is temporarily gained by being a source of ostracism, but then over time the ostracism starts to take control of the source.

Self-Esteem

Self-esteem is another need that was hypothesized to be under attack when a person is ostracized. The reason behind this is that ostracism often signifies punishment for some undesirable act, or, conversely, for not doing something that was desired. Hence, when ostracized, targets may assume they did something wrong. Also, because ostracism often comes without explanation, targets may ruminate over the various things they may have done wrong, thus making salient to themselves a virtual "laundry list" of acts that provide grist for self-derogation. Because we had agreed to be ostracized during the week, and we supposedly knew the reasons why it was being done, we felt that self-esteem would not be severely shaken. Nevertheless, even in these circumstances, there were still a few entries that suggested that target's self-esteem was fragile during ostracism. Ms. Yellow (a target) wrote, "When I cracked a joke I automatically turned my head to Dr. Brown [a source] whom I expected to laugh, as usual. But he too didn't laugh and it made me feel pretty stupid." Dr. Black (a source) observed of Ms. Pink (a target), "I think it's interesting that Ms. Pink felt motivated to do this [hand in her revision of the method section] today, as though she's more concerned about receiving praise or feeling appreciated today more than other days." No evidence of self-esteem fortification was found in sources' entries.

Meaningful Existence

Ostracism was also hypothesized to affect the targets' sense of meaningful existence adversely, because the experience of being ostracized is a metaphorical reminder of what life would be like without the target. In anthropological and sociological accounts of ostracism, ostracism is often referred to as "social death." As a target, Mr. Blue wrote, "I feel like I am a ghost on the floor that everyone hears, but no one can talk to. I want to be noticed!"

A way to regain a sense of meaningful existence is to be recognized, regardless of whether people's impressions are positive or negative. Several entries documented such motivations. Mr. Blue (a target) wrote, "It is funny that I have begun using tactics to force them to acknowledge me. I don't care if I anger them; I just want someone to notice me." Dr. Black also seemed to care about being recognized more than creating favorable impressions. He wrote, "I'm seeing my goal today as trying to get people to recognize my existence, with good or bad evaluation—it doesn't matter." When they did something to get attention, they felt rewarded. Dr. Black wrote, "Oh, to be recognized! I felt victorious that I got them to acknowledge my existence."

SUMMARY OF FINDINGS

The aim of this study was to provide us with a substantive experience with ostracism. To this end, it was successful, perhaps more so than we bargained for. Prior to the week of the study, most of our colleagues expressed doubts that we would experience anything and suggested that it would be nothing more than an uninvolving role-play exercise that would yield nothing more than a few laughs. Contrary to these expectations, laughter was one of the rarer events. The ostracism affected the daily lives of all the individuals involved. It prevented some from doing their work, collaborating with their peers, being mentored, and receiving help. It interfered with the normal pleasantries and politenesses that lubricate the social fabric of a working group. It caused temporary emergence of group factions, displays of anger, embarrassment, concern, anxiety, paranoia, and general fragility of spirit. Attempts were made moments after midnight to seek reconciliation with the ostracized individual, even when it was quite apparent why the ostracism was taking place and that it was not personal. At the conclusion of the study, we decided that our understanding of ostracism was benefited at a phenomenological level, a theoretical level, and a methodological level.

Phenomenologically, we experienced what we were studying in the laboratory and what we were listening to in our structured interviews. Despite knowing the reasons for the ostracism, and knowing that a predetermined end was in sight, ostracizing was effortful for sources and unpleasant for targets. We questioned each other's motives, had difficulties carrying out our day-to-day duties, and felt disengaged from our friends and colleagues. As targets, we felt disconnected from the group, frustrated by our lack of control, uncertain of the value of our contributions, and unrecognized. As sources we felt a part of the group, empowered, and an increase in status, but also felt apologetic and eager to reunite with the target the next day.

The experience, while not an empirical test, lends credibility to my model and the needs-threat theory that I discuss in greater detail in the next chapter. We experienced several types of ostracism that varied across the four dimensions: visibility, motive, quantity, and causal clarity. Attributions were frequent moderators of the incidents and seemed to act as buffers or intensifiers. This was surprising because the attributions for the ostracism were quite clear (I discuss this in a little more detail below). Each need—belonging, control, self-esteem, and meaningful existence—was represented in the diary entries. And the immediate reactions of discomfort and unpleasantness were often converted to acts aimed at regaining the lost or threatened needs.

Methodologically, we learned that some questions about ostracism can probably be tested with role-play methods, whereas others may not be amenable to this technique. Even when knowing that motives for ostracism are under the control of the scriptwriter, ostracizing and being ostracized still had impact. This was probably more true of the targets—it feels almost immediately uncomfortable to be ignored in the presence of others, especially others who are friends. It takes little time to feel excluded, rejected, and ignored. Loss of control and wanting to regain control is particularly noticeable. Threats to self-esteem, however, seemed less affected than would happen without the consent of the individuals involved and their knowledge of the roles to be played. Also, the experiences of the sources were probably substantially different from those of actual ostracism sources who choose to ostracize for a reason. Usually, if we chose to give a friend the silent treatment, avoid eye contact with them, or do not invite them to a group activity, it would be because we were angry with them or they had hurt our feelings. Without this motive, sources are likely to feel uncomfortable and apologetic, as we did. On the other hand, the effort and difficulty in maintaining the ostracism may very well track the real world of experience of extended ostracism. In their structured interviews, long-term sources of ostracism, often claim that it is an all-consuming activity and is exhausting to keep up. As Dr. Brown so keenly observed: "A lot of effort was put forth to 'O' him during the meeting but I found that if I hyperattended to the task at hand and to everyone else in the room I could neglect him. Neglecting or ignoring is easier than actively 'O'ing. One qualification, ignoring is not quite the correct term because it was an ignoring 'act.' In fact, I processed everything Dr. Black said and contributed at the meeting but only attempted to communicate to him that I was ignoring him. So, in fact, I was endeavoring in deception. Perhaps this is partly responsible for the effortful nature of this. Deception is difficult to do. Maybe all this acting takes a lot."

Attributions

Causal attribution for ostracism seems not to have influenced its impact in the slightest. We all had the most clear and the most forgiving (self-serving) attributions for our sources and yet the impact was felt strongly. We couldn't have had a more face-saving context. Yet we still all bore the brunt of attributional confusion.

Attributionally, the participant observers had a clear schema through which to make and interpret observations and guide their expectations for sources' behaviors. Despite knowing the cause of the ostracizing behaviors to be external, targets nevertheless seemed tempted to consider (or perhaps needed to inhibit) internal attributions for sources' behaviors. This tendency is reminiscent of attributions made by participants who interacted with either a "friendly" or an "unfriendly" confederate even when they were informed that the confederate's behavior toward them had been intentional according to the experimental design (Napolitan & Goethals, 1979). It has long been known that the hedonic relevance of another's actions, particularly if it is negatively valenced for the perceiver, will increase the tendency to attribute those actions internally (Jones & Davis, 1965).

Stage theories of interpersonal perception (Gilbert, 1995; Jones, 1990; Trope, 1986) can be applied to the present context to suggest what might be occurring in the minds of the targets. Given a prior, clear, and strong expectation for ostracism, targets are primed (predisposed) to identify an act, or perhaps even a nonact, as an instance of an ostracism act. This will occur to the extent that such schemas are activated (i.e., salient) within the minds of the target. The diaries of our participants clearly showed that, while a target, the ostracism schema tended to be chronically activated as evidenced by the reported rumination and increased diary entries of all participants on their day as targets. This chronic activation predisposed targets to make ostracism-related identifications. Furthermore, targets and sources seemed to be experiencing high cognitive load during these interpersonal encounters with their attempts to compensate for the impediment to the normal flow of their social discourse. The added interpersonal burdens placed on targets may interfere with the subsequent inference and adjustment stages of the social judgment processes, thus causing internal ostracizing-related attributions to creep into their consciousness.

When the Rules Were Challenged

Van Ments (1983) wrote, "When people take a particular role they use a repertoire of behaviors which are expected of that role. . . . This behavior is often the result of internalizing the expectations developed by others—in other words doing what other people expect of that person in that role. . . . When people act out of role . . . they upset our expectations" (p. 18). Although it may not have been discussed, it would seem that each individual in the study held expectations about how targets and sources should respond to ostracism. That is, sources should not respond to the target and targets should passively endure ostracism. When sources challenged their role and failed to ostracize the target, targets responded both positively and negatively. Mr. Blue wrote, "I saw Ms. Pink in the hall, she forgot that she was ignoring me and we maintained eye contact for about 5 sec. which felt wonderful." Nevertheless, Mr. Blue continued, "She didn't ignore me very well during the interaction. I felt uncomfortable, because I wasn't sure how we were supposed to act and I just tried to get through the interaction quickly and end it." Dr. Black wrote of Ms. Pink's failure to ostracize him, "One part of me wishes she'd ostracize me, the other part appreciates the interaction."

Targets challenged their role by seeking recognition, attempting to provoke a reaction from sources. Source reactions to such tactics were overwhelmingly negative, tending to center on their perceived loss of control. As mentioned earlier, when Dr. Black, as a target, beeped his horn at Dr. Brown, who reflexively waved back, Dr. Brown reported feeling quite angry with himself. But this anger could also be turned toward the provoking target. On Dr. Black putting the "O" on his head, Dr. Brown wrote, "Normally, it would have struck me as being really funny and perhaps it was and did, but I could not nor did I want to be humored by him so I fought the urge. What is extremely interesting is that I managed to sincerely change or manipulate my affective response from one of laughter to one of annoyance and irritation. . . . I genuinely achieved a state of irritation and annoyance and was sincerely ordering him to knock it off. Stop with the pranks. Apparently, when I'm 'O'ing somebody it's annoying to me for them to attempt to humor me or make me feel good. Altruism, warmth, compassion, and good humor actually is responded to (by me) with irritation, annoyance, and anger. It's as if I'm saying, 'No, don't be nice to me. I don't want to be nice to you. If you try I'll get angry at you.' Offhand, I can't think of any other instance where I get angry at somebody for being nice and friendly."

Revelations

We may have also learned something about ourselves—and about each other that we did not know before. As Dr. Brown observed, "Each 'O'er is unique. It does not feel like the same phenomenon with each person. 'O' comes in many varieties. People handle it differently." Indeed, Dr. Black and Mr. Blue sought recognition, Dr. Brown introspected and avoided aversive situations, Ms. Pink was defensive, and Ms. Yellow was resigned. None of us was able to predict our own idiosyncratic reactions prior to the study. Future research efforts on ostracism would benefit by taking into account the personality differences of both sources and targets of ostracism.

CONCLUSIONS

Engaging in and experiencing a week like this was both revealing and uncomfortable. We have recently learned (from a participant in one of our structured interviews) that an organization in the United Kingdom begins its orientation week by inducing its new members to join together and ostracize each member for a period of time so as to increase their sense of cohesion and commitment within their group! Having experienced this procedure ourselves, it is difficult to imagine that cohesiveness is the likely outcome. In fact, we feel that attempts to replicate this experience should be undertaken with caution. Despite this being a week of unanticipated powerful psychological effects, we were perhaps less affected than groups who would be less cohesive. Preexisting quarrels, hidden resentments, and competitive rivalries would almost certainly be magnified under the weeklong cloak of ostracism. As Ms. Yellow observed about the week, "Everything seems to have so much meaning." The meaning attached to ostracism episodes could be enlightening, but could easily be negative and hurtful.

Laboratory Experiments

The Ball-Tossing Paradigm

Many years ago, I took my dog, Michelob, to swim and play at a nearby lake. She loved to fetch sticks in the lake, and then take them still further away from me—she wasn't much at returning sticks, or even coming back to me when I called her. Anyway, I was sitting on a blanket when a Frisbee rolled next to me and stopped. I picked it up, turned around, and noticed two guys looking at me, obviously the owners of the Frisbee. I threw it back to them, and then, to my surprise, the guy I threw it to threw it back to me. So I threw it to the other guy, and he threw it back to me. I took this as an invitation, so I stood up and became the third point in a large triangle.

We tossed the Frisbee among us for several turns and then, without any warning or signal that I could detect, the two guys stopped throwing it to me. They just threw it between themselves, back and forth, turn after turn. At first, it didn't faze me, because it's fun to keep each other guessing as to whom is being chosen as the next recipient. But after five or six tosses, I suddenly grasped the idea that they weren't going to throw the Frisbee to me again. After about the fifteenth toss, I felt extremely awkward and left out. I didn't know these fellows, so it wasn't like they were my friends or anything, but the fact that I had once been "in" their group, however briefly, and now was being ignored and excluded, hit me more powerfully than I could have ever imagined. I wasn't sure what to do, so being a male, I started looking around for things that would send these two guys the message that there were other things more important to me than this stupid Frisbee game, and so I slinked back to my blanket, called Michelob, and when she came back (a surprising relief!) gave her a hug. I still belonged to her, and she to me.

I had been interested in studying the phenomenon of ostracism ever

125

since 1977, when I watched a TV movie about James Pelosi, who had been "silenced" by his cadet peers at West Point for 2 years. But I didn't know exactly how to study ostracism in a controlled laboratory setting until this day at the lake. I wanted some means to bring the psychological drama of ostracism from the real world in to the laboratory, where, although simplified, it would still retain the psychological impact of being ignored and excluded.

Suddenly it hit me. I could arrange it so that a participant would show up where two other "participants" were waiting, but in fact these two would be working for me as confederates, playing the role of participants. I could get them to start throwing a ball to each other, with some sort of clever cover story. Then, after the first few tosses, the two confederates would stop throwing the ball to the participant for the remainder of the session. I would compare the consequences of this "ostracism" condition with those of a control condition, in which participants were included in an equal exchange of ball tossing. So, in 1982, I ran a study with the assistance of Steve Predmore that did just that. I wasn't exactly sure what sort of "consequences" I was thinking of, so I simply asked participants afterward if they wanted to work on the next task alone, with the other two people, or with a new group of people. I figured that those who were ostracized would prefer to work with a new group of strangers rather than working either alone or with the two individuals who had just ostracized them. This was all rather atheoretical though; it was just a hunch.

As each participant showed up, I made sure that one confederate was already in place; to make things more believable, I had the second confederate show up a minute later. I told all three that I was interested in studying reaction time in physical tasks. I would be asking them to do a variety of such tasks and I would frequently measure their reaction times by dropping a yardstick between their fingers. As soon as I let go of the yardstick, they were to grasp it as quickly as they could, and then I would write down in my record book the inch line where they had grasped it. Participants were misled to believe that this was a legitimate measure of reaction time. I gave this explanation to each individual in a room where he or she was out of sight of the other two. Then I told them their first task was to toss a racquetball among themselves, quickly and in a way such that no one could anticipate if he or she was going to get the ball next. That is, they shouldn't throw it in a predictable sequence. These instructions were reasonable, given that the goal was to increase their hand–eye coordination and reflexes, which would then improve their "yardstick reaction time" measure.

At this point, I left the room, but gave an unobtrusive signal to the confederates, indicating to them what condition was being run, based on a random assignment sheet that I had prepared earlier. If it was the inclusion condition, they were to toss the ball to each other in a random yet roughly equal manner, such that each person got the ball about a third of the time. If it was an ostracism condition, then after the first 30 seconds, the confederates were to stop throwing the ball to the participant, and just toss it to each other. In both conditions, the ball tossing lasted for 5 minutes. Afterward, I gave them each the reaction time measure again (out of sight of the others), and then gave them a short questionnaire, which basically asked them their preferences as to whom to work with on the next task: to work alone, with the same two they had just worked with, or with a new group of two individuals.

The primary results were that, compared to participants who were included, who said they wanted to work with the same two people with whom they had just played the ball-toss game, ostracized participants showed a tendency to prefer to either work alone or with a new group of two strangers. The effect was only marginally significant. I noticed, however, that some ostracized participants behaved differently than others during the game—particularly when they were being excluded during the ball-tossing exchange. After they noticed they weren't getting the ball thrown to them, some individuals just stood their, arms akimbo, and appeared to give up. Others would try to intercept the ball from the other two, sometimes successfully. But as soon as they threw it back to one of the others, they would again continue to be ostracized. So, for some participants, the game turned into a "keepaway" (or "monkey in the middle") game, and they seemed to be entertained by this. For others, it was clearly a negative experience that, from their expressions, seemed to last forever.

For several reasons, my initial attempt to study ostracism stopped at this point, and we settled for a conference presentation (Predmore & Williams, 1983). The feedback we got at the conference was that the obtained effects may have had nothing to do with the ostracism per se, but may have been the result of anticipated failure on the reaction-time task. Participants who had been ostracized, the argument went, were deprived of the pretask exercise that would likely have improved their reaction times. Hence, their expressions of displeasure and desire to work with others (or alone) stemmed not from being ignored and excluded, but instead from being prevented from succeeding at the subsequent reaction-time task. This was a good criticism, and something I had to take into account 12 years later when I began looking at ostracism again.

At the University of Toledo I was teaching a graduate seminar on small groups, and I wanted to lead a discussion about how one designs a study to investigate a question. I wanted to use a novel question so that the students would have to "start from scratch," so I asked them how we could examine the phenomenon of ostracism. I remember being faced with silence and puzzled looks. They seemed to be so confused by the topic I had selected that they couldn't even generate a hypothesis, let alone an experimental design. Clearly, I had to say more about "ostracism." After telling them the Pelosi story, and then my first attempt to study ostracism, we began picking apart the methodological problems with the ball-tossing paradigm I had developed. What emerged from our discussion was a new and improved ball-tossing paradigm, which then led to a series of experiments.

The new paradigm kept the essential features of the original one, while modifying some aspects so that we could remove the "task-failure" confound. Basically, what we had to do was to make the ball-tossing part of the experiment incidental—indeed accidental. This way, ostracized participants could not perceive their nonparticipation as impeding their performance on the experimental task. So the ball tossing would occur during a period of time while they were waiting for a fourth participant to show up. All this would require some convincing acting from my confederates. The three of them (my two confederates and the participant) would be seated in the room in roughly a triangular formation. A fourth seat, making a square, was left empty; this was the seat for the fourth participant who had not arrived yet. I told them that because the upcoming task involved interaction, it was important for them not to speak to each other while they were waiting. Then I left the room, and the confederates began their performance.

In the room with them was a small box of toys, above which was a sign that said "Children's Play Study." This box of toys and the sign were purposefully set up to give the appearance that their presence was legitimate. One of the confederates would look at the box of toys, look at the other confederate and participant, grin, and pick out a racquetball. He'd bounce it, look at the other confederate, and throw it to him. The second confederate would then look at the participant, who was almost always grinning and looking back, and throw the ball to him. All the participants caught (or attempted to catch) the ball, and all of them threw it to one of the confederates. This was almost always accompanied by grins and maybe even stifled laughter. Apparently, participants felt that they were getting away with something: the experimenter told them not to talk, and they weren't talking. But they were throwing a ball—something they probably thought the experimenter would not approve of. Just before I left the room, I had given a signal to the confederates, indicating whether the condition was ostracism or inclusion.

If I gave them the inclusion sign, they gleefully continued tossing the ball among themselves for the 5 minutes I was away. Often, the ball tosses would get more and more inventive—they would use the walls and ceiling to ricochet the ball to each other. When they heard me returning (I was talking loudly enough to the fourth participant—another confederate—for them to hear me), they quickly stopped throwing the ball and returned it to its box. If I gave my confederates the ostracism sign, they would behave the same as they did in the inclusion condition for the first 20 or 30 seconds. Then, without warning or any apparent reason, they would limit their throws to each other. As with the inclusion condition, the confederates would continue to get more and more clever with their throws, but they would make sure that the ball would not fall into the hands of the participant. In addition to not including the participant in the ball tossing, they also would not look at or respond in any way to the participant, in case the participant said something to them. Interestingly enough, hardly any participants initiated conversation or tried to intercept the ball. Perhaps this "apathy" occurred because the game was incidental and not something on which they were being evaluated, or maybe it was simply because they were seated rather than standing. One participant out of about 250 picked up the ball when it accidentally rolled to him, at which point he sat on it—thus ending the ball tossing for all.

EXPERIMENTS 1 AND 2. EFFECTS OF OSTRACISM ON THE LOSS AND RECLAMATION OF CONTROL

According to the model outlined in Chapter 3, control is one of four fundamental needs that are threatened by ostracism. In the short term, the model predicts that individuals subjected to ostracism will attempt to regain or repair whatever need is threatened. Therefore, in our first experiment using the ball-tossing paradigm, we hypothesized that individuals who were subjected to ostracism, and therefore deprived temporarily of a feeling of control, would, if given the chance, try to reassert that sense of control. So we arranged things such that when the last confederate arrived, the participant was paired off with him and moved to the next room (supposedly, the other two "participants" were paired off together, but in reality they remained in the same room to trick the next participant). In this new room, the experimenter explained that he was interested in the ability of people to transmit nonverbal information from the right and left sides of their faces. At the University of Toledo, a good deal of research was being conducted on hemispheric laterality, so most introductory psychology students had already participated in at least one study in which the left–right distinction was of interest to the experimenter. So this cover story seemed plausible. They were then told that one of them would be looking at a series of playing cards that were hidden from view from the other person. The participant who would be looking at the cards was called the "transmitter"; the other participant would be called the "guesser." Through a rigged drawing, the actual participant drew the slip of paper that was labeled "guesser." The guesser's task was to look carefully at the face of the transmitter and after gauging whatever he could from the transmitter's facial expression, he was to guess whether the card the transmitter was looking at was red or black, at which point he would be given false feedback that worked out, over the series of guesses, to lead him to believe that he had guessed correctly 50% of the time. He was told that because certain subtle nonverbal information may be transmitted better from either the left or the right side of the face, the guesser could, prior to each guess, request that the transmitter turn his head as often as the guesser desired.

This fairly complicated and convoluted cover story was created in an attempt to give participants the opportunity to exact behavioral control over another person. It is important to note that the person who was being controlled was not someone who had been involved in the previous ball-tossing game. This meant that the participant was not merely retaliating against a former ostracizer by making his head spin. What this head-turning option meant to us was that ostracized participants, because they needed to regain a feeling of control, would direct another person to turn his head more times than would included participants, who presumably would have no need to regain a sense of control.

To make things even more interesting, we decided to cross the ostracism/inclusion manipulation with another variable that we thought would influence whether or not ostracized participants exerted more control. The actual participant arrived at the experiment after the first confederate was already there. After the participant arrived, the second confederate arrived. At this point, for half the sessions, the two confederates appeared to not know each other, as though they were complete strangers. In the other half, however, one confederate would say to the other, "Hey, Jim, how's it going? You heading up to the cabin this weekend?" The experimenter would quickly intervene, telling the two that it was important not to talk at the beginning of the experiment. But the desired message had already been sent: the participant had been signaled that these two other guys were friends. According to the model, the nature and magnitude of the impact of ostracism should depend on the target's attributions for the ostracism. For instance, being ignored by another passenger sitting next to you on a train is not likely to threaten your needs in any meaningful way. That sort of behavior is expected and normative, so it is easily discounted. We reasoned that if targets can easily dismiss their ostracism as the result of the other two individuals being good friends, then targets would be less affected by the ostracism, and hence would request fewer head turns. If, on the other hand, there was no convenient excuse for the ostracism, as would be the case in the stranger condition, then ostracism should have the most impact, depriving them of control, which would lead them to request more head turns. That was our thinking at the time, anyway.

After the experiment, participants were debriefed and dismissed. Participants in the ostracism condition were reintroduced to the confederates during the debriefing session, and extra measures were taken to ensure that all of the participants understood that they were randomly chosen to be ostracized. We found that the process of reintroducing the confederates to the participants benefited all parties involved. The confederates were slightly uneasy and anxious about ostracizing the participants, and felt more comfortable when afforded the opportunity to talk with them after the experiment. During this phase of the debriefing, the confederates and participants interacted freely, and the experimenter played a secondary role. The debriefing also allowed participants to talk out their feelings about being ostracized. This appeared to reduce any residual anxiety caused by the ostracism.

We tested only 27 males. The paradigm was a human resource nightmare in that we needed four people to run one participant (one experimenter and three confederates). The participants were undergraduates enrolled in introductory psychology. We observed and also videotaped the sessions through a one-way window. The videotaping was done in order to later assess nonverbal reactions to ostracism.

Our first observation was that the 5-minute seemingly emergent ball-tossing game was quite successful. All included participants chose to go along with the game, and all appeared to enjoy themselves doing it. Our second observation was that it was unexpectedly painful and difficult to watch the sessions in which ostracism occurred. Ostracized participants would, at first, smile and wait expectantly for their next toss. Then, as time and several ball tosses passed, a realization came over the participant that he was not going to get the ball again. Then two sorts of reactions occurred. Ostracized participants either slowly disengaged by slumping down in their chairs and looking downward (and dejected), or they would engage in various activities that we interpreted as being motivated by wanting to save face. These face-saving activities included searching through one's wallet, combing one's hair, standing up and walking around the room, or reading whatever they might have brought with them to the room.

It was then time to separate them and engage them in the card-guessing task. No one questioned the cover story, or the rigged drawing (subsequent measures of suspicion revealed no concerns about this task). All participants seemed to take the task seriously, closely examining the face of the transmitter. All but two participants requested at least a couple of face turns. After we tallied up the total number of face turns per conditions, we found that the number of head turns depended not only on whether participants had been ostracized, but also on whether the two confederates had appeared to be friends with each other or not. But the pattern of the interaction was not in the expected direction. Participants exerted more control only when they had been ostracized by two individuals who were perceived to be friends with each other. Participants in the friends/ostracism condition requested almost twice as many head turns as those in the other three conditions. I will come back to this unexpected pattern of results in a moment.

After the card-guessing task, participants filled out a questionnaire. Our manipulations appeared to be successful: confederates in the friends condition were perceived to more likely be friends than those in the strangers condition; participants in the ostracism condition reported receiving the ball fewer times than those in the included condition (this was one of the last questions, because it clearly "gave away" the purpose of the study). When asked why they didn't receive the ball, they gave all sorts of interesting answers. The first participant said, "After I bent down to tie my shoe, they stopped throwing the ball to me." We reran the videotape of this individual and were surprised to find that he had never bent down to tie his shoe. Others claimed the two confederates were jerks (or worse). Others said that the confederates could tell that they (the participants) were not interested in continuing to play. The only psychological question that differed reliably between conditions was how frustrated they felt: participants reported feeling less frustrated if they had been waiting with two people who were friends with each other, regardless of whether or not they had been ostracized! Clearly this result was not consistent with our predictions or with the behavioral data.

The results of our first study were encouraging, on the one hand, and confusing, on the other. The paradigm seemed to work well in all respects. It was engaging, they were not suspicious, they looked dejected or acted strangely when ostracized, and we found that ostracized participants tended to request more head turns. But, contrary to our prediction, it was the participants who were ostracized by two people who appeared to be friends with each other who were responsible for requesting more head turns. Why did this occur? Our first thought was that it was a fluke and not a reliable finding. Then David Buss told us the results were consistent with an evolutionary psychology position because people should only react negatively to being ostracized by attractive groups; this would be the most adaptive response, because there would be no selection value for individuals to feel badly about being excluded from undesirable groups. We weren't so sure, though, that two friends were perceived to be a more attractive group than two strangers.

We would have to replicate the study. Before I could replicate it, however, I changed jobs, moving to Sydney, Australia, to take up a position at the University of New South Wales (UNSW). So the replication would necessarily be different on several dimensions: it would involve a different culture, and, because nearly 80% of our introductory psychology students were female, a different sex. Furthermore, because no one was conducting hemispheric laterality experiments at UNSW, I deemed that my previous cover story would be implausible. So Helen Lawson Williams and I preserved the ball-tossing aspect of the experiment and the friend/stranger manipulation, but instead of waiting for a fourth participant to show up, participants were told to wait quietly until the experimenter had finished setting up the laboratory for their upcoming task.

Fifty female undergraduates participated. The confederates were also females. After the ball-tossing game, they were told that their first task was to individually fill out a short questionnaire and then to watch a videotape. We separated them and gave the participant the questionnaire. Among other things, embedded in the questionnaire was a scale that measured desire for control (modified from Burger's [1992] trait measure for desire for control). We reasoned that ostracized participants should report higher scores on desire for control, and that such scores might be dependent upon whether or not the two confederates had appeared to be friends with each other (but this time we weren't so certain about the nature of this dependence). We then had participants view the videotape from their ball-tossing exchange and report on their thoughts and feelings during the game.

Again, the paradigm seemed to work successfully. The female participants all took part in the ball-tossing game and seemed to enjoy it. Once the ostracism occurred, we saw nonverbal signs of engagement, followed by dejection. The female participants watched the other two closely, as though they were watching a tennis match. But once they realized the ball was not coming their way, they slumped down in their chairs, looked downward, and had sad expressions on their faces. There were very few instances of the "face-saving" activities we observed with the males. When asked to describe how they were feeling, the participants were more likely to admit feeling excluded and dejected, and were more likely than not to accept the blame. "I'm not a very good ball thrower" was a common response.

The paradigm seemed to work just as well in Australia with females as it had in the United States with males. More importantly, however, was what influence the ostracism had on participants' desire for control.

Would the same pattern emerge? The answer was yes. Scores on the desire for control scale were significantly higher for those participants who had been ostracized by two females who had appeared to be friends with each other. For the other three conditions, their desire for control scores were lower, but not different from each other.

In two experiments, run with different sexes and from different cultures, using a different measure for regaining control, we observed the same unexpected pattern of results. The idea that this pattern was a fluke was becoming less plausible. Why might people desire (or exert) more control only when two people who were friends with each other ostracized them? Our questionnaire in Study 2 provided some hints: when we asked how much they felt they belonged to the group, ostracized participants reported lower levels of cohesiveness than included participants, regardless of whether the two others were friends with each other or not. On two questions tapping into their perceptions of meaningful existence, however, they felt most meaningless (feeling unworthy and low in contributing something meaningful to the experiment) in the context of being ostracized in the friends condition, consistent with our original predictions. These different patterns opened our eyes to the realization that need for control may be affected differently than needs for belonging or meaningful existence. So, what is it about being ostracized by two individuals who are friends with each other that causes males to claim behavioral control over a new individual, and females to express a higher desire for control?

Our tentative conclusion, and one still under investigation, is that individuals who are in a situation in which they are surrounded by other people who are friends with each other (but not with the individual) already feel awkward and limited in their personal control. Sometimes we refer to this situation as feeling like we are "fifth wheels," unnecessary, redundant, and generally in the way. What control do we feel we have in this type of situation? The other two have a common language and common interests. There is too much past history between the two friends for a new individual to know how to behave or what to say. Thus, they already may feel less control. If those two individuals suddenly include the new member, however, all is well. The individual is back in control (not necessarily having more control than the others, but having a feeling of personal control that is standard for the individual). But when the others ostracize the individual, then that control threat manifests itself into a real and palpable construct. In this case, what is potentially awkward becomes actually awkward, and for 4½ minutes the individual must endure this awkward, out-of-control feeling. We think that this is why in only the ostracism-by-two-who-are-friends condition do males choose to request 48 head turns of a new participant, and females report the highest levels of desire for control.

EXPERIMENT 3. EFFECTS OF OSTRACISM ON BELONGING AND REINCLUSION INTO THE GROUP

A few studies have examined ostracism and its effect on people's behavior with and toward the ostracizing group members, but their results are conflicting. Some studies found that ostracized individuals disliked and preferred to avoid the ostracizers (Geller et al., 1974) or that excluded individuals were less likely than included individuals to want to work with the rejecting group in the future (Pepitone & Wilpizeski, 1960), particularly if they are low in self-esteem (Dittes, 1959) or high in public self-consciousness (Fenigstein, 1979). As I mentioned earlier, Predmore and Williams (1983) found that socially ostracized males were more likely to want to be with a different group of people, rather than staying in the same group or being alone. However, other evidence suggests that the desire for group membership does not decrease when a rejecting group is viewed as highly attractive (Jackson & Saltzstein, 1957).

In the following experiment, Kristin Sommer and I asked participants to work together on a thought-generation task (Williams & Sommer, 1997). But prior to working on the task, they had been waiting with each other and some of them were subjected to ostracism. The participants in this study, unlike those in previous studies, did not have an option to exit, could not choose who their workmates were, nor could they directly punish the ostracizers (without also punishing themselves). Under these conditions, we expected that ostracized participants would do whatever they could to maximize their chances for reinclusion. There were two types of work tasks: coactive and collective. In *coactive* groups, individuals work in the physical presence of each other, but do so independently and expect individual evaluation. In *collective* groups, they are also in the physical presence of each other and they work independently, but they expect their contributions to be pooled with the contributions of the other members. Previous research on social loafing (Latané, Williams, & Harkins, 1979; see Karau & Williams, 1993, for a meta-analytic review of the social loafing literature) has shown that individuals are less motivated and are less productive when working collectively than when working coactively (males more so than females). Williams and Karau (1991) found that in certain circumstances, individuals would do the opposite of social loafing: social compensation. When participants expected poor performance by their coworkers, and when the task was important to them, they would work harder collectively than when working coactively, presumably to carry the group to an acceptable performance.

We thought that another occasion for social compensation might be when an individual wanted to gain reinclusion into the group. To work especially hard on a coactive task would not achieve this goal because individuals alone would garner the accolades for their own good performance. Good individual performance would not reflect well on the group, and may even make the other group members look bad by comparison. But to be especially productive when working collectively could accomplish reinclusion. Individual performance would not be assessed, and the group as a whole would share the credit for a good performance. This would suggest the ostracized individual was a good "team member" and should create a feeling of group cohesion.

Once again, we expected that attributions for ostracism were likely to affect its impact on people. Snoek (1962) had groups reject individuals by not talking to them, either because they were not worthy of group membership (personal reason) or because the group was too full (impersonal reason). He found that when participants were strongly rejected for impersonal reasons, their desire to affiliate with the group decreased; but when they were rejected for personal reasons, people maintained their desire to belong. Snoek concluded that personally rejected individuals possessed a "need for social reassurance" that could be fulfilled only by remaining in the group. These results suggest that the attributions generated by ostracized individuals may mediate their subsequent desire for group membership. Because the participants in this study were not provided with any explanations for their ostracism (i.e., causally unclear ostracism), we thought they would be likely to engage in attributional processing in order to make sense of the ostracism. Without making specific predictions, we explored our participants' attributions in the present study.

In this study we sampled both males and females. A total of 177 undergraduates (96 males and 81 females) from introductory psychology classes at the University of Toledo participated and produced useable data. One participant and two confederates (of the same gender as the participant) arrived for an experiment entitled "Brainstorming." The laboratory was divided in half by two large cloth partitions. In the first phase of the experiment, the participant and confederates sat in the half of the laboratory with an observation window, the same one used in Experiment 1. They were told to sit quietly while the experimenter made some last-minute arrangements. The ball-tossing paradigm was used during the waiting period, with the addition of a no-ball-toss control group, who simply sat quietly for the 5 minutes without any interaction whatsoever.

When the experimenter returned, participants and confederates were led to the other half of the room and seated in a circular configuration. Three desks were separated by 6-foot-high cloth partitions, so participants and confederates could neither see nor speak to one another.

Each person received a sheet of instructions that was read aloud by the experimenter. The instructions noted that they would be generating as many uses as possible for a given object, and that quality or creativity was not important (these are standard instructions used in social loafing experiments).

They were randomly assigned to either the coactive or the collective condition. In the coactive condition, the experimenter explained that she was interested in individual performance and that each person's output would be compared to that of the other group members. Coactive participants heard that they would receive feedback about their individual performance at the end of the experiment. A container with three small slits in the lid was removed from the center of the room and shown to each person. The container was divided into three sections by cardboard. The experimenter noted that individual responses would be separated and evaluated. In the collective condition, the experimenter explained that she was interested in the group's performance and that the group's total output would be compared to that of other groups. Participants also believed that the group's output would be reported to them at the conclusion of the experiment. The experimenter showed participants the same empty container (without partitions) and noted that their responses would be combined there.

After answering any questions regarding the task, the experimenter replaced the container at the center of the room and said, "You have 12 minutes to generate as many uses as you can for the object 'knife.' " She then started a stopwatch and left the room. Responses were written with red felt-tip pens on slips of paper and inserted into slits positioned directly in front of the participants. Confederates simply wrote their names or scribbled on each slip, so that the experimenter could easily separate the participants' responses from those of the confederates (especially in the collective condition). The confederates inserted about 23 slips of papers into the bucket regardless of condition.

The experimenter stopped the task after 12 minutes. She handed each participant a questionnaire, noting that the questionnaires would be completed in separate rooms. The experimenter "arbitrarily" chose the real participant as the one who would remain in the laboratory and suggested that the other two come with her. The questionnaire first probed for suspicion by requesting participants to describe any thoughts they had regarding the purpose of the study. Several questions were then asked to assess the effectiveness of the work condition and ostracism/inclusion manipulations. Additional items assessed the participants' self-reported effort on the task, their feelings toward their partners, their mood, and their attributions for why others stopped tossing the ball to them. Afterward, they were fully and sensitively debriefed.

Once again, our observations suggested that the paradigm was successful. We noticed that most participants reacted positively to the initial exchange of ball tosses. Often their enthusiasm escalated, resulting in trick bounces, throws off the wall or ceiling, and suppressed laughter. In the ostracism condition, however, a very different pattern of behavior emerged. First, participants laughed or smiled when they noticed they weren't being thrown the ball. Then they looked at the confederates in order to make eye contact. As seconds passed, and neither their eye contact nor the ball was returned, participants displayed various signs of displeasure and disengagement. These reactions were rather unpleasant and disturbing to observe, even after dozens of experimental sessions. From our casual observations, then, it again appeared that something quite negative was happening as social ostracism occurred.

Postexperimental questionnaire data indicated that the manipulations were effective. For example, participants in the included and ostracized conditions were asked an open-ended question, "Why did the others stop throwing the ball to you?," near the end of the questionnaire. None of the ostracized participants denied that this occurred, and all of them offered some sort of explanation for their ostracism. In contrast, 82% of the included participants said that the confederates never stopped throwing them the ball. Responses to the question, "How much interaction did you have with your partners?" revealed the highest scores in the inclusion condition, followed by the ostracism condition, and then the control condition. Perceptions of group cohesion followed the same pattern. Feelings of acceptance versus rejection took on a different pattern: those participants who were ostracized felt most rejected, whereas those who were included felt the most accepted.

The work condition manipulations were also perceived as intended. Compared to participants who worked collectively, those who worked coactively were more likely to believe that the experimenter would know how many uses they generated for a knife. Additionally, collective participants felt significantly more responsible to their groups than did coactive participants. Females reported feeling significantly more responsible to their groups than did males. Last, collective participants reported having less control over their group's performance than did coactive participants.

When asked to report on how hard they tried, there were no overall differences between those working coactively and those working collectively. However, included participants reported working harder coactively than collectively, whereas ostracized participants reported working harder collectively than coactively. Participants' feelings toward their partners were most positive in the inclusion condition.

The primary measure of interest to us was the mean number of uses generated by participants in each condition. This measure represented a behavioral response to an effortful task in which participants had to come up with as many uses for a knife as they possibly could in 12 minutes. Previous research has shown that low motivation on this task corresponds with low productivity. When sex of subject was not factored into our analysis, no effects emerged. But when we examined the pattern of results with sex as a factor, two clearly different patterns emerged. First, let us consider the control condition. This represented a replication of a typical social loafing paradigm, in which comparisons are made between participants working individually, but in the presence of other coworkers, and individuals working collectively, who combine their inputs with that of their coworkers. The usual result is less productivity in the collective task condition, hence the term "social loafing." In the control condition of this experiment, males tended to socially loaf, whereas females did not. Other research has shown that although females do exhibit social loafing on a variety of tasks, the effect is smaller and less reliable (Karau & Williams, 1993). Second, based on previous research suggesting reduced or eliminated social loafing in cohesive groups, we expected and found no differences on collective versus coactive tasks in the inclusion condition (Karau & Williams, 1993, 1997). Third, and most importantly, we expected social compensation by those who were in the ostracism condition. Indeed, females socially compensated, working harder collectively than coactively. Males, however, continued to loaf even if they had been ostracized.

There were also sex differences in participants' attributions for the ostracism and in their nonverbal behaviors while being ostracized. Overall, participants were more likely to blame the reason for being ostracized on their partners rather than themselves. But females were more likely than males to attribute the ostracism to their own poor character. Compared to females, males tended to attribute the ostracism to their own disinterest or to the fact that they did not appear to the others to be interested in bouncing the ball (regardless of whether they were truly interested in playing). With respect to nonverbal behaviors, included participants showed more engagement (e.g., leaning forward, maintaining eye contact) than ostracized participants, but this effect was significant only among ostracized females. Included participants smiled and laughed more than ostracized participants. Finally, ostracized males were more likely than any others (included males, ostracized females, or included females) to manipulate objects in their environments—a behavior we interpreted as a strategy to save face.

The results of this experiment complimented and extended the results of Experiment 1. Ostracizing or including people in the ball-tossing paradigm was again effective in producing differences in nonverbal responses, self-reports of feelings and thoughts, and behaviors. And these differences were largely consistent with the theoretical predictions. Ostracized participants showed fewer nonverbal signs of pleasure and engagement, reported liking their partners less, and tried to make sense of being ostracized by either blaming the others (males, in particular, did this) or blaming themselves (females were more likely to do this). Males also appeared to try to save face during the ostracism by examining or manipulating objects or looking otherwise occupied. When given an opportunity to work with the other two people in the group, males did nothing to improve their reinclusion—they continued to socially loaf when they combined their efforts with their copartners. Females, however, were more likely to behave in ways that could increase their likelihood for reinclusion—by actually working harder when combining their contributions with the others than when working individually. This latter finding is consistent with the hypothesis that ostracism threatens the need to belong, which causes individuals to attempt to regain that need. Clearly, however, the males did support our hypothesis. Indeed, males blamed the others more, showed signs of disinterest, and did nothing that could reinclude them in the groups. It appears to us that although males did not like being ostracized, they tried hard not to show that it bothered them. This suggests that if the need to belong is active in our males, it may translate into trying to preserve a good public image (and perhaps a good private image). This is consistent with Leary's (e.g., Leary et al., 1995) sociometer hypothesis, which claims that self-esteem is in the service of belonging: maintaining high self-esteem and projecting that image to others increases one's attractiveness and hence inclusiveness to others.

CONCLUSIONS

The ball-tossing paradigm, despite having no verbal interaction and a minimal context, seems to extract the essence of the drama of ostracism. Within a very short period of time (less than 5 minutes), ostracism has powerful and fairly consistent effects. Emotions and feelings become more negative, attributions for blame are engaged, and strategies are employed to cope with the threat that ostracism poses. These strategies include exacting control over another individual or working harder for the group than for the self. Gender of participants guides the strategies: females are more inclined to do things that will get them back into the group, whereas males try to project a confident and positive self-image. Observing the ball-tossing paradigm also convinces me that it is powerful. Despite having watched hundreds of sessions, I still find it difficult to watch the interaction live. I wince, avert my gaze, and talk myself into simply watching the videotapes. The confederates go through an interesting transition as well. Initially, they are very bothered by the ostracism manipulation. They feel badly and mean. They can't wait till debriefing when they can reunite with the participant and let him or her know that random assignment, not their desires, guided their behavior. But, in a similar vein to doctors distancing themselves from their patients and resorting to gallows humor to cope with dealing with human suffering, our confederates often come to take a strange delight in producing noticeable effects. Perhaps, then, this paradigm might also be used to study sources of ostracism in addition to targets.

There are, of course, costs and disadvantages to the ball-tossing paradigm that need to be considered. First, it requires the use of confederates (at least two) and an experimenter, which is sometimes difficult to accomplish and to coordinate. Second, although the fact that there is no verbal communication may be considered an elegant and simple means to produce ostracism effects, its generality to real-world types of ostracism may be questioned. Although the idea stemmed originally from a real-world event (the errant Frisbee tossed my way), most ostracism probably involves the loss of verbal communication. It is possible to add a verbal component to this paradigm, but perhaps it is simpler to manipulate ostracism in a conversation paradigm, in which the target suddenly is ignored and excluded in the context of a group discussion.

More Laboratory Experiments

The Train Ride

It takes me 2 hours to commute to work each morning, and another 2 hours to return home in the evening. For 3 of those 4 hours, I ride the train. I like the train; I get a lot of work done, because for the most part I can work uninterrupted (in fact, I am writing this chapter on the train). But occasionally I find myself in a configuration of seats facing each other, and often the other three commuters begin to talk to one another. Sometimes they are friends, but other times they are strangers who strike up a conversation. At that point, I am in a bit of a dilemma. Do I join them, doing my bit to be sociable in a normally unsociable context, or do I keep my eyes glued to my papers or laptop? And then another thought creeps in: Why don't they try to include me? Why are they happy to keep the conversation to themselves? What's wrong with me? Why can't I enjoy their friendly conversation too? Okay, I admit it. I have ostracism on the brain, but the setting intrigued me, as it did my PhD student, Lisa Zadro, who also rides trains and buses regularly.

Of course, one expects to be ignored by strangers on a train. But it feels surprisingly unpleasant when two or three people are paying attention to each other, but not to you. Indeed, my collaborators and I have felt the effects of ostracism in the most innocuous settings. Take the Scarlet Letter Study, for example, a case of preplanned ostracism. We knew why we were doing it and how long it would last, but we still felt excluded, ignored, and uncomfortable. We went to great lengths to get noticed, even if noticed unfavorably. And consider what happened when we were developing the ball-tossing paradigm. During pretesting, the person playing the role of the target felt awkward and left out even though he or she knew the other two participants were only playing a role and the ostracism only lasted for 5 minutes. Based upon these contrived, yet potent, experiences and our train-riding observations, we thought that it might be possible to examine the effects of short-term ostracism in a role-playing paradigm. To give a context to this role-playing paradigm, we adopted the train-ride context. We set up our laboratory to resemble a makeshift train. About 10 rows, three seats to a row, comprised the train. We tape-recorded the sounds heard by passengers in a train and played the tape in the background. We also placed signs on the walls similar to those found on our local trains (No Smoking, No Placing Feet on the Chairs, etc.). Our intent was to provide cues to the train-riding context, not to fool people into thinking they were actually riding a train.

An additional benefit of this paradigm was that we could also begin to tap into the psychology of being an ostracism source. Our previous paradigms focused on the targets of ostracism, but in the train ride participants were randomly assigned to play the roles of targets or sources. How did it feel to ostracize another individual? Was it empowering, as our Scarlet Letter Study suggested? Did it increase the strength of the bonds with the other source, as the anthropological literature suggested, thus making the dyad feel more cohesive?

Participants were randomly assigned to their seats. They were all issued booklets that contained scenarios, role-playing instructions, and a series of measures at the end. They were instructed to read only the scenarios and the role-playing instructions, and to ask any questions prior to the whistle that signaled the train was leaving the station. They were asked to play their roles until they heard a second whistle and the announcement that the train had arrived at its destination. At that point, they were instructed to answer the questions at the end of the booklet. After the last person completed his or her answers, all participants were debriefed. Many of the participants were high school students visiting our campus to learn more about the sciences. We spent considerable time with them discussing not only our interest in ostracism, but in the usefulness of various methods, including role play, to study it. Every participant was given a lollipop as he or she left our laboratory, so that at the very least they left with a sweet taste in their mouths (other research suggests that this may have also lifted their moods).

The details of the scenarios varied across studies, but common to all was that the individual was commuting on the train and that he or she was seated in a row with two other individuals. The two commuters on the outer seats of each row were always given the role of sources, and the individuals in the middle seat of each row were always assigned the role of targets. In many instances, the flanking sources proceeded to ostracize the sandwiched targets. We could then assess both the targets' and the sources' subsequent feelings, attitudes, and, in some cases, behaviors after an ostracism episode. But with whom would we compare their answers? Clearly, the answers of targets would differ from those of the sources, either because targets and sources would truly be affected differently or because they were merely providing us with plausible answers demanded by the transparent situation. We were more interested in comparing targets to targets and sources to sources. Unbeknownst to the participants, triads in other rows were involved in different scenarios, in which they had different roles. In some cases, the sources were told to include the targets in their conversations. In other cases, sources were told to argue with the targets. Still other conditions involved manipulating the motives for the ostracism. In this way, we felt fairly confident that if we observed differences between targets of various conditions, or between sources of various conditions, the results could not easily be chalked up to demand characteristics.

STUDY 1. OSTRACISM CAN CAUSE TARGETS TO OVERESTIMATE CONSENSUS

The aim of our first study was to replicate previous effects of lower reports of need levels for ostracized individuals, and, more importantly, to demonstrate effects that are consistent with our theory, but that are not easily explained from a demand characteristics interpretation. We were overly ambitious in our first study and attempted to manipulate too many factors related to the model that had not yet been put to the test.

All targets were ostracized. Sources were told either that they were friends or strangers to each other, and their targets were also told the same information about the sources' relationship to each other. Sources ostracized targets for *punitive* (i.e., because they saw the target knock down an old lady when getting on the train), *defensive* (i.e., they were told to imagine that the target looked scary), or *oblivious* (i.e., they were told that they were to carry on an intimate conversation with the other source and that they were so involved in their conversation they didn't even notice the person in the middle seat) reasons. All targets were instructed to imagine that in their rush to get on the train, they had accidentally knocked down an old lady and then had been pushed forward into the train before they could help her up. Targets who were punitively ostracized were told that the other two people in their row had seen them knock over the lady; targets in the defensive and oblivious conditions were led to believe that the other two individuals in their row had not seen the incident. Targets were instructed to try to carry on a conversation with the other two people.

There was only one effect for the manipulation of the sources' relationship to one another. Targets reported lower levels of self-esteem when both they and the sources believed the sources to be strangers rather than friends. It stands to reason that if two friends ostracize an individual, it would be easier for that individual to attribute the ostracism to the relatively innocuous explanation that friends may simply not pay attention to strangers. When, however, strangers pay attention to each other while at the same time ignoring a third stranger, then all that is left for targets to surmise is that they are somehow undesirable to the sources.

There were no effects for our manipulation of motives for ostracizing. Perhaps the act of ostracism overpowered the assigned motive. Or, because our participants were not trained in method acting, they may not have immersed themselves deeply enough into their roles. For whatever reason, studying the impact of different motives will either require stronger manipulations or another method.

Large effects were shown on all measures between sources and targets. Targets reported feeling less belonging, control, and meaningful existence levels than did sources. On a single-item measure of self-esteem, targets reported lower levels than sources, but there was so much variation on this measure that the difference was not statistically reliable. Overall, these differences in need levels were interesting, but could indicate compliance with demand characteristics. Participants could have guessed that we would expect sources to have higher levels of belonging, control, self-esteem, and meaningful existence needs than targets. Our observation of their nonverbal behaviors, however, reminded us of our targets of ostracism from the ball-tossing paradigm. They showed initial interest and eye contact, and even attempted (unlike participants who do not get the ball thrown to them) to break into the conversation. But, within a minute or so, they fell into the familiar slump, gazing at the floor and looking dejected. Our sense was that despite the fact that our participants were merely playing a role, they were also feeling the effects of being ostracized. Our primary interest, however, was to demonstrate an effect derived from our theory, but one that could not so easily be attributed to participants merely seeing through a transparent manipulation. By demonstrating a nonobvious effect, we could be more confident that the train ride was a useful paradigm to study the impact of ostracism.

To make our nonobvious prediction, we borrowed the theoretical rationale provided by Pyszczynski and his colleagues (1996) in their clever study testing the self-threatening consequences of mortality salience. *Mortality salience* refers to instances in which individuals are reminded of their own mortality; usually, stimuli related to death, like coffins and skeletons, invoke such an effect. In two field studies, they interviewed passersby about their attitudes toward a controversial local issue. They reasoned that individuals would be most likely to cope with ego threat by incorrectly overestimating agreement with their own position only when they were in the attitudinal minority (Marks & Miller, 1987). This reasoning is consistent with the theoretical position taken in this book: that reactions to any sort of needs threat are initially aimed at repairing or regaining what was threatened. The ego threat they employed was mortality salience—in their case, whether the passersby were asked the question directly in front of a funeral home or not. In support of their hypothesis, both studies showed that only attitudinal minorities—those whose opinions are not widely held by others—who were asked in front of a funeral home overestimated the population's agreement with their position.

Our rationale was much the same as theirs. We proposed that ostracism threatens four fundamental needs: belonging, control, self-esteem, and meaningful existence. To cope with these threatened needs, individuals who were already in the attitudinal minority would be expected to overestimate others' agreement with their position. Why? To increase their inclusionary status, as hypothesized by belongingness researchers, individuals could convince themselves that their attitudes are more the norm than they actually are. Believing that one holds a normative position probably also affords individuals a sense of efficacy and control. One's self-esteem is likely to be raised by holding a more popular position. Finally, meaningful existence works hand-in-hand with motives to buffer mortality salience. To the extent that ostracism is a metaphor for social death, then it, like a funeral home, could be construed as another means to trigger mortality salience.

Therefore, we asked our participants about their views concerning the then controversial topic of Australia becoming a republic. Public polls at the time showed a clear preference for changing to a republic (i.e., no longer being a monarchy with Queen Elizabeth as titular head of state). This position was even stronger among students. Indeed, the majority of our participants showed a clear preference for Australia becoming a republic. After the train ride, we asked them to indicate their own position and to estimate how many people in the voting population agreed with their position. For the most part, everyone estimated correctly how well the population's views mirrored (or did not mirror) their own. There was one exception: participants who held the minority position (favoring keeping Australia a monarchy) *and* who were targets of ostracism overestimated the population's agreement with them.

Thus, using an indirect and nontransparent measure of ostracism's impact, we found support for our prediction that ostracism is threatening and can lead individuals who already hold a minority position to buffer their exclusionary status by reporting that more people agree with them than actually do.

STUDY 2. CAUSALLY UNCLEAR OSTRACISM IS WORSE THAN CAUSALLY CLEAR OSTRACISM

Another aspect of the model that we were interested in testing using this paradigm was the causal clarity of the ostracism. Causal clarity is highest when sources announce their intention to ostracize the target, or when targets are restricted in terms of the attributions they can make for the cause of the ostracism. Causal clarity would be lowest when the reason for ostracism is not announced and when multiple attributions for its use are reasonable.

Previous research using a triadic conversation paradigm found that when targets were not given a reason for being ostracized they were more likely to work harder on a subsequent group task than when it was clear why they were being ignored (Ezrakhovich, Kerr, Cheung, Jerrems, & Williams, 1998). Participants in the causally clear condition were led to believe that they were late, thus delaying the completion of the experiment for the other participants. Ezrakhovich et al. concluded that when ostracism was causally unclear, targets had to engage in attributional speculation about why they are being ostracized, and during this process were likely to generate derogatory self-attributions. Because of this, they were more likely to attempt to rehabilitate themselves in the eyes of the others. Similarly, Sommer et al. (in press; discussed in Chapter 4) found that, when they content-analyzed narratives by individuals who had been given the silent treatment, narratives that were coded as being low in causal clarity were also coded as showing lower levels of belonging and self-esteem. However, low causal clarity narratives were less likely to show evidence of targets attempting to regain these needs.

In the present study, we predicted that targets would report lower needs when the cause of ostracism was unclear compared to when it was clear. We predicted that sources should report higher levels on the four needs when they had a clear reason for ostracizing the targets because they would feel more justified for employing ostracism.

Thirty-four male and female high school students participated in the study. They were once again randomly assigned to seats. Those in the middle seats were assigned the role of targets; those on the outer seats were assigned the role of sources. Participants were then given scenarios to read that either supplied a reason for the ostracism (high causal clarity) or did not (low causal clarity).

In the high causal clarity condition, sources were instructed to ostracize the target because they had not been invited to the target's birthday party. In the low causal clarity condition, sources were told to ostracize the target for no particular reason ("Why are you ignoring T? There seems to be no reason. . . . "). Similarly, targets in the high causal clarity condition were told that "[the sources] must have found out that you didn't invite them to your birthday party next weekend," whereas targets in the low causal clarity condition were told that "there seems to be no reason why they are ignoring you."

Once again, our primary measures assessed the participants' reported levels for the four needs. As in Study 1, targets reported lower needs than sources for belonging, control, and meaningful existence. Reports of self-esteem, however, were in the same direction but did not reach standard levels of significance. More importantly, in accordance with our predictions, targets in the low causal clarity condition reported lower levels on the belonging and self-esteem measures than all other participants. Unexpectedly, however, sources reported lower levels of self-esteem when ostracism was high, rather than low, in causal clarity. We have no ready explanation for this source effect. Perhaps they felt the birthday party explanation did not justify the treatment, and when left to enact ostracism without a supplied reason they conjured up their own to help justify their actions.

Nevertheless, Study 2 demonstrated that targets who were ostracized under conditions of low causal clarity were more negatively affected, replicating previous research. The train-ride paradigm reveals patterns of data similar to those found in the other experiments, giving us more confidence in its use as a method of understanding the processes and consequences of ostracism. Despite drawbacks associated with role playing, we are able to conduct studies with larger groups of individuals in each session, with less deception, and were able to examine the impact of ostracism on sources as well as targets.

STUDY 3. OSTRACISM IS WORSE
THAN ARGUMENT

The two previous studies indicated that the role-play train-ride paradigm allowed us to replicate and extend our knowledge of ostracism. One benefit of this paradigm is that it allows us to investigate effects of ostracism on both sources and targets. Because of this, we turned our attention to reactions of targets and sources that were unique to ostracism. Specifically, we were interested in comparing the differential effects of engaging in social ostracism rather than an argument.

Interviews with long-term users and recipients of the silent treatment have indicated that social ostracism (most often the use of the silent treatment in close interpersonal relationships) often alternates with verbal and/or physical abuse (Williams & Zadro, 1999). Yet many targets have stated that they would prefer to be argued with or even hit than ostracized. In fact, many long-term targets of ostracism have related experiences in which they deliberately tried to provoke the source into an argument, preferring negative acknowledgment to no acknowledgment at all. We observed similar reactions of targets of ostracism in the Scarlet Letter Study (Chapter 5), in which two of us continually sought to provoke some reaction, even if it were negative. We would have rather been argued with than ignored. Yet there has been no research examining whether the psychological ramifications of being either a target or a source of social ostracism differs from being a target or a source of other forms of interpersonal conflict—this was our primary aim in Study 3.

We hypothesized that there would be differences in self-reports between sources and targets concerning the interpersonally aversive interactions. But we predicted that the self-reported differences between sources and targets should be greater in the ostracism condition than in the argument condition. For targets, the negative impact of being ostracized should be worse than being argued with; for sources, the benefits of ostracizing should be greater than the benefits accrued through arguing.

Why? Let's start with targets. Compared to targets of ostracism, targets of argument are included, recognized, attended to, and have an impact on what is being said. Despite the aversiveness of the argument experience, targets of ostracism, therefore, should still maintain a sense of belonging, control, and meaningful existence. Their self-esteem, however, may suffer. What about sources? Sources of argument must contend with the arguments of the target. Sources must work together so as not to contradict each other. Their arguments may not be as strong or as articulate as the target's arguments. Therefore, they may not stand to benefit much from the argument episode. Sources of ostracism, however, need not worry about the target's reactions. They need not worry about justifying their actions. They need only attend to each other. Hence, they should feel empowered and superior, while at the same time enjoying a tighter connection with their cosource. This final prediction bears a strong resemblance to the proposed explanations put forth by anthropologists and comparative psychologists regarding the functionality of ostracism: it increases feelings of cohesiveness among the ostracizers.

Thirty-five high school children, 26 females and 9 males, participated. As in Study 1, they were randomly assigned to seating position, and then read the scenarios. In these scenarios, all participants read that the sources were angry at the target for not inviting them to the target's birthday party. Sources in the ostracism condition were then instructed to ignore the words and actions of the target, whereas sources in the argument condition were instructed to argue with the target for the duration of the ride. Targets were not informed about the tactic of aversive influence that the sources would take, but were simply instructed to strike up a conversation with the sources. After the train ride, they were asked to fill out the questionnaire, which was similar to the one used in Study 1.

Observation of participants while the train was "in motion" suggested to us that our paradigm was once again engaging the participants in an active psychological drama. However, there was marked contrast between targets in the argument versus the ostracism conditions. Targets in the argument condition generally tried to meet the sources' accusations and strenuously tried to defend their actions. In contrast, when targets in the ostracism condition began to perceive that their attempts to join the conversation were unsuccessful, they became quieter and gradually disengaged. Their comments became less frequent and their attempts to engage the sources through eye contact, facial expressions, and body posture were curtailed to the point where (after about 2 minutes of ostracism) they remained seated with arms folded, staring off in the distance, utterly silent and nonresponsive to the noise and laughter that continued around them. There were a minority of targets who, when faced with ostracism, began to try harder to engage the sources' attention (e.g., by imposing themselves prominently in the sources' line of vision, by loudly answering questions that the sources directed to each other). However, by the third minute of ostracism, even these targets began to withdraw. Interestingly, targets were often the last to leave the train ride, demonstrating signs of lethargy and sluggishness.

Looking at our quantitative data, we first noted that the act of ostracism was successfully enacted: targets in the ostracism condition reported lower levels of inclusion than all other participants. More importantly, as predicted, we found that there was a larger spread between targets and sources of ostracism than for argument for the questions on the extent to which they were currently experiencing the four fundamental needs. Sources had higher scores on these needs, targets lower scores. These differences, however, were more pronounced in the ostracism conditions than in the argument conditions. This pattern held up for each need, but less so for self-esteem.

The results of this study were intriguing. Argument and ostracism are two ways in which people react to anger, yet these two methods appear to have very different effects on those who employ them and on those who receive them. As we suspected, ostracism rather than argument was more likely to negatively affect targets' reported levels on their psychological needs, in particular belonging, control, and meaningful existence. Our measures of self-esteem yielded no differences between targets of ostracism and targets of argument. At the very least, the different pattern that emerges between belonging, control, and meaningful existence, on the one hand, and self-esteem, on the other, suggests that participants were not simply relying on a response bias when making their reports. But we suspected that self-esteem would be similarly threatened for both ostracism and argument. In both situations, it was clear that someone was angry at the target because the target failed to invite friends to his or her birthday party. As a result, they felt badly about themselves, regardless of the tactic that was used.

Sources of ostracism enjoyed more positive benefits than did sources for argument. In particular, they reported higher levels of control and a stronger bond with the other source. Perhaps because it is easier to coordinate mutual ostracism, ostracism sources felt more effective, and hence more powerful. Making the target appear disengaged and discouraged may have also led to enhanced feelings of power. Perhaps also these gave the two sources a special sense of efficacy that they interpreted as effective teamship. In any case, we found support for the contention that ostracism is worse for targets than argument, and that ostracizing makes sources feel more cohesive.

In the next study, we wanted to replicate our basic effects, and extend our measures of impact to measures that are related to health—specifically, anxiety and stress. If targets of ostracism experience lower levels of three of the four proposed needs, would they also report higher levels of anxiety and stress? One additional change was made in the design. To determine whether a portion of the negative response from our targets was due merely to the fact that they were in the middle seat and had to contend with interacting with individuals on both sides, we added an inclusion control group. This group also allowed us to see if the act of ostracism actually increases the cohesiveness of the sources compared to when they are including the individual in the middle seat.

STUDY 4. EFFECTS OF OSTRACISM, ARGUMENT, AND INCLUSION ON NEEDS, STRESS, AND ANXIETY

How should ostracism, compared with argument, affect levels of stress and anxiety? Targets of both tactics must endure an aversive episode, so compared with sources they should report higher levels on both measures. However, because the previous studies showed that targets of ostracism were affected more negatively on measures of belonging, control, and meaningful existence, we expected that they would report higher levels of anxiety and stress.

How does this prediction fit with the notion that reactions to ostracism pass through three temporal stages? The first stage represents targets' immediate response to ostracism. This reaction is hypothesized to be aversive because fundamental needs are threatened. In the next stage, targets are hypothesized to attempt to regain, repair, or rehabilitate the needs that were lost or threatened. For example, if belonging is threatened, there should be an attempt to regain a sense of belonging. If control is threatened, targets should try to exert control. But what opportunities are available to our targets in the 5-minute train ride? They cannot join new groups, they have little option to conform or to exert control over someone else. Instead, they are left to stew in their unsatisfactory state without recourse. Without opportunities to regain deprived needs, targets may begin to enter the third stage.

In the third stage, if attempts to regain threatened needs are thwarted, then targets will begin to internalize the consequences of reduced levels of belonging, control, self-esteem, and meaningful existence. Although the third stage was originally postulated to account for targets of long-term ostracism, we further postulated that instances of internalization might occur in the short term. This would be most likely for targets who have no opportunities to rehabilitate their needs, which may typify the train-ride context. Thus, we expected a mild internalization of the deprived needs, which we hypothesized would be represented as greater reports of anxiety and stress. Because targets of argument have fewer needs threats, they should report less stress and anxiety than targets of ostracism.

Absent from the first two studies was the standard control condition we had used in previous experiments, that of being included. How aversive is being argued with or being ostracized compared to being included in a nonaversive conversation? Do sources experience any benefits when ostracizing compared to when they argue with a target or even when they include the target? It was also possible that targets of either argument or ostracism felt uncomfortable merely because they were playing the middle-chair role. After all, they were seated between two others and had to constantly move their heads from left to right in order to interact with and acknowledge the contribution of each of the sources. For these reasons, we added an inclusion condition. Finally, we altered the scenarios so that for the first minute, all targets were included, and then (after the first whistlestop), sources would commence ostracizing. This change, similar to that used in our ball-tossing paradigm (e.g., being included initially, then being ostracized), was thought to make the ostracism more salient (i.e., targets could compare what they had to what they had lost).

Our basic prediction for reported levels of needs follows a fanning pattern as depicted in Figure 7.1. Differences between inclusion targets and sources should be minimal. These differences should increase for targets and sources of argument, and should be most pronounced for targets and sources of ostracism.

Once again, our observation of the train-ride participants reinforced our impression that even in this role-play context, participants' nonverbal behavior and levels of engagement were consistent with previous observations in non-role-play contexts. Inclusion participants (even the targets in the middle seats) were lively and communicative. They maintained eye contact throughout the exercise, and generally seemed quite happy. The argument participants engaged in heated communication, never letting up. Sources were enthusiastic and highly involved. The targets maintained eye contact and did not disengage, although there were far fewer observations of them showing enjoyment or engaging in laughter. The ostracism participants showed marked differences between the behaviors of targets and the behaviors of the sources. Sources of ostracism looked much like sources of inclusion; they were communicative, engaged, and happy. Targets of ostracism, however, showed initial engagement, and sometimes even a bit of provocation by placing their heads in the line of sight between sources. But within a minute or two, they assumed what we are now calling the *ostracism pose*: slumped in their seats, gazing downward, and looking disengaged.

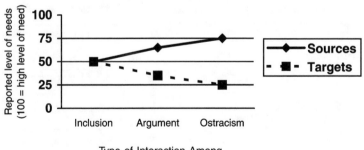

FIGURE 7.1. Expected fan-like pattern of results as a function of being the source or target of inclusion, argument, or ostracism.

Their reports on the postexperimental questionnaire for each need are presented below in Figure 7.2.

For each need, the fan-like pattern emerged. Sources and targets of inclusion reported no differences across the measures. For argument, sources and targets began to diverge, with targets reporting experiencing lower levels of the needs. Sources reported levels similar to those in the inclusion condition. Especially for belonging and control, it was worse to be the target of an argument rather than to be included. However, the most dramatic differences emerged in the ostracism condition. After ostracism, we see the widest separation of reported needs between sources and targets. In some cases, sources actually increased their reports of how much they experienced fundamental social needs. In most cases, targets showed significant decreases in how they experienced these needs.

For most of the questions related to needs, the "action" of the fan-

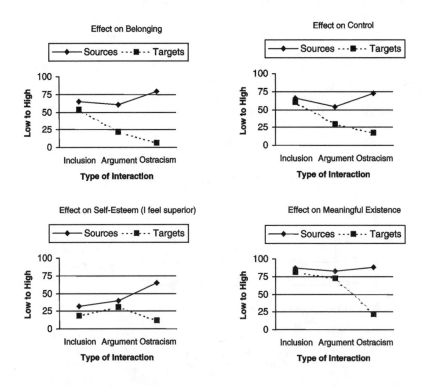

FIGURE 7.2. Obtained reports on each of the four needs, as a function of being a source or target of inclusion, argument, or ostracism.

ning was attributable to the targets. As we progressed from inclusion to argument to ostracism, targets reported lower levels of belonging, control, and meaningful existence. Note that the fanning action began for meaningful existence only between argument and ostracism. This suggests that however unpleasant the interaction was for targets of argument, they still felt noticed and recognized; targets of ostracism, however, felt invisible.

Only in the case of feeling superior, did we observe any increases in sources' reports, and this occurred only for those engaged in ostracism. Like our earlier finding in which sources of ostracism increased their bondedness with each other, they also apparently felt more superior. Neither feelings of bondedness nor feelings of superiority increased for sources of argument. Here, then, is the clearest indication that engaging in ostracism can be beneficial to sources.

But what about the effects of inclusion, argument, and ostracism on anxiety? To determine this, our participants filled out the Spielberger (1983) State-Trait Anxiety Inventory (STAI). Several weeks before they showed up for the experiment, they filled out the trait part of the form. Then, after the train ride, they filled out the state part of the form. In this way, we could calculate the effects of their experiences on the train ride compared to their typical state of anxiety. Our hypotheses were similar to those that we posited for the effects on their four needs. We expected that being sources or targets of inclusion would have little impact on their anxiety levels, and that whatever impact it had, it would be experienced similarly for sources and targets. For argument, we expected increases in state compared to trait anxiety, because argument is an aversive interaction. We expected that targets of argument would be more anxious than sources of argument because targets were engaged in defending an inappropriate action on their parts, whereas sources were on the offensive. For ostracism, we expected substantial differences in anxiety for our sources and targets. Because sources gain certain benefits from ostracizing (i.e., belonging, control, and superiority), we felt they would be experiencing little if any anxiety. Targets of ostracism, however, because their needs were threatened, and because their potential to influence the sources was limited, would experience the greatest increase in anxiety. The results for anxiety are shown in Figure 7.3.

The bars in Figure 7.3 represent the difference between participants' earlier reports of their trait anxiety levels and their reports of their current state of anxiety after the train ride. Bars below the zero line indicate less anxiety than normal, bars above the zero line indicate more anxiety than normal. There are several interesting results. First, and consistent with theories of belonging (Baumeister & Leary, 1995) and the sociometer hypothesis (Leary et al., 1995), being included in a friendly con-

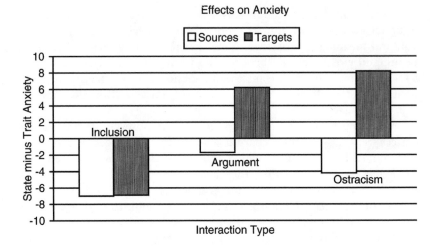

FIGURE 7.3. Effects of inclusion, argument, and ostracism on sources' and targets' anxiety scores.

versation is a positive experience. Indeed, both sources and targets of inclusion reported feeling less anxious than they normally did. Second, sources of argument and ostracism did not experience more anxiety from playing their roles. Indeed, both were slightly under the zero line. Thus, our anticipation that engaging in an argument with a target would cause mild anxiety was not supported. Perhaps this is because sources had allies (each other), and were able to diffuse any negative effects between them. Most interesting is the reported levels of anxiety for our targets of argument and ostracism.

As predicted, targets of argument and ostracism experienced more anxiety compared to their normal trait levels. Ostracism targets, however, experienced more anxiety than argument targets. The difference between levels of anxiety was significantly greater between sources and targets of ostracism than between sources and targets of argument. Higher levels of anxiety for ostracism targets could not be attributed simply to the strenuousness of their activities. Indeed, targets of argument were more fully and continuously engaged and had to do more work than targets of ostracism. Apparently, having to sit and stew about being ostracized, about being ineffective in getting the sources' attention, caused more anxiety than having to fend off sources.

This study was the first to show potential differences between two types of aversive interpersonal interactions, argument and ostracism, as they compared to a nonaversive interpersonal interaction: inclusion. The pattern of results is largely consistent with our hypotheses. Inclusion is a pleasurable event that appeared to fulfill social needs and reduce anxiety. Argument was unpleasant for targets; it reduced their levels of belonging and control, and it increased anxiety. But, as unpleasant as argument was for targets, ostracism was worse. Ostracized targets reported the lowest levels of needs and the highest levels of anxiety. Interestingly, despite the effort and attention it took to engage in ostracism, sources of ostracism experienced no increases in anxiety, and actually reported higher levels of belonging and superiority than even sources of inclusion. Engaging in an argument, however, provided little benefit to sources.

STUDY 5. EFFECTS OF OSTRACISM AND ARGUMENT ON STRESS, MOOD, AND EATING

Our final train-ride study examined further the possible differences between the psychological experiences of argument and ostracism. In addition to assessing participants' reports on their need levels, we examined the effects of these two methods of interpersonal conflict on sources' and targets' arousal and stress levels, mood, and eating behavior (see Oliver, Zadro, Huon, & Williams, 2001).

In this study, sources and targets engaged in only two types of interaction, argument and ostracism. Instead of using the STAI, we used the Stress-Arousal Adjective Checklist (SACL; Mackay, Cox, Burrows, & Lazzerini, 1978; modified by King, Burrows, & Stanley, 1983). This 20-item scale consists of two 10-item subscales, one assessing stress (e.g., tense, worried, apprehensive) and the other assessing arousal (e.g., active, energetic, vigorous). This measure purports to show a distinction between arousal and stress. Arousal can be viewed as a functional physiological reaction to any challenging circumstance, whereas stress can be viewed as a dysfunctional reaction to psychological threat (Blascovich & Mendes, 2000). With this measure our primary question was, Do targets of ostracism show stronger stress reactions than targets of argument?

We also assessed mood. We asked participants to respond to how they felt on the following bipolar scales: happy/sad, discontent/content, pleasant/unpleasant, ashamed/proud, good/bad, and unconfident/confident. Previous research has shown that ostracized targets experience depressed moods compared to included targets. We wanted to replicate this finding with the train-ride paradigm, while also assessing the moods of sources. Finally, we wished to determine if targets of ostracism showed depressed moods more than targets of argument.

Finally, after the train ride, participants were told that another researcher was conducting some taste tests for a perception experiment, and asked to give their opinions about some food they would taste. Research reported in the eating disorder literature suggests that depressed mood, as well as removal of perceived control, can cause excessive eating in *high disinhibitors* (people who are prone to overeat) but reduced eating in *low disinhibitors* (Herman, Polivy, Lank, & Heatherton, 1987). We wondered if our low ostracized targets would be especially more (in the case of low disinhibitors) or less (in the case of high disinhibitors) likely to eat than would the other participants in our experiment.

Fifty-seven university students participated. Weeks previously, they had filled out an eating disorder inventory. The scenarios followed those used in Study 4: they were randomly assigned to seats in rows of a simulated train, were given scenarios to read, and then were asked to act out the roles they were assigned. Targets sat in the middle seats of the rows, sources on the outer seats. After the 5-minute train ride, they filled out postexperimental questionnaires that contained items related to their needs, anxiety and stress, and mood. Finally, they were each given a small plate of countable savories and sweets. They were then debriefed, encouraged to ask questions, and finally dismissed.

We were again struck by the nonverbal differences between targets of ostracism and the rest of the participants. Sources of argument and ostracism, as well as targets of argument, were thoroughly engaged and lively. They maintained constant eye contact, and talked for the entire 5 minutes. Targets of ostracism, within 2 minutes, assumed the ostracism pose. The most noteworthy observation was that when they were offered their plates of food morsels, sources and targets of argument left their train chairs and went to larger tables at the room's periphery so they could more easily write down their reactions to the taste of the food. Targets of ostracism remained seated in their chairs, eating their morsels and writing their responses.

Analyses of the needs again revealed several significant differences. Compared to sources, targets of both types of aversive interaction showed lower levels on all needs measures. For measures of belonging, self-esteem, and meaningful existence, these differences were larger between sources and targets of ostracism than between sources and targets of argument. Compared with targets of argument, targets of ostracism reported lower scores on belonging, meaningful existence, and self-esteem. Oddly, participants (sources and targets, combined) role playing the ostracism scenarios scored lower on meaningful existence than those role playing the argument scenarios. Needs scores were slightly higher for sources of ostracism than for sources of argument, but did not reach standard levels of significance.

Mood scores showed some similarities to needs scores, but also

showed some differences. Across and between the argument and ostracism conditions, targets had more depressed mood scores than sources. When compared against each other, however, targets of argument reported about the same levels of mood as targets of ostracism. There were no source differences on mood between the argument and ostracism conditions. These results indicate that, first, mood scores do not necessarily follow our obtained scores on needs, which at least argues against a simple response bias interpretation. Second, they suggest that being a target of either type of aversive interaction puts one in a worse mood compared to the reported moods of the sources, but that targets of ostracism were not in a worse mood than targets of argument. These results argue against a simple mood interpretation for our results on needs and anxiety.

On our measurements of arousal and stress, we found that targets of ostracism had the lowest arousal scores combined with the highest stress scores. The higher stress levels for targets of ostracism in this study are compatible with our findings that ostracism targets had higher anxiety levels in Study 4. Arousal, as measured in this study, refers to general activity levels (e.g., active, energetic, and vigorous). Our observations suggested that our ostracism targets were lethargic, not active.

Finally, we found that low disinhibitors (people with normal eating habits) who were targets ate significantly fewer sweets than sources, but there were no differences in amounts of food consumed between targets of ostracism and targets of argument. At best, this suggests that being ostracized and argued with were unpleasant and aversive, causing normal eaters to reduce their intake.

CONCLUSIONS

The results of these five train-ride studies point to several important conclusions. Perhaps more than any specific finding, we were pleasantly surprised by our observations of the power of the paradigm. Despite its artificiality and the fact that participants were merely playing roles, their roles and the scenarios visibly affected them. For the most part, individuals playing one particular role in one particular scenario—targets of ostracism—behaved differently than all the rest. Targets of ostracism disengaged within 2 minutes of the ride, stared unsmilingly at their feet, and remained seated after others had left the "train." It was as though they had been hit with a stun gun. All others, including targets of argument, were lively, engaged, maintained eye contact, and interacted throughout the ride.

The paradigm also generated significant differences in self-reports

of needs, mood, anxiety, arousal, and stress. Most differences indicated that targets of ostracism were specifically disadvantaged, whereas sources of ostracism were, if anything, benefiting from the interaction. Some predicted and obtained effects were so psychologically complicated that the results challenged any simple demand characteristics explanation. That we only saw an overestimation of consensus among attitudinal minorities who were also targets of ostracism is a case in point.

Third, the train-ride paradigm gave us an efficient means to study some effects of ostracism on sources. Admittedly, ostracizing someone in order to play out a role is different from ostracizing someone out of anger or fear or resentment. Thus, this paradigm went only so far in illuminating the psychology of the ostracism source. Still, we caught a glimpse of ostracism's lure. Participants playing out the role of sources of ostracism felt more connected to their cosource, more empowered, and superior.

Fourth, we were able to show unique effects of ostracism over another commonly used aversive interpersonal behavior: argument. Both argument and ostracism are means to deal with others with whom we are angry. Both are unpleasant for the targets, while enabling the sources to vent or to show their anger. But here the similarities end. For some effects, ostracism simply brought more unpleasantness to the targets. This was the case for feeling less belonging and less control. For other effects, the differences were of a categorical nature. Compared to inclusion targets, targets of argument did not feel more invisible, and did not report lowered self-esteem, but targets of ostracism did. These results are consistent with what targets of long-term ostracism have told us in their interviews: they would rather argue than be ignored. We also showed unique benefits for sources of ostracism compared with sources of argument. Compared with sources of argument, sources of ostracism feel higher levels of belonging, control, and superiority. These results are consistent with observations by anthropologists who claim that ostracism is functional because it increases the group's cohesiveness.

Despite using a relatively innocuous means to study ostracism (i.e., role play), we were even able to detect the potentially deleterious effects of ostracism on measures related to psychological health. In Study 4, ostracized targets, more than all others, had the highest anxiety scores; in Study 5 they had the highest stress scores combined with the lowest arousal scores. Both sets of results suggest that targets of ostracism, compared to participants in the other conditions, are least able to cope with the demands of their situation.

Our results are also consistent with research conducted in other laboratories. For example, Stroud, Tanofsky-Kraff, Wilfley, and Salovey (2000) found affective, physiological, and behavioral responses to the

Yale Interpersonal Stressor (YIPS). Their interpersonal stressor combined actively deriding, then ignoring targets. They found that being exposed to the YIPS (in comparison to those who worked on a nonsocial task of searching for randomly typed letters on a sheet of paper) caused targets to experience greater levels of negative affect and lower levels of positive affect. Further, they reported restrained eaters ate more following the YIPS than did nonrestrained eaters.

Restrained eaters are often also high disinhibitors. We too found that our high disinhibitors ate more than our low disinhibitors following being targets of either argument or ostracism. But, for our sample, it was clear that this difference was primarily because low disinhibitor targets ate less than the sources, rather than because high disinhibitor targets ate more. Review of Stroud et al.'s (2000) data suggests that it is possible that their primary effect was due to the fact that their low restraint eaters ate less than those in their control group. In either case, it is not clear from either program of research whether ostracism per se has a differential effect on eating, beyond that from any unpleasant interpersonal interaction.

Finally, aside from its use in investigating effects of ostracism on sources and targets, this paradigm might be the most easy and efficient means for psychology instructors to demonstrate the power of ostracism in the classroom. With minimal cost and resources, we were able to capture within 5 minutes the drama of interpersonal ostracism. Postexperimental debriefing sessions were lively and informative. Our high school participants reported that social ostracism was rampant among the cliques within their classes. Still others saw direct connections between being ostracized and becoming violent or suicidal. We were amazed at how participation in this exercise triggered so many ideas. This alone makes the train-ride paradigm worthy of attention.

CHAPTER EIGHT

Cyberostracism

Getting Silenced on the Internet

A woman contacted me a few months ago in response to an ad we had placed in a women's magazine. We were looking to talk with people who had "long-term" experience with the silent treatment, either giving it or getting it (as discussed in Chapters 2 and 10). What made her call stand out from the rest was that she claimed to be a target of the silent treatment over the Internet. Specifically, she had "met" a man in a chat room and had developed over the course of a year or so a relationship with him. Most of their relationship took the form of Internet communications, in chat rooms and via e-mail, although they had had a few weekend face-to-face rendezvous. But the silent treatment occurred in the Internet communications rather than the face-to-face meetings, and it caused her to feel great frustration, demoralization, and fear that their relationship would terminate. We were halfway through the interview before she hesitated, then told me she had not revealed the whole story. She said that for us to make sense of her predicament, she needed to confess a few more contextual details. I urged her on, and she said, "He's my master and I'm his slave." Basically, he would demand that she do various behaviors (she admitted most were sexual but didn't go into details), and she would either do them or not and then tell him about them. She was happy with their master–slave relationship and made it very clear that it wasn't role playing. Apparently, her refusal to perform an occasional act was not the cause of the silent treatment. Instead, during their Internet discussions she would occasionally say something that would "disappoint" him. That word usually tipped her off that she would soon be getting the silent treatment from him. It would start with shorter phrases, then shorter words. Instead of typing, "okay," he would type "k." Some words would simply sound shorter or less friendly—as

162

when he would type "yep" instead of "yes." Then he would stop typing altogether, sometimes leaving the chat room, other times not. No matter what she would type, how apologetic she tried to be, he wouldn't respond, sometimes for a few hours but other times for up to a few weeks. She said it drove her crazy. She would become depressed and despondent. I asked her why getting the silent treatment, in the context of being asked to do many embarrassing acts, was so bad? Wasn't it just another way for him to exert his "mastery" over her? She said the degrading requests were okay, it was what their relationship was about, but the silent treatment "wasn't fair."

We happened to also interview the "master" in this relationship. His accounts of what happened were remarkably consistent with her accounts, even in his description of how he gave the silent treatment. When he was disappointed with her, he would knowingly use the silent treatment to let her know how disappointed he was—he viewed it as punishment and as a means to rehabilitate her. He also said he used it on his wife and with past Internet relationships.

Lest we jump to the conclusion that being ignored over the Internet is reserved for a somewhat unusual and relatively small portion of the population let me share an anecdote. I had lunch with one of my academic colleagues just last week. She had received an e-mail message from an old friend (and former lover) saying he was thinking of taking his sabbatical in her city (he lived in a distant country) and wondered how she thought he would like it. She was a bit curious about his motives for selecting this particular sabbatical site, but responded encouragingly. She also added a bit of what she thought was good-natured teasing. The next day, she was surprised and disappointed that he had not yet responded. A week passed without an answer to her e-mail. She figured he could be out of town or his computer network might be down. As more weeks passed she generated an ever changing list of innocuous reasons for his lack of response. But having heard nothing back from him for a month, she e-mailed him again, and asked him why he hadn't replied. She wrote that she hoped he hadn't taken any offense at her offhanded humorous remark. Again, she received no reply. Days, weeks, and months passed and she did not hear from him. She told me that she couldn't believe how upset she was becoming because he hadn't replied. She said she would have much preferred if he would have been angry with her, sarcastic, or otherwise confrontational, as long as he gave her *some* response. She told me the Internet silence started to intrude on her thoughts, that she worried about why he didn't answer ("Was he dead?," "Did he change jobs?," "Is he really that angry with me?," "Will he ever talk with me again?"). Her intrusive thoughts started to affect her motivation at work and her general mental health. She confessed that before this incident, she would have laughed at the idea that getting no response from an e-mail could be that upsetting. She even went so far as to say that for some reason that she couldn't really understand, getting no response via e-mail was worse than getting the silent treatment in person. She said that at least in person she would have gotten some visual feedback, and she would have known that her correspondent was alive and well.

The number of people using the Internet now is astoundingly large and growing exponentially. Claims that Internet users are a "special" population are becoming less and less plausible as more and more people use it. Research by Matrix Information and Directory Services (1997) revealed that there are 57 million users of computers who can access the World Wide Web (WWW) and 71 million users of e-mail as of January 1997. In fact, e-mail has started to outnumber conventional postal mail, numbering 95 billion versus 85 billion deliveries, respectively, in 1996 (Cowley Internet, 1997). The Internet is rapidly becoming an extension to our social universe. Over the Internet, people participate in activity traditionally considered social, such as conversation, competition, shopping, gambling, meeting new acquaintances, attending concerts, and even partaking of psychotherapy. Moreover, users actually initiate or maintain social relationships over the Internet. Parks and Floyd (1996) recently examined the formation of personal relationships resulting from online communication. This study revealed that over 60% of respondents to an electronic mail (e-mail) survey had formed new acquaintances, friendships, or other personal relationships because of participation in Usenet newsgroups.

Communication between respondents and their partners was also found to be frequent: nearly one-third (29.7%) corresponded with their partners three to four times per week, while over half (55.4%) did so on a weekly basis. Moreover, relationships initiated on the Internet often broadened to include other channels of communication. Nearly two-thirds of respondents (63.7%) had used communication channels other than the computer with their computer-initiated relational partners. From these findings, Parks and Floyd (1996) surmised that people may not draw clear boundaries between their Internet-based and real-world social activities. It is therefore important to extend social psychological research to include those interactions and relationships conducted over the Internet.

The sheer number of people using the Internet, then, demands the attention of social scientists. Most people use the Internet for some form of communication, using one or a combination of options: e-mail, chat rooms, or MUDs (multiuser dungeons, which involve fantasy role play). Despite this active (and interactive) use of the Internet (as compared with the passive activity inspired by TV), Kraut and his colleagues

(1998) found in a longitudinal study that individuals who made more use of the Internet for just a year or two were more likely to become depressed and lonely. As a result of frequent but shallow interactions, they claim, the quality of interaction decreases, resulting in feelings of loneliness, depression, and a lowered sense of belonging.

Recently, Rintel and Pittam (1997a, 1997b) observed that Internet users often perceive that they are being ignored. They viewed chatters' responses to noninteraction as particularly difficult, because of the chatters' need to defuse carefully the "hostility of silence" (p. 510) while gaining the attention of another interactant. They acknowledged the particularly ambiguous nature of silence over the Internet Relay Channel (IRC), in that the silence can be interpreted on a spectrum from deliberate to nondeliberate. Therefore, chatters may feel they are being ignored whether or not they really are.

Taken together, all this information indicates that we have a widely used medium of social interaction that predisposes people to be depressed and lonely and to perceive frequent episodes of ostracism. With this information, we were naturally drawn to study ostracism on the Internet. Our interest in this phenomenon serves various functions. Most obviously, because ostracism occurs over the Internet, we are interested in its affects. Should we expect that this sort of ostracism, in comparison with social or physical ostracism, similarly deprives targets of their needs for belonging, self-esteem, control, and meaningful existence? Or, because of the greater physical distance involved and the absence of visibility, should the effects be negligible? If there are fundamental differences between cyber- and other forms of ostracism, we can compare them to understand these differences. But if they are more similar than different, then we can use the Internet as another useful paradigm in which to test hypotheses stemming from the model. Finally, there may be distinctive features of the Internet paradigms that are more amenable to answer certain questions. For instance, at some point we hope to track peoples' physiological responses to ostracizing and being ostracized, but it is difficult to do this if the participant moves too much or speaks. Thus, the ball-tossing or conversation paradigms are problematic. It may be possible, however, to use the nonspoken and relatively inactive form of behavior that occurs through Internet ostracism to assess physiological responses.

CYBEROSTRACISM

We have now begun several programs of research into *cyberostracism,* by which we mean acts (perceived or real) of ostracism that occur over media such as the Internet, telephone, fax, and even surface mail. Acts of ignoring over the Internet may be perceived as deliberate and punitive, as when a group of MUD or chat-room users choose to ignore members who violate the group's norms (e.g., by straying from the topic or by being profane). Experienced chat-room users may not bother to acknowledging the existence of Internet newcomers (called "newbies"), thus giving the newbies the impression that they are not worthy of attention. Or, newbies may infer that general inattention is to be expected with their newcomer role. Thus, they may interpret the silence as role-prescribed. Defensive ostracism is also a possibility, as was the case with the woman whose interview opens this chapter. When the "master" initially gave her the silent treatment, she would retaliate defensively with her own (short-lived) silent treatment. Internet users can also consider several other possibilities that might explain why they receive no responses to their e-mail messages or chat-room inputs. Silence might indicate any number of real-life distractions to those with whom they are communicating (e.g., when one must temporarily leave the computer to attend to a crying child or to answer the doorbell). It might also indicate that there are technological problems with the Internet connection, such that their messages or the messages of the others were either delayed or lost in cyberspace. If ambiguity can fuel the aversive impact of ostracism, then it would seem that targets of cyberostracism might be particularly vulnerable.

In this chapter, I present in detail one new paradigm that we have used in our "virtual laboratory" to study the effects of cyberostracism. Two online experiments were conducted with this paradigm in collaboration with Christopher Cheung and Wilma Choi (Williams, Cheung, & Choi, 2000). These experiments, like those in our actual laboratories, involved random assignment to manipulations of ostracism or inclusion. The type of social interaction was a virtual metaphor of our ball-toss paradigm, in which participants were led to believe they were interacting in a triadic "cyberball" game with two others who were simultaneously logged on. Finally, I end the chapter with some ongoing research from two chat-room paradigms that we are currently testing.

THE ONLINE FLYING DISC AND CYBERBALL EXPERIMENTS

Conducting experimental research over the Internet presented challenges and opportunities. To date, surveys are the primary means to collect data over the Internet. For instance, there are online surveys investigating romantic relationships (Snell, 1997), effects of war experience (Robbins & Hunt, 1997), and new Internet user behavior (Roberts, 1997).

Nevertheless, experiments can also be conducted through online experiments.

In online experiments, as with laboratory experiments, participants are randomly assigned to conditions. Cover stories can be presented and augmented with engaging animated visuals. Missed answers can be dealt with by reminding participants to complete all questions before moving to the next screen. Likert scales, open-ended answers, and reaction times can be collected. Data can be collected 24 hours a day, 7 days a week, and can be downloaded directly into statistical programs. Large numbers of people from all over the world can participate. Students at small colleges or even high schools, who do not usually have opportunities for research participation, can learn about research methods by being encouraged by their teachers to participate in online experiments (in which informed consent, extensive debriefing, and opportunities to contact the experimenter via e-mail are provided). Tests of cross-cultural differences are also easier to implement.

There are potential methodological shortcomings to Internet experimentation as well. People can pretend to be who they are not, they may attempt to participate multiple times, and researchers have no control over who or what is in their immediate environment while they participate. Any method has its advantages and disadvantages, so triangulation with other methods is always advised (and is a central theme of my research program on ostracism).

Overview of Current Paradigm

The two studies were conducted on a website on the World Wide Web, and are based upon the laboratory ball-tossing paradigm described in Chapter 6, in which two confederates encouraged each participant to engage in an impromptu game of catch. In the inclusion condition (no ostracism), participants were given the chance to catch and throw the ball, and were included by the confederates for the full 5 minutes. In the ostracism condition, however, participants did not receive the ball again after the first minute, and their attempts to engage in interaction with the confederates were ignored. The current research tried to capture the drama of the ball-tossing paradigm in virtual reality. Participants were asked to visualize tossing a flying disc or ball with two other participants who were ostensibly simultaneously logged on to the website.

The experiments were set up so that when the participant had the flying disc or ball, he or she could throw it to the player of his or her choice by selecting a graphic on the screen. The result of the throw was then reported, stating the player who last tossed the flying disc or ball, and to which player it was thrown. When the participant was neither the thrower nor the receiver, he or she was shown a report stating that the flying disc or ball had been tossed from one player to another, along with an animated visual depicting a successful or unsuccessful throw.

The first three turns of the game were standardized such that the player would start with the flying disc or ball and each player would have tossed and received the flying disc or ball once. Thereafter, the probability that the participant would receive the flying disc or ball again was manipulated in accordance with his or her assigned experimental condition.

It is acknowledged that this paradigm presents a relatively impoverished social environment. This was done purposefully. It allowed us to test the relatively pure effects of ostracism minus the supplemental information that targets may use to explain its occurrence (as might occur if there was verbal interaction). It also allows for the controlled addition of other variables in future studies, and as such facilitates examination of each of these variables in relation to ostracism, its antecedents, and effects.

Experiment 1. Virtual Flying Disc Game

The first goal of Experiment 1 was to test a new paradigm for studying ostracism, specifically cyberostracism. Our hope was that through a relatively short and seemingly innocuous triadic interaction, we could successfully manipulate inclusion and ostracism such that participants would perceive differential levels of inclusion, and would have temporary negative psychological reactions to ostracism.

Second, we wanted to examine the impact of varying quantities of ostracism on the participant. In the model, one of the taxonomic dimensions is quantity. Ostracism can range from very subtle to complete. All forms of interaction can be eliminated, such that no eye contact is made, no discussion is initiated, and no questions are answered (or even responded to). Often, however, ostracism is less obvious than that; perhaps fewer words than normal are exchanged, or less eye contact is made. Although partial ostracism may be particularly ambiguous (and hence frustrating) because targets may wonder if it is really happening, we felt that complete ostracism would be more aversive than partial ostracism. People show remarkable ability to construe interactions in a self-enhancing light. When ostracism occurs in low quantities, targets may misperceive the lack of attention, denying that it is occurring.

Furthermore, some have argued that being a target of ostracism is essentially the same as being the target of focused attention—that both cause anxiety in the form of self-awareness (Carver & Schier, 1978). If so, then participants who are overincluded within the interaction, that is, who feel conspicuously attended to, should react similarly to those who are conspicuously unattended to. Although plausible, we felt that being the object of inattention was not the same as being the object of attention. Therefore, we hypothesized that overinclusion would not be aversive, whereas ostracism would be.

Finally, we examined trait self-esteem as a potential moderator of reactions to being ostracized. Research has identified several differences between high and low self-esteem individuals that should influence the way each is affected by ostracism differently. First, Schneider and Turkat (1975) reported that those with high self-esteem are less dependent upon the evaluations of others in determining their sense of self-worth. Because being ostracized can be perceived to be a negative social evaluation, this finding suggests that those individuals with low self-esteem would be more severely affected by ostracism. A recent study by Nezlek et al. (1997) found that individuals scoring low in self-esteem and high in depression felt less accepted when they believed others personally rejected them in the group. Moreover, Baldwin and Sinclair (1996) suggest that low self-esteem individuals hold negative cognitive schemas, which predisposes them to interpret socially ambiguous responses as rejection. We predicted that there would be a main effect for self-esteem, such that those with lower levels of self-esteem would report higher levels of aversive impact. We also hypothesized that there would be a significant interaction between self-esteem and quantity of ostracism. If low self-esteem individuals are predisposed to perceive negative feedback, then they should be more likely to perceive and react negatively to partial ostracism than those with higher levels of self-esteem.

Quantity of ostracism was manipulated and self-esteem was measured prior to the interaction. The study was conducted on an Internet website, and the data were collected over 15 months.

We had 1,486 participants who took part in the entire study. They accessed the site through various avenues. About half were undergraduate students from various universities; others were recruited though listservs, newsgroups, or links on relevant websites. The participants came from 62 different countries, with the majority from the United States, followed by Canada, Australia, and others. More females (64%) than males participated, and ages were spread out evenly from young to old. Forty percent of the participants indicated that they had had 2 to 3 years experience with the Internet. When asked about weekly use, the largest single response (37%) was that they used the Internet to communicate between 2 to 4 hours weekly.

Cover Story

The experiment was conducted under the guise of research into the utility of the computer as a tool in mental visualization. Participants were informed that recent studies found mental visualization of an action or task had proven to be beneficial in real-world performance, and that this study evaluated the use of the computer as a tool in aiding mental visualization. The welcome message also notified the participant that he or she would be interacting with two other players, who were participants like themselves, in a virtual flying-disc game. In this way, they were given the impression that they would be interacting with real people. In fact, the other players were computer-generated.

The preexperimental questionnaire asked participants for standard demographic information, such as age, sex, level of education, employment, whether English was their first language, and amount of experience using the Internet (in years). Participants were asked to indicate their e-mail address for two reasons. We used the address as an identifier so that data from the preexperimental and postexperimental questionnaires could be calibrated, and to discourage participants from accessing the study more than once. Thereafter, the participant completed Rosenberg's (1965) self-esteem scale.

Participants were then given an overview of the experiment. Each was told that there would be two other players and that they should all visualize themselves throwing and catching the flying disc according to the messages that were shown on their screens. Further, participants were informed that they could choose to "quit" at any time and move on to the last part of the study. In fact, the "quit" option was presented only after the sixth throw to ensure that the ostracism manipulation was perceived. Thereafter, the participant picked one of seven colors to represent him- or herself in the game. This color choice was confirmed and then the participant was informed which colors the other players had chosen (in fact, the computer randomly assigned the other players' colors). This was the only information provided about the other players.

For each turn a message and an animation was presented on the screen, detailing what had happened. The message and animation varied according to who threw and who caught the flying disc, as well as whether the throw and the catch were successful ("good"). The message had the following structure; "[Thrower] threw the flying disc to [receiver]. It was a good [bad] throw. [Receiver] caught [did not catch] it." "Thrower" and "receiver" were replaced with the respective player's chosen color in the appropriately colored word. In cases where the participant was either the thrower or the receiver, then "You" (in the participant's chosen color) was placed appropriately in the message. To keep things interesting, there was a one-in-10 chance that throws and catches were bad. This feedback was accompanied by animation of an errant throw or missed catch.

When participants received the flying disc, they had the choice of whom to throw to next by selecting that player's color. On each of the turns that participants were not in possession of the flying disc, they were simply notified of what had happened during the previous turn, and given the option to continue. The computer-generated players' throws were controlled by an algorithm. The probability that they would throw it to the participant was programmed according to the quantity of ostracism condition to which the participant was assigned. To make the computer-generated players seem more like real people, their response times would vary systematically with the player.

The game began with participants in possession of the flying disc. They were asked to whom they would like to throw the disc. During the first three turns of the game, the course of the interaction was common to all participants. Each player was given a chance to throw once and catch the flying disc once. Thereafter, the participant was randomly placed into one of four conditions that varied in the quantity of ostracism (overinclusion, none, partial, and complete). Quantity of ostracism was manipulated by controlling the probability that either of the computer-generated players would throw it to the participant. In an unbiased situation, any particular player would expect to have possession of the flying disc (and the decision of whom to throw to next) one-third (33%) of the time.

In the no ostracism condition, the program set the probability for participants being thrown the disk so that they received the flying disc for approximately 33% of the turns. In the partial ostracism condition, participants received the flying disc only 20% of the turns. In the complete ostracism condition, the computer-generated players threw only to each other and the participant was not thrown the flying disc again. In the overinclusion condition, the participants were thrown the disc about 67% of the time.

The game continued indefinitely until participants chose to quit, at which point they proceeded to the postexperimental questionnaire and thought-listing option. Thereafter, participants were provided an extensive debriefing that outlined the aims of the study and reassured them that the other players were in fact computer-generated and were programmed to include or ostracize. They were provided a link to the experimenter's e-mail address if they had any further questions.

Analysis indicated that the ostracism manipulation was successful. Participants who were overincluded believed they were thrown the disc more about 50% of the time; included participants reported receiving about 35% of the throws; partially ostracized participants said 26%; and completely ostracized participants reported receiving only 12% (keep in mind, all participants were tossed the disc at least once). There was no effect for self-esteem, nor was there an interaction between self-esteem and quantity of ostracism. The success of the ostracism manipulation was echoed by several participants who chose to comment on their experience in a "thought box" provided at the end of the questionnaire. One participant wrote:

> "I visualized us playing on a big open-spaced park, with a small fence surrounding it. I visualized each disc thrower throwing their disc. Mr. Brown appears short; Mr. Green seems lanky. They formed a conspiracy against me. I began to get disinterested when I was not included."

Another wrote:

> "Felt like I was having fun. Then I didn't get the disc back and felt left out, ignored."

Still another wrote:

> "Surely green is trying to appear nice with purple. . . . I assume he 'wants' to please 'her' and disregard my feeling about her! . . . As I leave I'm somewhat happy their behavior will surely make them guilty when they will notice I went away. As I leave I remember it is quite the same in my real life . . . and this is the most painful!"

Aversive Impact

An aversive impact index was designed to measure the general negative consequences that ostracism had on participants. We calculated an index based upon the composite of scores on items that measured mood, intensity of ostracism, needs threatened, and perceptions of low group cohesiveness. Higher index scores meant participants were more negatively affected (scores ranged from 12 to 108). As shown in Figure 8.1, participants who were low in self-esteem reported higher levels of aversive impact. Increasing levels of quantity of ostracism corresponded with higher levels of reported aversive impact.

Individual analyses were conducted on each component of this index indicating that we generally obtained the same pattern of results as we did for the aversive impact index. All measures were sensitive to self-esteem effect, in that higher levels of self-esteem resulted in self-reports that were more negative, but higher levels of the quantity of ostracism resulted in negative reports for all measures except for control and meaningful existence.

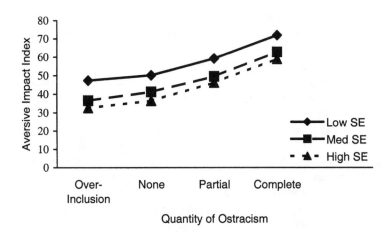

FIGURE 8.1. Mean aversive impact index scores at different quantities of ostracism for low, medium, and high self-esteem (SE) participants in Experiment 1: virtual flying disc.

Behavioral Measure: Turns before Quitting

The number of turns the participant played before quitting the game was taken as a behavioral measure of enjoyment of the interaction. The average number of turns played before quitting for the entire sample was 13.17. Those in the complete ostracism condition quit the game earlier than did those in the other conditions. Curiously, partially ostracized participants persevered the longest, perhaps an example of the large number of trials needed to extinguish a response when under conditions of partial reinforcement.

Summary of Experiment 1

Our main goal was to determine whether or not we could use the Internet successfully to study the effects of cyberostracism. The results were very encouraging in this regard. First, we drew a large and diverse sample of participants. In fact, we found our experiment endorsed on a teaching of psychology electronic "listserv." Possibly because of this endorsement, we enjoyed a large sample size. Second, our check of the ostracism manipulation was successful and fairly accurate. The participants who were overincluded reported being overincluded, and those who were not ostracized believed they received the flying disc an equal portion of the turns. The participants who were partially ostracized thought they received the disc about 25% (instead of the actual 20%) of the turns, and those who were completely ostracized reported receiving the disc for only 12% of the turns (they did in fact receive one toss at the very beginning, so their higher-than-zero estimate reflects this). Third, subjective states assessed after the game were significantly influenced by the ostracism conditions in the predicted direction. Aversive impact followed roughly linearly across the four ostracism/inclusion levels. Those who were overincluded or included reported the least aversive impact, those who were partially ostracized reported more aversive impact, and those who were completely ostracized reported the highest levels of aversive impact. We were also able to show that the conspicuousness of ostracism was reported as aversive, whereas the conspicuousness of overinclusion was not. Being overincluded, however, did not have any positive effects beyond that of being equally included.

This experiment also sought to explore the differences in the way that low, medium, and high self-esteem individuals reacted to different quantities of ostracism. We thought that perhaps individuals with lower levels of self-esteem might be particularly sensitive to ostracism, even when it was performed partially. This prediction, based on research by Nezlek et al. (1997) and others, was not supported: there was no interaction. Nevertheless, the online measurement of self-esteem appeared to be successful because lower levels of self-esteem resulted in higher levels of aversive impact.

Overall, our results were encouraging, both in terms of developing a new paradigm to examine ostracism, and in supporting the theoretical predictions of the model. Still, we were left only with self-reports as measures of impact. Can the impact of cyberostracism as manipulated through a virtual toss game affect behaviors as well? In Experiment 2, we explore a plausible behavioral consequence of cyberostracism: conformity. If cyberostracism deprives its targets of a sense of belonging, will they try to regain a connection to others by subsequently agreeing with an incorrect unanimous majority?

Experiment 2. Cyberball

In a study on group processes, Schachter (1951) observed that when attempts to change the view of the nonconformist in the group failed, the group ceased to regard the nonconformist as one of its members, and the individual was no longer considered eligible for any role within the group. He was rejected and excluded. Later, in his influential book *The Psychology of Affiliation*, Schachter (1959) documented his intention to conduct an experiment investigating the nature of variables affecting the affiliative tendency. Specifically, he was interested in examining the effects of social deprivation and isolation on conformity. Unfortunately, Schachter's intentions were never realized: the ethical constraints of physically isolating individuals could not be surmounted. We believe that the psychological state of isolation can be achieved even when individuals are in the presence of real (or virtual) others, as in the case of social and cyberostracism. If we are correct in this assumption, Schachter's question can now be investigated.

We have argued that ostracism deprives people of a sense of belonging to others—a need that is argued to be not only emotionally desirable, but also evolutionarily adaptive. As Baumeister and Leary (1995) asserted, the need to belong, defined as frequent, affectively pleasant, and stable interactions with a few others, is a powerful, fundamental, and extremely pervasive human motivation. They reviewed myriad studies that showed a link between the absence of affiliation and a variety of physical and psychological illnesses, including depression, anxiety, loneliness, stress, and relationship problems. Baumeister and Tice (1990) postulated that human beings function to minimize social exclusion by engaging in achievement-oriented behaviors (demonstrating their ability and willingness to contribute to the group), accommodating to group standards (i.e., conforming), and behaving in socially desirable ways. Likewise, Moscovici (1980) argued that when majorities exert social influence, they produce compliance. Individuals will publicly accept the majority view while privately retaining their initial view, motivated by a desire not to appear deviant or to risk possible negative sanctions from the majority, such as ostracism or ridicule.

In Experiment 2, we hypothesized that cyberostracism threatens participants' need for belonging, creating a need to reestablish bonds with other individuals by conforming to their group norms. Furthermore, we examined the strength of ties between the target and the sources as a potential moderator of ostracism's impact.

Group composition (as defined by the strength of ties between the target and sources of ostracism) could alter the attributions and consequences of ostracism. Presumably, it should be more hurtful and threatening to be ostracized by others with whom one has something in common than with others with whom one lacks a common bond. In our study, we manipulated group composition such that two in-group members, two out-group members, or a mixed group (one in-group member and one out-group member) ostracized participants.

Depending on the group composition, targets could attribute the ostracism differently. Specifically, when ostracized by out-group members, targets could easily diffuse the negative impact of ostracism through the use of external, group-level attributions. The motive for ostracism is relatively clear. For example, targets may think "those people are ostracizing me because the group to which they belong is rejecting the group to which I belong." They should simply care less about being ostracized by people with whom they have weaker ties.

According to social identity theory (Hogg & Abrams, 1988; Tajfel & Turner, 1986) and self-categorization theory (Turner, Hogg, Oakes, Reicher, & Wetherell, 1987), social influence results from a process of self-categorization whereby individuals perceive themselves as group members, and thus desire to possess the same characteristics and attitudes as other in-group members. The theories also postulate that feelings of belonging strengthened by in-group identification are central to the maintenance of self-esteem and a positive self-concept. Consistent with the reasoning of Baumeister and Leary (1995), ostracism by in-group members ought to be more threatening than ostracism by out-group members because evaluations by in-group members are more meaningful and important to individuals. Furthermore, ostracism by in-group members should be more ambiguous and less easily attributable to differences in group membership. Targets of in-group ostracism should be more likely to make internal attributions that are self-blaming. They may think "we are all in the same group and they are ostracizing me, so there must be something wrong with me."

We predicted that ostracism by a mixed group would be the most threatening condition. When ostracized by a mixed-group, targets should be less likely to make group-level attributions because an in-group member is also ignoring them. Perceptions of betrayal by the in-group member should be particularly keen, because the in-group member has colluded with an out-group member to mutually ignore a fellow in-group member. Therefore, targets of mixed-group ostracism may be led to make more internal, self-blaming attributions for the ostracism—for instance, "I am such a loser that even an in-group member is choosing to play with someone from the out-group."

First, we hypothesized that, compared to included participants, ostracized participants should show higher levels of conformity. We also hypothesized that a significant interaction between ostracism and group membership should emerge such that participants ostracized by a mixed group would show the highest level of conformity, followed by those ostracized by in-group members. Ostracism by out-group members was expected to have minimal impact on conformity.

In Experiment 2 we changed the flying disc game to a ball game we called "Cyberball." This new game differed from the flying disc game in several respects. First, we increased the level of animation of the tossing game in order to increase psychological engagement in the game. Second, we retained only two levels of the ostracism manipulation: no ostracism and complete ostracism. Third, we chose not to allow participants to continue the game indefinitely, because it didn't appear to add any value to the analysis, and it added unnecessary variability to the experiment. Thus, all participants (with the exception of those in the control groups) played the game for 10 turns, the first three of which were standardized as per Experiment 1. Finally, online "bubble thoughts" were added so that participants could enter their thoughts about their experience while it was happening.

In addition, Experiment 2 went beyond examining self-reports to testing the behavioral consequences of the effects of ostracism. After engaging in Cyberball, participants were asked to respond to several perceptual comparisons after viewing the responses of five other people with whom they were performing the perception task (all computer-generated users). Conformity was measured on the critical trials in which the others gave unanimously incorrect responses.

Two opposing groups of computer users, PC and Mac, were chosen to serve the purpose of the in-group/out-group manipulation. We felt this was a nice real-world analogue to typical laboratory studies on minimal group effects (Tajfel, 1970), in which arbitrary assignment to groups induce in-group favoritism. At this point in time, Macs and PCs are probably more similar than they are different. Yet intergroup stereotypes of Mac and PC users are felt intensively, commonly shared, and universal. Heated controversy exists and persists, both online and offline, regarding whether the PC or the Mac is the superior computer platform (Schlack, 1995). Despite the numerous articles documenting the increasing similarities between the two dominant types of computer in the present computer market, a simple online search using the AltaVista search engine yielded 784 matches to anti-PC and 1,008 matches to anti-Mac sites. Some of these sites are specifically designed to degrade or mock the rival make. The severity of the intergroup conflict between PC and Mac users reaches the extent to which generalizations are made concerning the personality traits of the two groups of computer users—for example, typical quotes on various Mac or PC sites include, "unlike PC owners, Mac users are pioneers, a temperament suited to the vast frontier of online potential" and "M.A.C. stands for Morons At Computers."

Participants were randomly assigned to a group: in-group, out-group, or mixed, and to an ostracism condition: inclusion or ostracism. There were two additional control groups: a conformity control group and a perception control group. The study was conducted via a website on the Internet. Data were collected over 5 months.

Of the 501 Internet users who initially logged onto the study, 270 did not complete the study and 18 were correctly suspicious about its exact nature. Although we cannot know precisely the reason for such a high dropout rate, we did receive feedback from several participants and teachers who said their modem speeds were so slow that the time needed to complete the experiment was intolerably high. The final sample consisted of 213 participants, 87.3% of whom were PC users, and 12.7% of whom were Mac users. Most (81.7%) participants indicated that they had used their type of computer for 1 year or more. Fourteen different countries were reported as the location of access to the study, with the majority of participants accessing the study from the United States (58.7%) and Australia (31.9%). The overall sample consisted of one-third males and two-thirds females, whose modal age range was between 19 and 25. Most participants indicated they were university undergraduates who had been using the Internet for 1 to 4 years.

Participants in this study were recruited in several different ways. Psychology students at the University of New South Wales, Monmouth College (in Monmouth, Illinois), and the University of Toledo (in Toledo, Ohio) were invited to participate in the study to gain credit for their courses. Posters were put up in an Internet café at the University of New South Wales to encourage participation in the study. Internet users were invited through the use of advertising on various psychology websites (e.g., American Psychological Society and Social Psychology Network), anti-PC and anti-Mac websites, and through banner sharing. Finally, the website itself was made "searchable" on several popular Internet search engines so that those who "surfed" the Internet could locate and access the study.

The website consisted of a series of pages such that participants had to click on the icon "Next" to move onto subsequent pages. Participants were first presented with a brief description of the study, described as comparing perceptual abilities of PC versus Mac users. Participants were requested to fill in a preexperimental questionnaire that included a question about which type of computer they used and an open-ended question asking them to list three traits of Mac users and three traits of PC users (to strengthen the in-group/out-group manipulations). Then, they were instructed on how to participate in our Internet Cyberball game. Emphasis was placed on having them mentally visualize the tossing of the ball between interactants. Participants were then told whom the other players were (PC users, Mac users, or both) in their group. They then played the game for 10 ball tosses. Afterward, participants moved onto the second part of the study, which involved a perception task. Participants were ostensibly randomly assigned to be the sixth person in a new six-person group who would be asked to make judgments on six perceptual comparisons. Afterward, participants filled in a postexperimental questionnaire and then were debriefed.

Ostracism Manipulation

As in Experiment 1, each of the 10 throws was accompanied by a message and animation informing participants what had just happened. In addition, a thought bubble also appeared at every "throw" to allow participants to enter any thoughts they had during that part of the game. The first three throws were held constant for all conditions. The game always started off with participants in possession of the ball and every player was given the chance to throw and catch the ball once. On throw #4, participants were once again in possession of the ball and had the chance to throw it to either of the two computer players. From the fifth turn onward, we randomly assigned participants to be either ostracized or included. Those in the inclusion condition continued to receive the ball for a third of the throws, whereas those in the ostracism condition were not thrown the ball again. At the end of the tenth turn, the game was terminated; participants were thanked for completing the first part of the study and were asked to move onto the perception task.

Perception Task

Participants were informed that they were to participate in the perception task with five new online users, and that they would indicate their decisions consecutively. The computer program assured that participants were always respondent number 6. Their task consisted of six trials; on each they were to indicate which of six complex geometric figures contained a target stimulus, shown briefly prior to showing them the six alternatives. An overview of the task was given together with an example (shown in Figure 8.2). Each of the six trials consisted of a different set of stimuli. Trials 1 and 2 were designed to be easier than the ones that followed to familiarize participants with the demands of the task. Trials 3, 4, and 6 were the critical trials in which the computer was preprogrammed to display unanimously incorrect responses by the other five users. All the other trials displayed unanimously correct responses by all other users.

Measuring Conformity

Degree of conformity was the primary dependent variable. It was operationally defined as the average percentage of critical trials on which participants selected the same incorrect response as the unanimous majority. Twenty participants were randomly assigned to a conformity control condition in which they were asked to complete the preexperimental

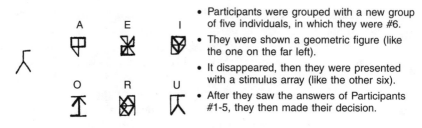

Perception Task to Measure Conformity

- Participants were grouped with a new group of five individuals, in which they were #6.
- They were shown a geometric figure (like the one on the far left).
- It disappeared, then they were presented with a stimulus array (like the other six).
- After they saw the answers of Participants #1-5, they then made their decision.

FIGURE 8.2. Example screen with perceptual judgment task following the Cyberball game.

questionnaire and were then directed immediately to the perception task. They were neither informed of, nor played, the game. This condition provided a baseline for the conformity measure to determine whether simply playing a group game prior to making judgments would influence conformity. Twenty-four participants were also randomly assigned to a perceptual control condition. Like the conformity control condition, participants did not know of or participate in the game. After completing the preexperimental questionnaire, they were directed to the perception task. However, they were not part of a group so that we could assess to what degree participants made errors on the perception task without group influence.

Postexperimental Questionnaire and Debriefing

On completion of the perception task, participants filled in a post-experimental questionnaire that measured other dependent variables of the study such as manipulation checks and belonging. Participants were then thanked and given a detailed debriefing. As before, participants were encouraged to e-mail the researcher if they had any questions or comments regarding the study.

Participants in all conditions were fairly accurate in estimating how often they were thrown the ball, except for those who were in the in-group, ostracism condition. These particular participants reported receiving the ball about one-third of the time, which would reflect approximately equal participation. On the face of it, it would appear we unsuccessfully manipulated ostracism for the in-group participants. However, as we shall see, analysis of their conformity scores suggests otherwise. I will return to this paradox later.

To assess whether the PC/Mac distinction was an effective in-group/out-group manipulation, participants' descriptions of the average PC user and the average Mac user were rated according to their negativity. Examples of negative quotes included: "PC users are pedophiles," "Mac users are wimps," "PC users are Microsoft's milking cows," and "Mac users are dorks." Examples of positive quotes include: "PC users are cool," "Mac users are friendly," "PC users are the mainstream," and "Mac users are one of a kind." PC participants tended to describe PC users more positively than the average Mac user, whereas Mac participants tended to describe Mac users more positively than PC users.

We compared responses of the two control groups to determine whether participants were as likely to choose the same incorrect responses even without social influence. No one chose these stimuli when making the judgment alone, but almost 17% did when the unanimous majority made incorrect judgments. Merely playing Cyberball had no overall effect on participants' likelihood to conform. Participants in the ostracism conditions were more likely to conform than participants in both control groups.

Conformity

Overall, 55% of the participants in the experimental groups did not conform at all; 31% conformed once to the incorrect unanimous majority on the critical trials, 7.7% conformed on two critical trials, and 6.5% conformed on all three critical trials. As predicted, ostracized participants conformed more than those who were included. Although those ostracized by their in-groups tended to conform more than those who were ostracized by mixed groups or out-groups, this was not statistically significant.

Ostracized participants reported that they experienced lower feelings of belonging than those who were included. Feelings of belonging were differentially affected according to the group membership condition, and mirrored the pattern of results for how often participants thought they were thrown the ball. Participants who were ostracized by either the out-group or the mixed group reported correspondingly lower senses of belonging than their included counterparts. Participants who were ostracized by in-group members, however, reported similar levels of belonging to those who were included by in-group members.

Bubble Thoughts

Online thoughts were captured in thought bubbles (there were a total of 10 potential thought-listing bubbles for each participant). Ninety percent of the participants listed thoughts in at least one thought bubble during the Cyberball game. The thoughts listed varied widely from (a few) complaints about not being thrown the ball to (more) comments on the quality of the website or (still more) thoughts unrelated to the experiment altogether. We had hoped that this measure would provide us with a glimpse of how participants perceived the situation, but it seemed simply to provide participants with something to do while waiting for the next screen.

Summary of Experiment 2

Our first goal was to extend the results of Experiment 1 (the virtual flying disc) by examining whether cyberostracism would decrease targets' sense of belonging and increase their likelihood to conform. Rather than giving targets the opportunity to conform to (or deviate from) the ostracizing group, we tested their likelihood to conform to a new group for whom they would have no preordained reasons to impress or offend. Both predictions were supported. Targets of ostracism had lower levels of self-reported belonging and were more likely to conform to the unanimous incorrect judgments of a new group. These findings lend support to the notion that ostracism serves an important function for sources because its aversiveness influences targets to behave in ways that will make them more acceptable to the group (Gruter & Masters, 1986b). It also supports the early speculations of Schachter (1959) that a psychological sense of isolation will increase affiliative tendencies.

We also examined strength of ties between participants and their sources on their reports of belonging and subsequent conformity. We predicted that participants who were ostracized by out-group sources would report less impact on their sense of belonging and would be less likely to conform than those who were ostracized by in-group sources. Conformity was greatest when individuals were ostracized by in-group members, but the difference was not significant. The reports for belonging, however, ran counter to our expectations. Participants were more likely to conform to a new group if their in-group had ostracized them. However, they reported that their sense of belonging was least affected when their in-group had ostracized them. This pattern was further buttressed by their self-reports of what percentage of the time they were thrown the ball. Whereas in every other condition the estimates were fairly accurate, those participants who were ostracized by their in-group overestimated their inclusion to the point that they seemed to be denying being ostracized at all. It appears as if in-group ostracized participants did not want to admit (to themselves or to us?) that their in-group had ostracized them even though it had an effect, which was revealed in their higher likelihood to conform. Being ostracized by in-group members may have increased targets' need to view their in-group and their status within that group favorably. This is consistent with the social identity and self-categorization postulations that feelings of belonging are central to the maintenance of self-esteem and a positive self-concept (Hogg & Abrams, 1988; Tajfel & Turner, 1986; Turner, 1984; Turner et al., 1987). At this point, these inferences are speculative and will require further experimentation to validate. By adding questions that will be sensitive to these processes we may be able to explain the apparent paradox that those most likely to conform were least likely to report perceiving or feeling the ostracism.

Finally, we had hoped to capture targets' online thoughts by supplying them with thought bubbles in which to type their thoughts. Occasionally, participants gave us insightful comments. One wrote, "Oh, I feel bad, PC1 and Mac1 are leaving me out of the ball throwing. I want to play with the ball. No one likes me. I feel really rejected and sad." Another wrote, "Why are they only throwing to each other? Okay, this is getting irritating. This is crazy!" And still another revealed, "Are they ignoring me? What the hell?!?" Unfortunately, most bubble thoughts were empty, and the filled ones contained comments about the quality of the website (mostly positive) or thoughts unrelated to the experiment. Perhaps making participants believe that their thoughts could be read by the others would increase their use and their degree of self-disclosure.

Summary of Cyberball Studies

An analogy of real-world aversive social behavior was successfully examined on the Internet. It is indeed rather astounding that despite the fact that our participants did not know, could not see, could not communicate with, and were not anticipating future interaction with "virtual others," they felt ostracized when these others neglected to throw them a virtual ball. Cyberostracism elicited worsened mood; declines in senses of belonging, control, and self-esteem; and increased conformity. Further, these results were largely consistent with our theoretical model of ostracism. Ostracism was hypothesized to threaten targets' fundamental needs, including belonging, self-esteem, control, and meaningful existence. Except for our measure of meaningful existence, the results supported the model. When given an opportunity to regain a sense of belonging, ostracized individuals were more likely to conform, especially if other individuals with whom they had felt stronger ties had ostracized them.

The larger implications of this research, if replicated and extended, would point to concern for those who routinely use the Internet. In addition to recent findings indicating that such usage results in increased feelings of depression and loneliness (Kraut et al., 1997), Internet use may also predispose its users to perceive that others are ignoring them, perhaps even when they are not. Our findings, in conjunction with Kraut et al.'s, suggest that Internet users, even (or especially) those who use the Internet primarily for interaction, may be unintentionally setting themselves up to be alienated, lonely, and depressed.

CHAT-ROOM PARADIGMS

The Cyberball paradigm, like the ball-tossing paradigm, has many advantages. It is simple, efficient, and—if we wish—free of context. But, as we discussed in Chapter 6, we also developed a laboratory conversation paradigm so that we could study ostracism in a more realistic situation in which context was an essential element, and in which we could assess verbal as well as nonverbal reactions. The best Internet analogue to small-group face-to-face conversations is probably the chat room. In chat rooms, two or more individuals log on to a room site and talk to each other. Often, the content of the chat room is indicated by its name (e.g., alt.Olympics), but other times by some characteristic of the users (e.g., newbies). Discussions are relatively free-flowing and simultaneous. While one person types in his or her comments, other chat-room members might also be keying in their comments. The comments are then listed for all to see in order of input.

With Vanessa Croker and Alby Lam, I have begun two approaches to studying ostracism in chat rooms. One way is through the use of (cyber)field studies, in which two or more students working on the project invite individuals who are already logged on to a chat-room network to enter their chat room. These unsuspecting participants are real chat-room users and could be logged on from anywhere in the world. Half of the invitees are included for approximately 5 to 10 minutes, whereas the other half are ostracized.

So far, we have only preliminary results from our chat-room paradigms, but the data we have encourage us to develop the paradigms further. For instance, in our (cyber)field studies, we have noted frequent attempts by ostracized users to confront the sources of ostracism. This "virtual courage" takes several forms. One form is to seek clarification from the others for their lack of responsiveness (e.g., "Hello? . . . What gives? . . . Can you hear me?). Another is to provoke a response, through teasing, insult, swearing ("flaming"), or "flooding." Flooding refers to attempts to block any communication among all chat-room members (e.g., by holding down the enter key). To illustrate the perception of being ignored and possible reactions to it, I offer a record of my first chat-room experience. I joined a chat room in progress, and the current members were named Cyndy and Sam. As will be apparent, Sam soon felt ignored, and he reacted in several ways.

"29/05/97 15:03:03","Kip","I'm male, 43"
"29/05/97 15:03:17","Cyndy","hey!!! someone my own age!!! :-)"
"29/05/97 15:03:31","Kip","Well, close enough!"
"29/05/97 15:03:40","sam","he's older"
"29/05/97 15:03:49","Cyndy","yeah but only by about 3 years"
"29/05/97 15:04:12","sam","I'm young"
"29/05/97 15:04:13","Cyndy","Kip . . . what do you do?"
"29/05/97 15:04:19","Kip","Sam, I'm in Sydney, where are you Cyndy?"
"29/05/97 15:04:24","Kip","I teach at a university"
"29/05/97 15:04:47","Cyndy","I'm in the US . . . Washington state"
"29/05/97 15:04:50","sam","bye"
"29/05/97 15:04:54","Kip","I used to live in Seattle"
"29/05/97 15:05:01","Kip","I'm American"
"29/05/97 15:05:08","Kip","bye Sam"
"29/05/97 15:05:19","sam","r u still there "
"29/05/97 15:05:26","Kip","who?"
"29/05/97 15:05:32","sam","kip"
"29/05/97 15:05:35","Kip","yes"
"29/05/97 15:05:46","Cyndy","did you teach at UW?"
"29/05/97 15:05:48","sam","who did u say bye to "
"29/05/97 15:06:10","Kip","I went to UW for my BS, then went back in '86 to teach for two years."
"29/05/97 15:06:34","Kip","sam, I thought you were saying goodbye, I got confused."
"29/05/97 15:06:56","sam","i thought you were going"
"29/05/97 15:07:17","Cyndy","so you guys are both staying, right?"
"29/05/97 15:07:19","Kip","Would you like me to?"
"29/05/97 15:07:24","sam","where in sydney do you live"
"29/05/97 15:07:37","sam","yes"
"29/05/97 15:07:40","Kip","In the eastern suburbs, near the university."
"29/05/97 15:07:47","Kip","I sort of got that feeling . . . "
"29/05/97 15:07:52","sam","I'm in Brisbane"
"29/05/97 15:12:42","sam","hello"
"29/05/97 15:13:03","Cyndy","hi sam :-)"
"29/05/97 15:13:13","Kip","So, Cyndy, you were asking about UW, did you go there? Are you in the western or eastern part of Washington?"
"29/05/97 15:13:43","sam","hey kip r u trying to crack on to this woman"
"29/05/97 15:13:59","Cyndy","I'm in eastern Washington . . . I work for the competition to UW"
"29/05/97 15:14:20","sam",",./;'[]"

"29/05/97 15:14:48","sam","abcdefghijklmnopqrstuvwxyz"

"29/05/97 15:14:57","Kip","Ah, WSU, yes. Hmm, new lingo here. Cracking onto this woman. Coffing. and then a bunch of characters. What's this mean?"

"29/05/97 15:15:04","Cyndy","wow sam . . . you're quite literate :-)"

"29/05/97 15:15:37","sam","well of cause i am don't be ridiculous"

"29/05/97 15:16:17","sam","i think old age is catching up with you kip"

"29/05/97 15:16:24","Cyndy","no it isn't . . . Do you get cable TV?"

"29/05/97 15:17:56","sam","now talk"

"29/05/97 15:20:26","Cyndy","[private] we can talk without Sam's seeing it at all :-)"

"29/05/97 15:20:44","sam","is anyone there"

"29/05/97 15:20:47","Kip","yes"

"29/05/97 15:20:53","Cyndy","yes I'm here"

"29/05/97 15:20:59","sam","good"

"29/05/97 15:21:13","Cyndy","[private] no it isn't"

"29/05/97 15:21:57","Kip to Cyndy","[private] Does everyone see this [private] designation, or just the persons who are talking privately?"

"29/05/97 15:22:19","Cyndy","[private] just the persons talking privately"

"29/05/97 15:22:24","Kip to Cyndy","[private] I did in the states, but haven't gotten it, yet. Trying to decide between Optus and Foxtel, or whether I really need it at all"

"29/05/97 15:22:36","sam","y is no one talking to me"

"29/05/97 15:22:43","Cyndy","[private] he can't see that."

"29/05/97 15:22:52","Cyndy","I am talking to you."

"29/05/97 15:23:02","sam","do you have cable tv"

"29/05/97 15:23:18","Cyndy","I have a satellite dish"

"29/05/97 15:23:47","sam","i have optus vision a cable network"

"29/05/97 15:24:00","Kip","I did in the states, but haven't gotten it yet. Trying to decide between Optus and Foxtel, or whether I really need it at all."

"29/05/97 15:24:50","sam","go for optus its the best thing this side of the sun"

"29/05/97 15:25:10","Cyndy","I hate watching TV"

"29/05/97 15:25:25","Kip","What's on Optus that's better than Foxtel?"

"29/05/97 15:25:33","sam","it's the best thing since sliced bread"

"29/05/97 15:25:36","Kip","Cyndy—you never watch TV at all?"

"29/05/97 15:25:47","Cyndy","rarely . . . I'd rather read"

"29/05/97 15:26:24","Kip","I like reading, too, usually always reading a book, one at a time . . . "

"29/05/97 15:27:12","Cyndy","I usually have a couple of books going at once."

"29/05/97 15:27:36","Kip","I can't do that . . . I get the books confused."

"29/05/97 15:28:03","sam","i have to go now bye"

"29/05/97 15:28:11","Cyndy","bye sam"

"29/05/97 15:28:16","Cyndy",":-("

"29/05/97 15:28:16","Kip","bye sam"
"29/05/97 15:28:25","sam","bye"
"29/05/97 15:29:21","Cyndy","sam is going to make us lose the connection"
"29/05/97 15:29:46","Kip","why"
"29/05/97 15:29:59","Cyndy","when he leaves he'll take you with him ... "
"29/05/97 15:30:11","Cyndy","because he initiated this conversation."

At first, Sam sought clarification (e.g., "is any one there?," "hello"), then he asked about not getting any responses directly (e.g., "y is no one talking to me"). Then he tried to provoke responses in a variety of ways (e.g., "hey kip r u trying to crack on to this woman," ",./;'[]," "abcdefghijklmnopqrstuvwxyz"), and finally he said "bye." Because he started the chat room, he was able to disconnect my conversation with Cyndy.

When we compare these responses to those made by ostracized individuals in the ball-tossing paradigm, we notice a fundamental difference in the targets' responses. Even in ball-tossing field studies that are more spontaneous and casual (and are not accompanied by experimenter's instruction to "not talk"), targets of ostracism rarely seek clarification or make any statements that might render them more interpersonally vulnerable. They either slump resignedly or act as though they have something better to do. However, on the Internet, they appear to have "virtual courage." What causes this virtual courage and why does it not happen in face-to-face encounters? Is it a healthier reaction? These are questions we hope to pursue with further research.

In our (cyber)lab studies, we recruit introductory psychology students and customers at the campus Internet café to participate in an experiment. Once they arrive, they are trained to communicate in a chat-room environment and engage in a 5-minute conversation with two others (who are confederates of the experimenter). Once again, half the participants are included and the other half are ostracized. The results of our pilot research suggest that, compared to individuals who were included, targets of ostracism perceive the ostracism, report feeling uncomfortable during the chat-room experience, and have worse moods (Williams et al., in press).

Because the Internet seems to supply people with more courage to provoke, we hope to use this paradigm to explore the possibility that being ostracized causes people to seek recognition at any cost. If relatively mild and innocuous attempts to get others to respond fail, will targets of ostracism escalate their provocations to the point of being verbally aggressive? Our interviews with long-term targets of the silent treatment suggest that aggression (verbal and physical) is an outcome of being ignored; the Internet chat-room paradigm will allow us to investigate this possibility in a causal and ethical manner.

CONCLUSIONS

Our research into cyberostracism has yielded a wealth of information. Not only are we able to successfully manipulate the experience of ostracism over the Internet within a very short time frame, but we see evidence of emotional, cognitive, and behavioral reactions that suggest that being ostracized over the Internet is emotionally aversive, cognitively challenging, and can be coped with by altering one's behavior in a group context. Furthermore, our chat-room research suggests that there may be some unique features to cyberostracism, especially with how targets react. Their virtual courage stands in stark contrast to the resigned or face-saving behaviors of their face-to-face counterparts. Perhaps we will learn from this how people can functionally cope with being ostracized.

Ostracism in and by Organizations

We recently received a letter from a worker in Melbourne who told us about how she and her coworkers were conspiring to ostracize their supervisor. She said that her boss was completely unreasonable and antagonistic, and no matter what she and her coworkers did nothing would change their boss's behavior. So they decided one day to give their boss the cold shoulder: none of them looked at their boss or initiated any conversation with her. If she asked them a question, they would answer it with a monotone short response. She said their tactic was working very effectively, and her boss was starting to show signs of cracking. They hoped to drive her out of the organization. She thought they would succeed.

Perhaps these workers would be more cautious if they knew of the Australian tradesman who was fired in 1997 for ignoring his boss. After failing to return his employer's morning greeting, he was dismissed. The boss explained, "[I told him that] I was sick of him ignoring me when I spoke to him and that he had done that on a number of occasions and I really can't continue to tolerate that attitude." The employee said that he had not heard the greeting and was taking his complaint to the Industrial Relations Commission (McKenna, 1997).

Ostracism in and by the organization is not uncommon. Most people can recall when their boss, coworkers, or employers ignored them; when coworkers looked away when they entered the room and made no attempt to include them; or when their questions or complaints to a company seem to fall on deaf ears. In this chapter, I present three lines of investigation that deal with these types of organizational ostracism.

The first set of studies involves a common response to whistleblowers when they return to their jobs: they are ostracized. Miceli and Near

189

(1992) report that workers are routinely ostracized after they have blown the whistle on their organization, coworkers, or employers for illegal or unsafe practices. In their groundbreaking book on the plight of the whistleblower, Miceli and Near attempted to codify the frequency and types of retribution that whistleblowers faced. They kept their definitions of retribution to those actions that would essentially leave a paper trail. These more tangible infractions included being dismissed, relocated, demoted, given menial tasks, or being victimized by physical acts of harassment. Thus, whereas Miceli and Near admitted that ostracism was the common response that all whistleblowers faced, they did not count ostracism as retribution. This is perhaps understandable, given that acts of ostracism are difficult to define or prove, and that to file a harassment charge, tangible evidence must be shown. This does not mean, however, that ostracism is not a real or powerful means to punish and drive whistleblowers out of the organization. In fact, because it is difficult for the whistleblower to prove harassment, ostracism may be the best way. Sonja Faulkner (1998) conducted the research reported here for her dissertation on "ostracism and the whistleblower."

The second part of this chapter deals with the phenomenology of being a temporary worker (i.e., a "temp"). Whereas whistleblowers most likely attribute their ostracism to some form of punishment, temps probably ascribe a different motive to their experience of feeling invisible. In the terminology of my model, it is likely that temps feel they are being ignored because of role-prescribed or oblivious motives. Temps report that other workers—sometimes, even employers—often do not look at or talk to them. They may figure that the other workers do not wish to invest time getting to know someone who will not be there the next day or the next week or maybe even the next month, so it is easier just to ignore them. A recent thesis by Sharon McInnes (1999) presents some interesting self-report data that describe the perceptions of the invisible temp worker.

Finally, we have probably all felt at one time or another that our attempts to get information from a large company go unrecognized. The relational approach in consumer behavior suggests that how we feel about and perceive organizations is much like how we feel about and perceive other people. Thus, if we feel frustrated and alienated by others who ostracize us, we may also feel these ways if companies do not respond to our queries. Chris Cheung, in his thesis (Cheung, 1999), examined how would-be consumers would feel about themselves and the company if they contacted a company by e-mail and got no replies.

As will be evident, reactions to being ostracized in the laboratory with strangers has much in common with how people feel being ostracized by coworkers and companies in the real world of being an employee and consumer.

OSTRACISM AND THE WHISTLEBLOWER

Whistleblowing may be defined as the reporting of illegal, immoral, or illegitimate practices to parties who can take action (Near & Miceli, 1987). Researchers have investigated tangible forms of retaliation against whistleblowers such as demotion and termination. Anecdotal evidence, however, suggests that ostracism may be the most frequently used form of retaliation on whistleblowers.

Whistleblowing appears to be on the rise (Ewing, 1983; Kennedy, 1987). As Miceli and Near (1992) explain, an opportunity to report wrongdoing occurs with every questionable activity; therefore, the potential for whistleblowing is vast. Unfortunately, there may be serious consequences for the whistleblower. Often whistleblowers stand alone against the larger and more powerful organization: a confrontation analogous to that of David and Goliath (Near & Miceli, 1987). Research has focused on how the Goliaths react to whistleblowing, what sort of retaliations the Davids experience, and how they cope.

Researchers agree that ostracism frequently occurs after individuals report wrongdoing (Miceli & Near, 1992; Parmerlee, Near, & Jensen, 1982). However, there is no empirical evidence to suggest how often ostracism occurs, or the conditions under which it is experienced as most aversive.

Study 1 assessed the frequency of ostracism among real-life whistleblowers after they had reported wrongdoing in their organizations. Guided by Latané's (1981) social impact theory—which states that social influence is a multiplicative function of the strength (or status), immediacy (i.e., physical distance), and number of influencers—we also investigated factors (e.g., strength or relative professional status of ostracizers, immediacy, and number of ostracizers) that might predict how aversive ostracism is for whistleblowers. Study 2 investigated two taxonomic dimensions of the ostracism model, visibility and motive, to determine if certain combinations of ostracism were more threatening to the target. Reactions in Studies 1 and 2 were restricted to self-reports. The other two dimensions, causal clarity and quantity of ostracism, were investigated in Study 3. In addition to assessing their self-reported reactions, we also observed the behavior of targets after a coworker had ostracized them. Our question was whether they would be more or less likely to help their coworker on a subsequent task.

Responses to Whistleblowing

Miceli and Near (1992) explain that the whistleblower could encounter a receptive, supportive, and even rewarding environment. For instance, a whistleblower might receive support from an ombudsman, outside agency, or coworkers who encourage and agree with his or her decision to whistleblow. This response typically occurs when the individual is viewed as credible and perhaps powerful in the organization. Conversely, whistleblowers who are seen as unimportant, wrong, or costly to the organization may face accusations, scorn, and retaliation. For example, the dominant coalition (defined in most studies as the top management group; Miceli & Near, 1992, p. 181) may resent the whistleblower for disrupting the environment at the office. Various forms of retaliation include lost telephone and parking privileges, being assigned to less important duties, losing out on promotions, being passed over for training, involuntarily being transferred to a different job or location, receiving poor performance appraisal reviews, being suspended, demoted, or terminated (Miceli & Near, 1992; Parmerlee et al., 1982).

Additionally, some coworkers may not approve of the decision to whistleblow because they fear that termination of the wrongdoing could cost them their jobs or benefits. Coworkers, for example, are often placed in a precarious position after a whistleblowing incident. They must assume two roles: both that of a coworker and an organizational member. These two roles may easily conflict, such that the strain created by one role makes it difficult to comply with the demands of the other (Beehr, Drexler, & Faulkner, 1997; Greenhaus & Beutell, 1985).

Whereas coworkers might agree that wrongdoing has occurred, many may not complain about it (Miceli & Near, 1992). They may feel that doing so would jeopardize the organization's performance and therefore their own job stability. Further, coworkers may resent whistleblowing in general because their lives may be made miserable due to increased workplace tension or probing by authorities or reporters, they may feel betrayed or even guilty for not having come forward themselves (Jensen, 1987), and coworkers might hesitate to report wrongdoing because of a general presumption that whistleblowing violates group norms (Greenberger, Miceli, & Cohen, 1987). Whistleblowers may receive praise from outside agencies or professional associations, but experience retaliation within the company.

Definition and Incidence of Retaliation

Miceli and Near contend that the incidence of retaliation is not as high as implied by media reports, but they only counted tangible forms of retaliation, which excluded ostracism. Nevertheless, researchers frequently allude to ostracism as a form of retaliation, and acknowledge that whistleblowers are often ignored (Miceli & Near, 1992; Parmerlee et al., 1982). Ostracism, however, can be quite effective in dealing with an unwanted whistleblower. Sheler (1981) offered an example of this point, describing an instance in which a secretary reported her boss's false expense accounts to top management. The boss was demoted and later resigned. The secretary, though commended by corporate chiefs, was labeled "the company fink" by coworkers and was ostracized and humiliated. She ultimately resigned (Sheler, 1981, p. 81).

Because current researchers do not consider ostracism a tangible form of retribution, there is no empirical evidence to suggest how often it occurs after one whistleblows, why coworkers and/or management would choose to employ this retaliatory strategy, and the subsequent effect this tactic has on the individual, the organization, and society at large.

Two arguments could be made that ostracism may occur more frequently than any other form of retaliation. First, anyone can ostracize another individual. One need not have power or authority within an organization to employ ostracism as a retaliatory technique. Second, because ostracism is not tangible, it is more difficult to document, and thus it is less likely to qualify as illegal retaliation. Other, more tangible forms of retaliation, such as a poor performance appraisal review or termination, may be contested in court, where they could cause employers further sanctions and penalties. Therefore, both management and coworkers may choose ostracism as a legally safe and relatively undetectable strategy to handle the whistleblower.

Ostracism in an organization would be difficult to tolerate for several reasons. Ostracism is likely to hinder the targeted employee's ability to accomplish his or her work because the required interdependency among people and tasks within organizations would be thwarted. The ostracized whistleblower may also be less likely to be promoted or given letters of recommendation. Ostracism may also go well beyond the immediate company—that is, many times whistleblowers are "blackballed" in their field, preventing them from finding employment elsewhere (Westin, 1981). Finally, ostracism may also hurt the whistleblower socially. Personal relationships are often an important aspect of the work environment (Schein, 1965). Thus, when ostracized, one may lose nonprofessional as well as professional affiliations.

Social Impact Theory and Its Relevance to Ostracism

Latané (1981) described social impact as "any of the great variety of changes in physiological states and subjective feelings, motives, and emotions, cognitions and beliefs, values and behavior, that occur in an individual, human or animal, as a result of real, implied, or imagined presence or actions of other individuals" (p. 343). According to Latané (1981), the amount of impact experienced by a target is a function of the target's perception of other peoples' strength, immediacy, and number. Latané defined *strength* as the salience, power, importance, or intensity of a given source to the target; defined *immediacy* as closeness of the sources to the target in space and time; and defined *number* simply as how many sources of impact there were (p. 344).

The effects of strength, immediacy, and number also depend upon whether these characteristics are describing sources of impact or co-targets of impact. If it refers to sources, then higher amounts of any of these characteristics cause higher amounts of impact. If the impact is negative (as would be the case for ostracism), then the impact of sources with higher levels of strength, immediacy, or number should be more negative. If, however, these characteristics are applied to cotargets (in our case, other coworkers who are also being ostracized with you), then higher levels of cotarget strength, immediacy, and number should reduce the potential negative impact. We also tested these propositions in Study 1.

Study 1. Incidence of Ostracism from Actual Sample of Whistleblowers

Study 1 attempted to establish the extent to which our sample of whistleblowers had experienced ostracism as a result of the whistleblowing. We also asked the whistleblowers to categorize the type of ostracism they were primarily receiving based upon the model's taxonomic dimensions. Finally, we tested the basic propositions of social impact theory by asking real whistleblowers to rate the three characteristics (i.e., strength, immediacy, and number) of the sources and cotargets (if any).

We provided 500 surveys to the Government Accountability Project in Washington, DC, to send out to its most recent contacts. Only 54 questionnaires were returned. We suspect there were two primary reasons for this poor response rate: these individuals have undoubtedly grown weary from being inundated with questionnaires and surveys from all sorts of government groups; and the questionnaire was too long (10 pages) and required a large commitment in terms of reading and completing it. Thus, we cannot claim that this sample is representative of whistleblowers. Nevertheless, as a real-world sample, we feel the information is interesting and potentially valuable. The majority of participants were male (73%), ranging in ages from 33 to 70. Most were Caucasian (86%). The majority were college graduates (62%), many with advanced degrees. Most of the whistleblowers described themselves as executives/professionals (66%). Finally, when asked how long they were employed at the company before they whistleblew, the majority reported more than 10 years (47%).

Respondents were asked if they experienced ostracism prior to or after whistleblowing. Twenty-four of the participants (44%) reported that they had encountered some form of ostracism within the organization prior to whistleblowing. The mean duration of the ostracism was about 7 months. All 54 respondents (100%) indicated that they experienced ostracism *after* whistleblowing. The mean duration of the ostracism after reporting the wrongdoing was 1,057 days, or almost 3 years.

After whistleblowing, however, respondents reported being ostracized by employees of all levels within the organization (supervisors, coworkers, and support staff). Sixty-seven percent thought that they were being punitively ostracized (i.e., "I became the enemy"). Sixty-three percent experienced defensive ostracism (i.e., "People were afraid to be associated with me—they thought they'd lose their jobs"). Thirty percent indicated that they were ostracized because of legal reasons, which we categorized as role-prescribed because the coworkers were instructed not to interact with the whistleblower. Fifteen percent reported being obliviously ostracized (i.e., "They don't even know I exist"). Five percent decided to label the ignoring and excluding behaviors of others as not ostracism (i.e., the others were simply preoccupied).

Respondents were also asked to what extent they experienced the following types of ostracism before and after they whistleblew: partial/social, partial/physical, complete/social, and complete/physical. All types of ostracism increased significantly from before whistleblowing to after whistleblowing, but participants reported that they experienced partial/social most frequently, followed by partial/physical, complete/social, and then complete/physical.

To test the predictions of social impact theory, we examined ratings of mood, perceptions of lost or threatened needs, and desire to regain lost needs to see if they increased with increases in source strength, immediacy, and number. For those respondents who indicated there were cotargets, we also looked to see if the strength, immediacy, and number of cotargets reduced the negative impact of ostracism.

The only source characteristic that predicted significantly increased aversive impact was the professional status of the ostracizers. The higher their professional status, the more likely the respondents were to report higher levels of overall aversive impact, feelings of lost control, and a desire to regain meaningful existence. With respect to the characteristics of their cotargets, only number of cotargets emerged as showing any potential relation. As the number of other ostracized whistleblowers (i.e., cotargets) increased, aversive impact decreased slightly. Thus, our attempt to use Latané's social impact theory as a framework to predict the magnitude of ostracism's negative impact on targets was only marginally successful. Whistleblowers reported being most negatively affected when higher status people ostracized them; and reported slightly less negative impact if they shared the whistleblowing responsibility with others.

Respondents freely volunteered a relatively large amount of information about examples of tangible harassment. These included examples of verbal harassment, having their phones tapped, being physically abused, and even having their family pets killed. Examples of being ignored or excluded were conspicuously absent. This was particularly surprising because all of our respondents reported being ostracized, and our questionnaire dealt almost exclusively with ostracism. Upon reflection, we wonder whether whistleblowers know that complaining about being ignored is fruitless; perhaps because it does not legally count as being harassed, they focus their complaints on those actions about which they can file charges.

Study 2. Effects of Ostracism Motive and Visibility on Target Reactions

In Study 2, we examined how variations in two of the model's taxonomic dimensions affected target's self-reported reactions. Specifically, we crossed manipulations of perceived motive (not ostracism, role-prescribed, defensive, punitive, and oblivious) with the three types of visibility (physical, social, and cyber), to see how it would affect reports of mood, need deprivation, attributions of responsibility, and desire to regain threatened needs. To do this, we used scenarios and asked employees of a large midwestern university to imagine themselves in the role of the whistleblower.

All participants read a story of an aeronautical defense industry employee who decided to whistleblow on his company because of its practices. Subsequently, this employee perceived that other employees were treating him (or her, depending on the sex of the university employee) differently. Combinations of the five motives and three levels of visibility created 15 distinct experiences for the target of ostracism. Information about visibility and motive was contained within the last paragraph. For example, in the cyberostracism condition, participants read, "Even though you see people walking around occasionally, something seems different. You're receiving considerably fewer e-mails and memos than normal from everyone—and, when you do receive e-mail or memos, they're all about business-related matters. There are no messages coming in from people talking about social or personal stuff anymore."

The perceived motive of the ostracism (not ostracism, role-prescribed, defensive, punitive, or oblivious) was manipulated in the last paragraph of the scenario after the clause: "When a group of employees are gathered at the water fountain one day, you overhear. . . . " Motive was manipulated in much the same way. Participants in the not ostracism condition read, "I'm so worried about getting everything done that I need to do before Friday!" "Me, too—I have more deadlines this week than I think I've ever had in my life!" For role-prescribed, participants read, "You know that we're not supposed to talk to him (her), right?" "Yeah, I know that—the company lawyers told us not to." Participants who were defensively ostracized read, "I think it's smart that we're disassociating ourselves with him (her)." "Yeah, me too—I don't want people thinking I'm bad news." Those who were punitively ostracized read, "I'm glad that we're punishing him (her) for what he (she) did!" "Me too—he (she) deserves it!" Participants in the oblivious ostracism condition read, "I'm not mad at him (her)—I just don't care about him (her)." "Yeah, he (she) doesn't even exist to me."

The primary dependent variables in this study were participants' hunches as to how much aversive impact they would experience because of their coworkers' behavior toward them. Similar measures were used in this study as in the previous one.

Participants included 384 employees of the University of Toledo. A total of 787 questionnaires were distributed, providing us with a response rate of 49%. Respondents ranged in age from 19 to 66 years old, and included administrators, academic and general staff, custodians and maintenance workers, and graduate students.

As expected, participants indicated that they would experience higher levels of aversive impact in the ostracism conditions than did those in the inclusion conditions. The results generally showed stronger effects for the motive manipulation than for the visibility manipulation. We predicted that social ostracism would be most aversive because it would be more salient, more ambiguous, and would uniquely threaten meaningful existence because, of the three levels of visibility, it is the strongest metaphor for invisibility or even death. There were, however, no differences in aversive impact among the three.

For motives, we predicted the highest levels of aversiveness for oblivious ostracism, followed by punitive ostracism. Both not ostracism and role-prescribed ostracism were predicted to have the least impact. As expected, participants in the oblivious ostracism condition reported consistently higher levels of aversive impact across all measures, with punitive ostracism close behind. Those in the not ostracism condition reported the lowest levels of aversive impact.

Why was visibility not predictive? Perhaps participants knew that they were being ostracized, and the perceived reason or motive behind the silencing was more important in determining how they reacted to it than the visibility. This may mean that motives overwhelm visibility, or that in this sort of scenario-based method, participants cannot appreciate the distinction between the three levels. The motive dimension was highly predictive of how participants would react to ostracism. Oblivious ostracism, for example, consistently elicited more aversive impact on all measures than any other perceived motive. Belonging, control, self-esteem, and meaningful existence deprivation were greatest under conditions of oblivious ostracism, as well as a desire to regain these needs. These results support my assertion that oblivious ostracism, unlike the other motives, attacks a sense of meaningful existence, perhaps because it is symbolic of one's social death and insignificance.

Although interesting, these findings should be viewed with caution because the scenario method employed is rather weak for producing experimental realism. We cannot be certain that participants would actually behave or feel the way they reported, or that they effectively imagined all the drama that would characterize such ostracism. Hence, in Study 3, we sought to experimentally induce whistleblowing, following it with inclusion or ostracism by the participant's coworker.

Study 3. Effects of Causal Clarity and Quantity of Ostracism

If ostracism is a negative interpersonal experience, there may be costs to companies if individuals exit the organization (e.g., for turnover, rehiring, and retraining) or if they stay (e.g., low morale, disengagement, loss of productivity, or even sabotage).

Study 3 was a laboratory experiment that examined the degree to which people were willing to assist a coworker. Except in the control condition, this coworker had just ostracized them for whistleblowing. Miceli and Near (1992) explained that it is very difficult to simulate conditions in a laboratory that organization members face, particularly the pressures that weigh on a potential whistleblower to act or not act. We attempted to make this study as analogous to the workplace as possible. Participants were asked to become acquainted, work together, and compete for a "bonus," just as they would in a company.

In an organizational context, there is often interdependency among tasks and people. If given the opportunity to help coworkers, what would an ostracized whistleblower do? Would she attempt to offer help in order to get back into the group's good graces, as we saw in the Williams and Sommer (1997) study; would she do nothing to contribute to the ostracizing coworker's performance; or might she even go so far as to undermine an ostracizing coworker's chance for a successful performance?

Study 3 attempted to answer these questions. Additionally, the aversive impact of the two remaining dimensions of the taxonomy, quantity and causal clarity, were examined. I have argued that the inherent ambiguity of ostracism is by itself potentially aversive. Because the quantity and causal clarity dimensions relate directly to the potential ambiguity of ostracism, this experiment could test this proposition. People generally tend to avoid ambiguous situations (Curley, Yates, & Abrams, 1986) because of a basic need to explain and understand their social and physical environment (Friedland et al., 1992). Causal attributions of events make the environment appear more predictable and controllable, and thus facilitate one's ability to cope with a given situation (Heider, 1958; Janoff-Bulman & Wortman, 1977; Rothbaum et al., 1982). Ambiguity, therefore, is threatening to many individuals, and often leads to high levels of negative emotional arousal such as stress, worry, and anxiety (Ladouceur, Talbot, & Dugas, 1997), reductions in perceptions of control (Keinan, 1994), and feelings of tension and dissatisfaction, somatic symptoms, and intentions to withdraw from the situation (Frone, 1990).

Two dimensions of my taxonomy relate directly to the potential ambiguity of ostracism. The first is causal clarity: reasons for the ostracism may be clear or unclear. This is best operationalized as whether or not there is a clear statement as to why the coworker refuses to talk to the participant. The second is quantity of ostracism. From the target's perspective, complete ostracism is easier to detect, easier to evaluate as a form of punishment, and easier to retaliate against. Partial ostracism, conversely, creates greater attributional ambiguity as to whether the target is really being ostracized, and makes it difficult to render clear interpretations and appropriate reactions. On the other hand, as I already discussed in Chapter 8, our findings up till now suggest that as quantity of ostracism increases from partial to complete, aversive reactions increase. Thus, quantity of ostracism, although containing elements of ambiguity, also contains elements of magnitude. Thus far, stronger ostracism is more unpleasant than weaker ostracism.

In this study, participants were induced to whistleblow on a confederate's wrongdoing (cheating), and were subsequently ostracized by the remaining group member. The ostracism was either causally clear or unclear, and the amount of the ostracism was either partial or complete. Whistleblowers were then presented with an opportunity to assist or hinder the performance of the group member who ostracized them. Measures of affect, need states, and desire to regain threatened or lost needs were also obtained.

Participants were 66 female introductory psychology students who received extra credit for their participation in a 1-hour experiment entitled "Problem-Solving under Time Constraints." The study manipulated the quantity of ostracism, partial versus complete, and the causal clarity of the ostracism, unclear versus clear. There was also a no ostracism control condition. Upon arrival, three individuals (one participant and two confederates) were asked to sit at a round table in a laboratory. After signing an informed consent form, the participant and confederates were told that the study was being conducted because of the admissions office's concerns with proficiency scores in math for incoming freshmen, which they were told were steadily declining. They were told that the Psychology Department was helping to find out the effects of time constraints on basic math problem performance. They were instructed that they would be given a list of basic math problems to work on for 10 minutes, and that they were to work as quickly and as accurately as they possibly could. They were explicitly told that they were competing against one another, and that the person who scored the highest would have his or her name entered into a drawing for $50 at the completion of the study.

But first they were given some rules. There was to be no talking during the test, nor were they to work together in any way. Finally, they were asked to leave all books, calculators, or anything else that could help them figure out the problems outside the exam room. They were then asked if any of them had any thing of this sort, and they all replied "No." All backpacks and books were removed, they were each given a sheet of scratch paper, the experimenter left the room, and they began the exam.

The participant and confederates turned the math worksheet over and began to work as soon as the experimenter left the room. After 30 seconds, the cheating confederate took a credit-card-sized calculator out of her pants pocket and said, "A friend of mine was in this experiment and told me that you had to take a math quiz, so I came prepared." The cheating confederate went back to work and easily finished all of the problems. After finishing the problems, she scribbled various numbers on the scrap paper to make it appear as though she had done the work. In the event that a participant asked to use the calculator, the cheating confederate was instructed to say, "No, there isn't enough time," but none of the participants asked.

After 10 minutes, the experimenter returned to the room and collected the worksheets and scrap paper. It was at this point that four (7%) of the participants whistleblew on the cheating confederate. When this happened, the experimenter said, "Thank you for notifying me of this transgression." For the remainder of the participants, the experimenter told them that she would be separating them into three different rooms, after which they would complete the second part of the study. Upon completion of that, they would once again be reunited in the exam room for the last phase of the experiment. One person was asked to remain in the exam room, while the other two followed. The noncheating confederate said she'd stay, so the participant and the cheating confederate followed the experimenter out into the hallway, where they were led to two separate rooms. Once situated, the experimenter handed the participant and the cheating confederate a questionnaire about their background and attitudes toward math, and their perceptions of their performance on the math exam. One item in the middle of the questionnaire specifically asked if any group member used any resources to help figure the math problems, such as fingers, mental imagery, or new math techniques. Participants were also asked if they themselves used any of these resources to help figure the problems. It was at this point that 46 (77%) of the participants whistleblew (in writing) on the cheating confederate. For those participants who still did not blow the whistle, the experimenter went through three consecutive probes: "One person did very well on the quiz . . . better than the two other people. Do you have any idea why that is?" (seven participants whistleblew at this point, or 12%); then, "Is there anything you'd like to tell me? Because something doesn't seem right" (one participant whistleblew during this second probe, or 2%); and finally, "I hate to put you on the spot, but one person did far better than anyone has ever done on this quiz. Are you sure that there's nothing that you'd like to tell me?" (One participant whistleblew at this third probe, or 2%). Only three participants refused to whistleblow, at which time the experiment was over.

Once the participant whistleblew, the experimenter asked that she finish the questionnaire if she had not already done so, and then to wait quietly until the experimenter came back to get her. After a couple of minutes, the experimenter told the participant to have a seat back in the original room (with the noncheating confederate). After the participant had gone back inside, the experimenter and the cheating confederate stood outside the original room, out of sight, but within listening distance of the noncheating confederate and the participant. At that time, the participant and the noncheating confederate overheard the experimenter talking angrily to the cheating confederate outside in the hall: "You obviously cheated, so you are disqualified and will not be eligible for the cash prize. In fact, I'm very upset about this, and I'd like you to leave." The cheating confederate then said, "I'm sorry, do I still get my extra credit?" The experimenter replied, "Yes, there's nothing I can do about that, but you're definitely disqualified from the $50 drawing, and I'd like you to leave." The cheating confederate said, "Can I get my bookbag?" The experimenter replied, "Have a seat in one of these chairs and I'll be with you in just a moment."

When the experimenter was scolding the cheating confederate outside in the hallway, the noncheating confederate, after hearing "You obviously cheated," said disdainfully to the participant, "I can't believe you told on her!" in the causally clear condition. In the causally unclear condition (and in the control condition), the noncheating confederate sat quietly and said nothing.

The experimenter went back into the original room and told the noncheating confederate and the participant that between the two phases of the experiment, there was another opportunity for them to earn even more extra credit by helping another experimenter out by engaging in a "get acquainted" task. This involved reading over a list of topics to discuss in order to get to know each other. They were told that while they were doing this, she (the experimenter) would have a chance to take care of "her" (nodding toward the cheating confederate) and get the materials ready for the next phase of the study. She then told them that she would be back in a few minutes to get them started on the next phase of the study. The experimenter then handed the list of topics to the participant and left the room for 5 minutes. The noncheating confederate then ostracized the participant in four out of five conditions. In the no ostracism condition, the confederate and the participant talked normally after the participant asked the first question, and the confederate included the participant in a friendly conversation. In the ostracism conditions, the quantity (partial vs. complete) and causal clarity (unclear vs. clear) of the ostracism varied.

Quantity of Ostracism Manipulation

In the partial condition, the noncheating confederate did not initiate any verbal interaction with the participant. She offered only very short responses, such as "Yes," "No," or "Maybe" if spoken to. Also, she did not make eye contact with the participant unless spoken to, and then only for the briefest moment. In the complete condition, the confederate completely ignored the participant. She made no eye contact, did not initiate any verbal interaction with the participant, and did not respond if the participant spoke to her.

Phase 3

After 5 minutes, the experimenter came back into the room and said it was time to do the last phase of the experiment, which would involve one of them constructing a math quiz for their partner to take. They were told that this aspect of the research dealt with problems people had in taking tests in front of others, among other things. Slips were drawn, but the drawing was rigged such that all participants were assigned the task of constructing the quiz. The experimenter then gave the participant a list of

60 potential quiz items, 20 of the which were grouped together and clearly labeled "simple," 20 labeled "medium," and 20 labeled "difficult" problems. After handing the sheet to the participants, the experimenter said that the participant was to create a quiz of 20 total items from this list of 60, and that she could choose whichever items she wanted.

The experimenter left the room and waited for the participant to finish selecting the quiz items for the confederate. Once completed, the experimenter went back into the room and said, "Thank you. I'll go give this to her, and while she's working on the quiz, I'll ask you to fill out this questionnaire. I'll come back in, get this from you, and you can be on your way." The participant then completed a questionnaire that assessed aversive impact while interacting with, and constructing the quiz for, their partner. Once finished, the participant was led to a debriefing room where the two confederates were waiting. An extensive debriefing took place with all four parties.

The results of the study were illuminating, if not totally predicted. First, the manipulation checks indicated that the participants perceived the manipulations as they were intended, indicating that they noticed that their partner either ostracized them or not, did so partially or completely, and that they either knew or did not know why they were being ignored. Although participants were not specifically asked on the post-experimental questionnaire why they thought they had been ostracized, many indicated during the debriefing session that it had been because they told on their partner.

A primary measure of the study was how participants would feel while being ostracized. This overall measure, called *aversive impact*, was an index of participants' threatened needs and current moods while interacting with the confederate. As hypothesized, participants in the ostracism conditions reported experiencing more aversive impact compared to those who experienced no ostracism. Additionally, compared with included participants, those who were ostracized expressed a greater desire to work with someone else in the future and a lower desire to work with the same partner again in the future.

Participants in the complete ostracism condition reported more aversive impact while interacting with their partner than those participants in the partial ostracism conditions. This finding replicated the Williams et al. (2000) results, and did not support the speculation that partial ostracism is more aversive because it is more ambiguous.

Contrary to predictions, the manipulation of causal clarity had no independent impact. However, causally unclear ostracism was particularly aversive (compared to all other ostracism conditions) when delivered completely. This provides some support for our hypothesis that causally unclear ostracism can be especially aversive.

Examining the questions the participants chose for inclusion on the quiz allowed us to assess the degree to which the participant tried to make life easier or more difficult for her coworker. Firstly, participants who were not ostracized helped their partner about the same as those who were ostracized. However, participants who knew their partners were angry with them (causally clear) were more likely to retaliate when they were partially rather than completely ostracized. Participants whose partner did not tell them they were angry (causally unclear), however, retaliated most when they were completely rather than partially ostracized. When the situation was most ambiguous (partial and unclear), participants appeared to be most reluctant to retaliate, maybe because they were unsure that they were really being ostracized. However, a low level of retaliation also occurred when the situation was least ambiguous. We could speculate that like those female participants in the Williams and Sommer (1997) ball-tossing study (described in Chapter 6), participants who knew their partner was angry with them and who were completely ignored behaved in a way that would give them the best chance for reinclusion. Clearly, however, more research is necessary to discover what mediated this effect.

In sum, this study was successful on several counts. We created a paradigm in which we could induce over 90% of the participants to whistleblow. Then we were able to subject them to ostracism in a plausible work-like situation. Furthermore, we found that higher quantities of ostracism were most aversive, and that causally unclear (and hence, ambiguous) ostracism was particularly aversive when it was delivered completely (i.e., with no verbal or nonverbal interaction).

Conclusions

A primary goal of this research was to determine if ostracism was a common retaliatory technique used on employees after they have whistleblown. Although whistleblowing researchers (Miceli & Near, 1992) have acknowledged that ostracism occurs after an employee reports wrongdoing, they do not consider it a tangible, or measurable, form of retaliation. Thus, there have been no data to this point that suggest how prevalent ostracism is after a whistleblowing event, why it is used by management or coworkers, or the subsequent effect it may have on the whistleblower, the organization, or society at large. Although our response rate in Study 1 was low, 100% reported that they were ostracized, for an average of over 3 years. Like researchers on whistleblowing, our respondents did not seem to dwell on ostracism, preferring to tell us about more tangible incidents instead. Although increasing numbers of ostracizers did not increase their reported aversive impact, higher status ostracizers did. The results of this study also support the proposition that all four fundamental needs are threatened by ostracism.

In Study 2, we found support for differential impact for different motives of ostracism. With university employees as our participants, we found that they said they would react most negatively to oblivious and punitive motives for ostracism. This is interesting because, behaviorally, the ostracism was the same for all conditions. But clearly the motives behind that behavior are important to participants' understanding of, and reactions to, ostracism.

Finally, Study 3 allowed us to examine actual responses to actual whistleblowing followed by ostracism. These participants experienced the drama and unpleasantness of agonizing over whistleblowing, and then having to put up with a coworker who ignored them. They found any sort of ostracism more unpleasant than being included, and complete ostracism more aversive than partial ostracism. Furthermore, the aversive impact was worse when the ostracizer did not clearly indicate she was angry, yet subjected the participant to complete ostracism. This study not only provided a good paradigm to study whistleblowing, but offered further insight into the differential effects of various types of ostracism.

This research supports our assertion that ostracism elicits profound, negative impact among its targets, with a variety of consequences. In organizations, however, these consequences go well beyond what is experienced at the individual level. Indeed, when a whistleblower is ostracized, the effect is detrimental to the entire organization because of low morale, low productivity, job turnover, and rehiring and retraining costs. The effects of ostracism may be harmful at the societal level as well. If employees anticipate ostracism as a consequence of whistleblowing, they may not report unsafe food, toys, or cars, or expose the dumping of toxic waste into rivers or oceans, for example. Ideally, organizations should have a system in place for employees to report wrongdoing without fear of retaliation. Minimally, however, companies should consider providing workshops, seminars, or training sessions for all organization members on the deleterious effects of ostracism in the workplace.

OSTRACISM AND THE TEMP

> In the company [I am assigned to], they make me feel so much like an outsider, a nobody. Whenever the whole office does something together, I am not included. It is as if I do not exist.
> —COMMENT MADE BY A TEMPORARY
> WORKER (in Feldman, Doerpinghaus,
> & Turnley, 1994, p. 54)

Downsizing, retrenchment, and the search for a flexible workforce have altered the labor landscape significantly over the past decade. Increasingly, temporary workers ("temps") work alongside permanent employees, where they could encounter support, encouragement, and inclusion, or hostility, indifference, and rejection.

Unfortunately, temporary employment represents an undesirable situation for many; a lack of benefits, job security, and recognition all feature prominently on the list of temps' complaints (Feldman et al., 1994). In addition, temps may be socially disadvantaged, even socially ostracized in the workplace.

The terms "just a temp" and "disposable workforce" imply that temps are somehow not as important as permanent workers (Henson, 1996). They are considered relatively insignificant human resources whose job satisfaction warrants only minimal attention. Researchers allude to temps being ostracized and acknowledge that temps may feel ignored or left out in the workplace (e.g., Feldman et al., 1994). Yet the importance of ostracism for these workers appears to be discounted, perhaps because, as I just noted with whistleblowers, ostracism is nontangible.

There are several reasons why ostracism of temps deserves serious consideration. As mentioned, temporary employment is big business, with the use of temps an increasingly common form of employment (Polivka, 1996; Von Hippel, Mangum, Greenberger, Skoglind, & Henemen, 1997). A recent Australian Bureau of Statistics (1997) study concluded that there has been a 50% increase in the number of temporary and part-time workers since 1991. Another reason is that the topic of temporary employment and equity has become hotly contested, with some concluding that a two-tiered workplace class system is emerging. In order to maintain flexibility and lower costs in the face of increasing competitive pressures, companies offer a privileged few secure work while marginalizing the rest of the workforce (Davis-Blake & Uzzi, 1993; Osterman, 1988). Finally, social ostracism has the potential to affect the organizations' "bottom line." Morale, productivity, team performance, and even sabotage are potentially related to the way temps are treated by their coworkers (Parker, 1994).

This study aimed to establish whether temporary employees are more likely than permanent employees to experience social ostracism in the workplace and, if so, to explore the effects of social ostracism on worker satisfaction, commitment, and stress. The opportunity for social interactions is one factor determining how happy a temp is in a job (Henson, 1996). Unfortunately, temps may be perceived as not worthy of social attention at all, as the following quote from a temporary worker illustrates: "It's really lonely. Eating lunch by yourself every single day. And no one ever asking you a personal question. Like the secretaries never, ever ask, 'where are you from?' or 'what have you been up to?' " (Henson, 1996, p. 87).

The type of ostracism that seems to be experienced here is quite different from that experienced by whistleblowers. Whistleblowers are vilified; temps are invisible. For full-time workers, temps are not *real* employees; it may not be worth getting to know someone who may be gone next week.

Feldman et al. (1994) surveyed 200 temporary employees and found that they were particularly unhappy with the impersonal and disrespectful manner in which they were treated at work. Temps routinely find themselves referred to as "the temp" rather than by name and excluded from work and social activities (Henson, 1996). Von Hippel et al. (1997) provided an excellent example of how temps were excluded. In a case study they described how permanent employees were so reluctant to train temporary employees that they "would not bother to learn their names." The organization reinforced this exclusion by issuing temporaries with "jumpsuits without their names on the pockets" (p. 99).

As with whistleblowers, the incidence and implications of ostracism for temps—a comparatively larger population that would appear to experience high levels of exclusion—have not been examined. Using a survey method, we hypothesize that temps will report higher levels of social ostracism than permanent workers. Second, we predict that exposure to social ostracism will be correlated with reports of lower satisfaction, lower commitment, and greater stress.

In the present study (conducted in Sydney, Australia), permanent employees and temps were asked to respond to a questionnaire about their perceived treatment in the workplace. A questionnaire was developed and distributed to more than 200 individuals from a variety of commercial and government organizations. One hundred and forty-one employees (65% female and 35% male) completed the questionnaire. The sample comprised 49 temps and 52 permanent workers registered or employed by nursing and administrative agencies, retail and investment banks, and within government and defense force organizations. Temps were defined as individuals who had neither an explicit nor an implicit contract for long-term employment (Polivka, 1996). Permanent employees were individuals in traditional and ongoing employment.

The remaining 40 participants were temporary part-time teachers working in an educational facility. They were not entitled to leave privileges, worked fewer hours than the permanent staff, and were not guaranteed hours. Although they could be considered temporary employees in the sense that they were not guaranteed hours, they had worked an average of 5 years in the organization and were less likely to have held other positions than temps—suggesting that they were a distinct group. To distinguish them from the permanent employees and the temps they are called "part-time employees."

The two-page questionnaire was developed using existing and specifically created items and scales to measure coworker treatment, causal attributions, personal control, work satisfaction, organizational commitment, and stress. Von Hippel, Mangum, Greenberger, Skoglind, and Heneman (1998) developed or adapted scales in their temporary employee research. These measures were heavily relied upon in the current research.

Participants were assured that all responses were confidential. All participants were provided with self-addressed and stamped return envelopes, and were instructed to think about their current temporary job or most recent placement. Respondents were asked to indicate how other employees generally treated them. Three items (general inclusion, inclusion in conversations, and eye contact) were used to assess ostracism. We also measured causal attributions for their treatment by coworkers, job satisfaction, extrarole behavior (i.e., doing more than was required), organizational commitment, and stress.

Our results were largely consistent with our hypotheses. The temp worker classification was positively correlated with higher levels of ostracism, and ostracism was negatively related to satisfaction and positively related to stress. In support of the model, feelings of belonging, control, meaningful existence, and self-value were all significantly negatively correlated with the ostracism measure.

Temporary employees reported more social ostracism than both permanent employees and part-time workers. Permanent workers did not report higher levels of satisfaction or commitment, or lower levels of stress than temps. But reported ostracism for temp workers significantly predicted lower satisfaction and commitment and higher stress, once age, gender, employment type, previous positions, and tenure had been controlled for. Among permanent workers, the relationships were quite different: reported ostracism did not significantly predict any of the dependent variables after controlling for the other variables.

When we performed a median split on the continuous measure of reported ostracism, and crossed that with employment type (permanent vs. temporary), we found that temporary and permanent workers differed in how they attributed their treatment. When ostracized, temps were more likely than permanent workers to attribute their treatment to their employment type. Alternatively, permanent workers who were ostracized were more likely than temps to attribute their treatment to "something they said or did." Thus, the negative impact of ostracism for temp workers emerged despite this apparent attributional buffer.

Overall, the results support our two hypotheses. As predicted, temps were more likely to report ostracism than permanent workers. They are also more likely than the part-time employee to report ostracism. Social ostracism was associated with lower levels of satisfaction and organizational commitment, and with greater stress. At least this was the case for temps. Ostracism did not predict permanent employees' satisfaction, commitment, or stress. This suggests that social ostracism is not only prevalent among temps, but also that it has unique consequences for them.

The qualitative descriptions provided on the questionnaire attest to the paucity of social interactions endured by some temps. One noted that "everyone goes to morning tea or lunch without asking me . . . [I'm] not included in general conversations let alone work-related ones." Another temp wrote, "They [coworkers] talk right over me. It is almost like I'm not there."

Implicit in this last statement is the notion that temps are unworthy of attention. This is consistent with the motive of oblivious ostracism. Targets of oblivious ostracism do not perceive any menace in the actions of others; rather, they simply perceive themselves as unimportant or unworthy of social attention. Sommer et al. (in press) note that "oblivious ostracism may be particularly prevalent in social or professional hierarchies wherein newcomers or those of a lesser status are not spoken to by higher ranking individuals."

Temps suffer two disadvantages: being newcomers and being perceived as lower status employees. Both disadvantages may lead permanent workers to perceive temps as being low in status, and preserve their feelings of higher status by ostracizing them. Additionally, permanent workers may rationalize that temps are unlikely to be around for long; therefore, it is a waste of time and energy to include them. Some of the comments made by permanent workers support this contention. One permanent worker wrote:

"There is an employee that started here whilst I was on holidays. . . . I haven't spoken to him since my return (4 weeks ago), I think its probably got something to do with the temporary nature of such employees that I haven't made the effort."

In contrast, part-time workers may identify, and affiliate more with, the core group of permanent workers than with the peripheral temps (Tansky, Gallagher, & Wetzel, 1997). Part-time workers are more likely to become long-term employees and may assume higher positions. This may explain why our part-time workers did not report significant differences in social ostracism when compared to permanent workers.

The Debilitating Effects of Ostracism

Despite common assumptions and a strong theoretical rationale (Oster-man, 1988; Pfeffer & Baron, 1988; Parker, 1994), we, along with others, found little evidence that permanent workers are more committed (Pearce, 1993; Tansky et al., 1995), or more satisfied (Lee & Johnson, 1991) than temps. The current study confirmed that employment type, in itself, is not significantly related to satisfaction, commitment, or stress.

However, social ostracism was related to self-reported satisfaction, commitment, and stress—but only for temps. It seems that, whether an employee is temporary or permanent per se is far less important than whether he or she is socially ostracized in that role. Further, temps not only are more likely to be ostracized, but may be particularly susceptible (less able to cope) to the effects of social ostracism. Alternatively, temps may experience or perceive a different, more insidious type of ostracism than that encountered by permanent workers. Full-time employees, when ostracized, may feel that it is some form of punishment. As such, they still feel important enough to warrant intended punitive ostracism. Oblivious ostracism, however, comes without intent or effort. One simply doesn't count enough to be noticed.

It is highly possible that some organizations will not be surprised or unduly concerned that temps experience more social ostracism than permanent workers. This could be considered an inevitable by-product of their employment. In some ways, managing temps takes considerable pressure off managers. Conveniently, temps do not need to be socially included. Coworkers don't need to expend energy building rapport with them, and no time is wasted trying to build interpersonal relationships with them.

Organizations should not assume that temps, simply due to the nature of their position, are less committed or less satisfied than permanent workers. It is not the distinction between permanent and temp that is important, but how temps are treated by their coworkers that largely determines their attitudes toward work satisfaction, commitment, and stress levels. Temps report being the targets of social ostracism more often than permanent workers, and also report that this ostracism is associated with less job satisfaction, lower job commitment, and greater stress on the job.

THE COMPANY OSTRACIZING THE CONSUMER

Our final excursion into the realm of the organization takes a different tack. What happens when a company ignores a consumer? We explored this question by means of e-mail queries directed to a mock company. The promise of the Internet as an avenue for commerce has prompted the creation of a large number of new Internet-based businesses and spurred established businesses to establish their own web presence. A recent survey reported 59% of business executives in the United States believe that the Internet provides the means to tackle key business issues and challenges, while 67% of senior managers have committed themselves to an Internet business strategy (International Data Corporation, 1999). For many of these organizations, the attraction of conducting business over the Internet lies not only in the capacity to deal across geographic boundaries, but also in the ability to eliminate the "middlemen" (e.g., retailers, suppliers, and agents) and interact directly with the customer. A corollary is that this promises customers direct access to the companies with which they are dealing. Hence, in return for our patronage, we expect that the business will provide services that are beneficial to us as customers—services that they are in the best position to offer. Often this includes product information as well as sales and technical support. Although a large proportion of these services can be dispensed via a website, there will invariably be situations in which customers require more specific or individualized information. For these people, electronic mail (e-mail) provides a direct method of contacting the company.

In a recent survey, a reported 85.2% of Internet users state that they have contacted businesses regarding their products or services (Graphics, Visualization, and Usability Center, 1998). This figure speaks to the fact that e-mail often represents a more economical and efficient method of making contact than traditional postal mail, facsimile, and telephone—especially for those customers who are geographically isolated from the business. Hence, regardless of how comprehensive and well designed a business's website is, it appears that we often find ourselves in the position of having to contact the company to satisfy pre- and postpurchase inquiries. One can surmise from this that many companies are inundated with e-mail regularly. Thus it should be no surprise that, on occasion, e-mail inquiries receive no response. What may prove surprising, however, is the prevalence of nonresponse. A study conducted by the Direct Marketing Association of the United Kingdom (Ockenden, 1999) found that the fulfillment of inquiries made over the Internet was poor for companies based in the United Kingdom. Specifically, over 40% of these requests for information or brochures were left unfulfilled after 3 weeks. There is little reason to assume that this phenomenon is isolated to the United Kingdom.

Up till now, we have considered ostracism to be primarily an interpersonal phenomenon. In considering the effects of ignoring customer inquiries sent via e-mail, we are extrapolating the concept of ostracism to the person–organization domain. That an organization and an individual can interact is by no means a new notion. Over the past decade, many marketers have embraced the concept of *relationship marketing*, which assumes that a business can not only interact with, but have an enduring relationship with, a customer (e.g., Gummesson, 1994; Morgan & Hunt, 1994). Hence, we have seen interpersonal constructs such as trust (e.g., Crosby, Evans, & Cowles, 1990; Garbarino & Johnson, 1999), commitment (e.g., Bettencourt, 1997; Kelley & Davis, 1994), and conflict (e.g., Ricard & Perrien, 1999) extended to commercial relationships between companies and their individual clients. It appears, then, that it is feasible to investigate ostracism in this context.

When a business allows e-mail inquiries to go unanswered, it is plausible that the company itself, rather than any particular individual representative of the company, is perceived to be the source of ostracism. Thus the company bears the burden of any resulting negative impressions. This is based upon the idea that when doing business with a company on the Internet, we rarely have the opportunity to identify the individuals with whom we are dealing. In traditional face-to-face interactions, we do business with a company representative who can be individualized through myriad qualities such as his or her name, appearance, voice, and personality. Even with the continually increasing prevalence of transacting business via telephone, the customer is given a slew of cues that enable the individualization of the representative on the other end of the line. In such instances, a nonresponse can readily be attributed to the representative with whom we deal. Consequently, at least some of the unfavorable attitudes that result can be directed at an individual representative rather than at the company as a whole.

In an online environment, however, companies are rarely afforded the buffer of frontline representatives. The design of company websites themselves frequently convey the preeminence of the organization as a whole over the individuals that make up the organization by identifying business units, corporate histories, products, and services while neglecting to identify individual employees. E-mail addresses in the form of "inquiries@company.com" and "techsupport@company.com" that enable customers to contact the organization are consistent with this impression.

This study examined the effects of being ostracized by a company through nonresponse to an e-mail inquiry, compared to two other typical responses. The desirable type of reply was responsive, quick, and fulfilled what was promised. The undesirable type was nonresponsive and did not fulfill the implied promise of service. Nevertheless, even this undesirable reply still recognized the consumer's existence. Our basic question was, Do consumers regard any response as better than no response? We go about answering this by examining what happens when an online company ignores us. Would it affect our self-perceptions like we have shown in our other studies by threatening our four fundamental needs? And, from the perspective of the companies, what effect would there be when a company ignored potential customers? Would it affect customers' impression of the company and their likelihood to do business with it?

Of the 93 participants who contacted the website and e-mailed a query to the company, 82 completed the study in its entirety. Participants were primarily recruited via a range of Usenet newsgroups and at various universities where participants were awarded extra credit for participation. The participants came from four countries, with the majority coming from the United States, followed by Australia. More females (78%) than males (22%) participated, and they fell mostly in the 19- to 25-year-old (81%) age group. When asked how long they had been using the Internet, 65% indicated that they had had 2 to 3 years experience with the Internet, with most spending between 2 to 4 hours a week online.

The study was conducted using two Internet websites and two e-mail accounts. One was used as the website for the research effort. An e-mail account was used by the researcher to provide instructions to and to communicate with the participants regarding matters to do with the study. The other website and e-mail account was used to provide the web presence of a mock company ("ShopLight"), and to communicate with participants under the guise of that company. Once they contacted the homepage of ShopLight, they were automatically assigned a participant identification number, and randomly assigned to condition.

Beginning the Study

The participants were invited to participate in a study concerning the "attractiveness, reliability, and speed" of company websites. Upon entering the research website, participants were met with a welcome page. This page introduced the study, announced that the study has been approved by the School of Psychology, University of New South Wales, and emphasized that data collected were confidential. Furthermore, participants were informed that participation was voluntary and they could discontinue at any time. They were also encouraged to e-mail the researcher at the address provided if they had any questions. The welcome page also included a summary of the tasks that the participants would be asked to complete.

Thereafter, participants were directed to another webpage where they could register by completing a registration questionnaire. They were required to supply their e-mail address and to answer several demographic questions and questions regarding their Internet usage habits.

Phase 1 of the ShopLight Experiment

Upon completing the registration questionnaire, participants were assigned a participant identification number (ID) automatically. This ID
was required each time the participant started a new phase of the study,
and assisted in the tracking of correspondence between the researcher
and the participants, and between ShopLight and the participants. Participants were asked to examine the ShopLight website, making sure that
they read at least part of the content in order to form an opinion regarding its attractiveness, reliability, and speed. Then they were instructed to
write an e-mail inquiry to ShopLight requesting a fee estimate for a job
that required research on three motor vehicles. Finally, they were asked
to complete a preexperimental questionnaire regarding their experience
with and impressions of the ShopLight website.

With the completion of the preexperimental questionnaire, the first
phase of the study was concluded. The participants were informed that
they would later receive a notice to complete the second and final phase
of the study.

ShopLight Shopping Services was described as a company that spe-
cialized in providing consumer research to enable clients to make better
purchasing decisions. Their services include, as stated on the website,
"traditional price comparisons, as well as assistance in choosing between different products." The website contained only five webpages,
entitled: "About Us," "What We Do," "How We Do It," "Clients," and
"Contact." Finally, to encourage the participant to e-mail the company,
the participant was notified that upon the receipt of any inquiries by the
company, a reply with a fee estimate for his or her approval would be
sent before work was started. This fee estimate was stated to be free of
charge. Thus, the participant was informed that he or she would not incur a fee by sending an e-mail inquiry to ShopLight.

Participants in two of the three experimental groups were sent e-
mail responses from ShopLight 2 days after their e-mail inquiry was received. Participants in the ostracism group were not sent any response.
Forms of response included a responsive message fulfilling the implied
promise of service ("responsive"), a nonresponsive message that acknowledged the customer's query but did not fulfill the implied promise
("nonresponsive"), and no response at all (ostracism).

Five days after the participant sent his or her e-mail inquiry to
ShopLight, the researcher sent an e-mail reminder to the participant to
complete the second and final phase of the study by logging onto another webpage. This phase consisted of a postexperimental questionnaire that included questions in common with the preexperimental questionnaire, in addition to manipulation checks, and a set of 12 questions

designed to measure the needs threatened. At the completion of the study, all participants were debriefed by an e-mail stating the purpose of the study.

Compared to the two response conditions, participants who were ostracized reported a lower sense of all four needs. The company's perceived trustworthiness, professionalism, and status or prestige were measured to provide general indicators of the effects that being ostracized by a company had on an individual's perception of the company. Participants' perceptions of the company's trustworthiness were negatively affected by ostracism, as were their perceptions of the company's professionalism and status or prestige. Ostracized participants also reported that they were significantly less likely to patronize the company compared with those who had been sent a response.

Participants who had been sent nonresponsive replies rated the company more poorly than did participants who had been sent responsive ones, but there were no general differences in the four needs between these two conditions. Finally, with regard to purchasing intentions, those who had received responsive replies were more likely to use the company than those who had received ineffective ones.

Compared with those who received the responsive reply, ostracized participants reported significantly lower levels of each of the four needs. Further, ostracized individuals reported significantly lower levels of belonging and self-esteem than did those who were sent the nonresponsive replies. They did not, however, report significantly lower levels of control or meaningful existence.

Compared with customers who had been sent responsive replies, ostracized customers' perceptions of the company's trustworthiness, professionalism, and status/prestige were rated lower. However, ratings of these attributes did not differ between the ostracized and the nonresponsive customers. The reported purchasing intentions followed a similar pattern. Ostracized individuals reported a lower likelihood to use the company than those who received responsive replies; however, ostracized customers' ratings did not differ significantly from those who had been sent nonresponsive replies.

Summary

This study aimed to examine whether being ostracized by an Internet company has similar effects upon an individual's fundamental needs of belonging, self-esteem, control, and meaningful existence compared with the findings in other studies in which ostracism was perpetrated by individual sources. Effects upon an individual's perceptions of a company and purchasing intentions were also investigated. The results showed that ostracism by a company does have similar effects to being ostracized by other individuals in that it attacks all four fundamental needs. An individual's perceptions of the company's trustworthiness, professionalism, and status or prestige were also negatively affected, and participants reported a lower likelihood of patronizing when ostracized by the company.

This suggests that, to some extent, individuals relate to companies in the same manner as they relate to other individuals. However, based solely on the present results, one can only speculate as to the degree these relationships are similar. Nevertheless, it is clear that when the participants did not receive a response to their inquiry, their perceptions of the source of the ostracism, in this case the company, were negatively affected.

One such perception, that of the company's trustworthiness, may be of particular note to relationship marketers. There is strong evidence that a customer's trust in the vendor is central to the success of marketing relationships (e.g., Fontenot & Wilson, 1997; Gwinner, Gremier, & Bitner, 1998; Morgan & Hunt, 1994). It is plausible that the lower level of trust reported by ostracized participants in the current study would result in a lower likelihood of purchasing the company's services, which was also evident. However, a nonresponsive reply also had a negative effect upon the participants' reported purchasing intentions. From the company's perspective, a nonreply is as bad as a nonresponsive reply. From the customer's perspective, a nonreply is worse. In one way, we might consider the nonresponsive reply as analogous to partial ostracism: it involves minimal recognition of the target, but without the expected level of interaction and attention. In this sense, complete ostracism was again (as in the whistleblowing Study 3) worse than partial ostracism, which, in turn, was worse than inclusion. Obviously, this was just an initial investigation into this domain. Follow-up research that involves real opportunities to purchase or recontact the company may reveal differences between these two less-than-ideal conditions.

CONCLUSIONS

Three programs of research investigated model-derived hypotheses regarding ostracism in and by organizations. Whistleblowers, temps, and customers can all be ostracized. Such ostracism reveals evidence of negative impact on the four fundamental needs. Whereas whistleblowers probably interpret the motives of their coworkers and employers as punitive, temp workers and customers probably regard the ostracism they receive as oblivious. When we have been able to make comparisons, it appears that oblivious is no better, and sometimes worse, than punitive ostracism. Targets of punitive ostracism at least know they matter enough for others to purposely try to ignore. This chapter represents an application of the ostracism model to organizational ostracism. The results provided substantial support for several aspects of the model, but also failed to support some assumptions. For instance, in Study 2 of the whistleblowing studies, the scenario method failed to observe different reactions to social versus physical versus cyberostracism. Clearly, other attempts should be made to examine the distinctions between these three levels of visibility. Nevertheless, these three programs of research not only inform our knowledge of ostracism and provide potential qualifications to the model's predictions, they also provide useful practical information concerning the workplace.

Everyday Ostracism over Days, Months, and Years

In the last several chapters we have focused our attention on the effects of relatively short-term, laboratory-constructed forms of ostracism. These methods have allowed us to observe the impact of ostracism, compared to inclusion, in controlled settings. They also permitted us to manipulate conditions of interest, particularly those aspects related to the taxonomic dimensions suggested by my model. We have discovered that even brief encounters with ostracism—those lasting only 4 minutes—are unpleasant for targets and empowering for sources. But what happens when we are ostracized, or when we ostracize others, in our own environment, at home, at work, or in the community. How do we react to ostracism when it occurs outside the confines of the laboratory?

In this chapter, I will summarize some of our current ongoing investigations that deal with the effects of ostracism in people's day-to-day life over longer periods of time. It is important to pursue longer term ostracism for at least two reasons. First, although there is considerable value and obvious advantages to investigating ostracism in controlled laboratory experiments, I am naturally concerned about if and how these effects occur in the world outside the laboratory. Second, in my model I predict that ostracism experienced repeatedly over time should have a different outcome to that which is experienced in isolated, short-term exposures. For targets, I propose that the four fundamental needs are threatened during both short- and long-term situations. However, a qualitative shift occurs in how we react to these threatened needs during long- versus short-term ostracism. In the short-term, I hypothesized that our functional and adaptive resilience to adversity would cause us to repair or regain those needs that were lost. If we were deprived of belonging, we would seek out others or try to strengthen our already existing bonds. If control was threatened, then we should subsequently attempt to exert control. But we can only react in this way for so long. At some point, depending upon the individual's persistence, self-esteem, and available options, targets of ostracism will succumb to the diminished levels of belonging, control, self-esteem, and meaningful existence. Then they will internalize these threatened needs, feeling alienated, helpless, depressed, and worthless.

For sources, the initial effects, while perhaps cognitively effortful, are empowering. Sources feel they have more control and power, as well as a stronger sense of belonging with other sources, than if they were acting in an inclusive manner with two others, or even if they and another source were arguing with a target. But what happens if sources of ostracism continue to ostracize over and over again? What if they develop a habit of ostracism in which it becomes their first line of defense rather than a method of last resort? Will they continue to feel in control and empowered?

My colleagues and I have taken two general approaches to begin the process of uncovering the answers to these questions. In the first approach, Ladd Wheeler, Joel Harvey, and I developed the Sydney Ostracism Record (SOR)—an event-contingent self-report booklet filled out during a 2-week period by over 100 paid volunteers. In our second approach, Lisa Zadro and I have conducted 1- to 2-hour structured interviews with over 40 individuals, some targets and some sources (and some who were both), who have experienced ostracism for long periods of time. Both approaches are still in progress, so our findings are preliminary and incomplete (Williams, Wheeler, & Harvey, 2001). But what we have discovered is interesting and provocative, and encourages us to continue with these sorts of less controlled, more qualitative investigations.

THE SYDNEY OSTRACISM RECORD

One way to find out about the frequency of ostracism incidences in day-to-day life and how we react to it is to monitor the behavior of individuals over time as they use or encounter ostracism. But how do we do this? Would we have to resort to creating an environment in which our participants were constantly under surveillance, like that in the movie *The Truman Show*? As tempting as that might be, after considering costs and ethical issues, we looked for another method that could be used to tap into day-to-day occurrences and effects of ostracism. We chose the event-contingent self-report method, commonly referred to as the "diary method." But our subjects don't use a diary in the normal sense of the word; instead, individuals keep a booklet with them during their waking hours, and every time an incident occurs that they, even for a moment, consider relevant to ostracism, they reach for their booklet and enter on one of its pages data about the incident.

The event-contingent self-report method has been previously applied in other domains within social psychology (see Reis & Wheeler, 1991, for a review). The best-known example of this method is the Rochester Interaction Record (RIR—Pietromonaco & Barrett, 1997; Reis & Wheeler, 1991; Wheeler & Nezlek, 1977). Subsequent records include the Rochester Social Comparison Record (Wheeler & Miyake, 1992), the Deception Record (DePaulo, Kashy, Kirkendol, Wyer, & Epstein, 1996), and the Iowa Communication Record, which measures dyadic conversation (Duck et al., 1991).

Compared to retrospective self-report questionnaires, there are several advantages to using event-contingent self-records. For instance, whereas self-report questionnaires can assess the occurrence and reactions to real-life instances, the particular incident selected for recall may be most readily available to memory (selection bias) and its content may be distorted (recall of content). Moreover, several events over time may be aggregated to form an overall global impression of the phenomena. As Reis and Wheeler (1991) state, questionnaires are "best seen as personalized impressions of social activity that have been percolated, construed, and reframed through the various perceptual, cognitive and motivational processes" (p. 271). The event-contingent self-report method, however, does not suffer to the same degree from selection bias because participants are instructed to record and describe *all* incidents that they encounter. Second, distorted recall of content is minimized because participants are encouraged to complete records as near to the incident as possible. Finally, incidents are not aggregated personally, but by computer analysis.

There are, of course, potential disadvantages to diary methods. One problem is that people may be so sensitized and vigilant that they overestimate the occurrence of ostracism episodes. Or the opposite may happen: the effort and bother associated with making entries may cause participants to skip making entries sometimes or even often. It is quite possible that these two opposing motives cancel each other out. Another problem is that individuals may differ in their degrees of vigilance and responsibility in carrying out their assignment. We tried to address this concern by conducting structured training sessions, giving participants many examples to make sure they were recording the episodes similarly, and having them return their filled-out records every 2 days. In this way, we were able to make sure that they did not fill them all out at the end, and if we spotted problems, we could address them before they affected that individual's entire set of data.

In two studies, we developed two similar event-contingent records: (1) the SOR-S (source), for recording instances of ostracizing others, and (2) the SOR-T (target), for recording instances in which individuals felt they were being ostracized. Individuals used only one type of record, either the SOR-S or the SOR-T. Both groups monitored their exposures and reactions to ostracism for 2 weeks.

Each episode was to be recorded using a structure derived from my model of ostracism including the four dimensions, needs that may be affected, and moderators that may temper the impact. Moreover, each entry required that the participant enter the date, time, and duration of the incident; gender of the target; the status of the target; the relationship to the target; whether the ostracism took place against a group; and whether the source was part of a group. Finally, the record contained a section in which participants provide qualitative information on the incident itself. Information desired included what actually happened, where the incident took place, whether this was the first incident of its kind, and further details on how it made the source feel. The time the record was completed must be entered to determine whether incidents are recorded soon after the event. Furthermore, in order to facilitate timely completion, the SOR was made to be pocket-sized, allowing it to be carried and retrieved easily.

The participants attended one of several 1½-hour training sessions on how to complete the SOR-S (or SOR-T). Participants were introduced as coinvestigators and were informed of the importance and value of the research in which they would actively be involved. A presentation was given detailing each section of the SOR, with particular time and care taken to ensure that all individuals in the group understood fully how to make an entry in an accurate manner. In order to facilitate learning and consensual agreement, numerous examples of different forms of ostracism were given and participants were encouraged to generate examples from their own life experiences. Moreover, written scenarios were compiled, conveying the different dimensions of the ostracism model, and participants had to code these accordingly. Reasons for their choices were also discussed in order to assess more fully their level of comprehension.

The participants were instructed that they had to complete the SOR over a 2-week period. Within these 2 weeks, participants were required to return their completed records, preferably in person, every 2 to 3 days. This ensured that entries were completed as near to the incident of ostracism as possible and allowed for any queries or concerns to be answered.

Methodological Issues

Before looking at the data sets for both source and target studies, I should mention briefly some of the methodological issues surrounding diary methods. Following the completion of the diary for 2 weeks, participants were asked to complete a short questionnaire providing details of their experience with the SOR. Participants were asked to indicate on 7-point scales how difficult it was to record incidents of ostracism, how accurate they perceived their records to be, and to what extent keeping the record interfered with their use of ostracism. Results indicated that participants found it fairly easy keeping the records, perceived their records to be accurate, and did not really think that keeping the record interfered with their use of ostracism.

Participants were also asked to indicate on scales whether their accuracy in recording changed as the study progressed and whether their use of ostracism changed during the study as a result of keeping a record. Participants felt that their accuracy increased slightly over time, whereas their reported use of ostracism decreased slightly. These results are in line with previous studies using event-contingent self-report methods (Reis & Wheeler, 1991).

THE SOR-S STUDY

Sixty-one individuals who answered advertisements posted within the community or in a local newspaper were recruited to participate in the SOR-S study. They were more heterogeneous than our usual psychology undergraduate samples, although the sample was still comprised of many university students. All participants were paid to cover their travel expenses. There were 23 males and 38 females and their average age was 27 years old (ranging from 17 to 56). The sample was diverse both in terms of occupational and martial status and in terms of religious and ethnic background.

Diversity of Episodes

The responses on the back of each completed SOR-S, shown in Figure 10.1, captured the diversity of ostracism episodes. They ranged from the innocuous to the extreme. For example, one entry that was recorded as being role-prescribed said, "I went for lunch with my close friend at a Chinatown restaurant. I ignored the waitress who served us food." Another involved physical ostracism: "[My boss] was very angry and yelled at me in front of other people in the shop. This upset me so much I col-

Date of incident _____   Your code # _____

1. What time did the ostracism occur?   Start _____   End _____

2. Whom did you ostracize (gender and initials)? M, F _____ M, F _____ M, F _____
   or groups greater than three: # Males_____   # Females_____

3. What was your relationship to the person(s) you ostracized? (Place the initials of
   the individual(s) in the space provided. If initials unknown, place a tick.)
   Stranger ____   Acquaintance ____   Ordinary friend ____   Close friend ____
   Relationship partner ____   Relative____

4. What was the status of the person(s) ostracized?   Inferior to you ____
   Your equal ____   Superior _____

5. Were you the only one who ostracized this person? Yes___ (go to #7)   No___
   If No, how many others were involved? ____
   Were you all part of a group/team ____   or strangers to one another ___?

6. What was your relationship with the other person(s) who were also ostracizing?
   (Place the initials of the individual(s) in the space provided. If initials unknown,
   place a tick.)
   Stranger ____   Acquaintance ____   Ordinary friend ____   Close friend ____
   Relationship partner ____   Relative____

7. What kind of ostracism was it? (Tick one option on each line.)

V Social___	Cyber___	Physical___		
M Not ostracism___	Role-prescribed ___	Punitive ___	Defensive ___	Oblivious___
Q Barely ___	Slight ___	Moderate ___	Substantial ___	Complete___
C Totally unclear ___	Pretty unclear ___	Moderate ___	Pretty clear ___	Totally clear___

8. The reason I ostracized the individual(s) was primarily because of:
   Me___   Them ___   Situation___

9. Compared to how you felt prior to ostracizing, how have your feelings changed as
   a result of ostracizing?

Lower on belonging	-3 -2 -1 0 $+1$ $+2$ $+3$	Higher on belonging
Lower on control	-3 -2 -1 0 $+1$ $+2$ $+3$	Higher on control
Lower on self-esteem	-3 -2 -1 0 $+1$ $+2$ $+3$	Higher on self–esteem
Lower on meaningful existence	-3 -2 -1 0 $+1$ $+2$ $+3$	Higher on meaningful existence
Less angry	-3 -2 -1 0 $+1$ $+2$ $+3$	More angry
Less apologetic	-3 -2 -1 0 $+1$ $+2$ $+3$	More apologetic

10. What happened? (*Write on back of page.*) Please describe the event. Where did
    it take place? If it is related to a previous ostracism or to ongoing ostracism, tell
    us about it.   Current date/time _____

FIGURE 10.1. Sydney Ostracism Record for sources (SOR-S).

lected my bags and walked out." Still another involved the oblivious, social ostracism of a relative. This entry read, "She has never been worthy
of my attention. I have ignored her on many occasions. She works in a
place where, unfortunately, I am forced to visit because of my work."

Frequency and Categories of Sources' Use of Ostracism

Over the 2-week period a total of 1,005 episodes were entered—about
16.5 entries per participant, or 1.18 entries per person per day. There
were no overall sex differences in the submission of completed records.
Males, however, were twice as likely to have ostracized males as they
were to have ostracized females, whereas females ostracized both sexes
equally.

The majority of ostracism incidents were coded as taking place
against strangers (30%), ordinary friends (25%), and acquaintances
(25%). Ostracizing close friends (10%), relatives (8%), and relationship
partners (6%) was less frequent. Sources regarded the vast majority of
their targets to be of equal status (78%), 11% of targets were regarded
as inferior, and 11% were deemed superior. About a fifth of the entries
reflected instances in which sources joined with at least one other source
to engage in the ostracism.

Most (62%) of the episodes were coded as instances of social ostracism, followed by physical ostracism (21%), and then cyberostracism
(17%). Of the five motives, a fairly even distribution was evident: not
ostracism led the list (26%), followed by role-prescribed (20%) and
punitive (20%), then oblivious (18%), and finally defensive (15%).

Deviations from these general averages revealed some interesting results. Not ostracism was least likely to be recorded with strangers
(19%); role-prescribed was least likely to occur with partners (4%) and
most with strangers (32%); punitive was observed in higher frequency
with partners (51%) and relatives (31%) and least with strangers (13%);
defensive was fairly consistent across categories of relationships, but
lowest with close friends (8%); and oblivious ostracism was least likely
to occur with partners (2%) and most likely to occur with strangers
(25%).

When participants categorized the quantity of ostracism that they
were exhibiting, 48% were regarded as slightly or barely, 23% as moderate, and 30% as substantial or complete. On the dimension of causal
clarity, most considered their behavior as being fairly ambiguous. Over
half (55%) regarded their ostracism episodes as unclear, 20% as moderate, and 23% as being relatively clear.

Attributions for the incidents were evenly distributed across self
(37%), target (30%), and situation (33%). Another way to interpret this

is that our sources deflected the responsibility for 63% of the incidences. Sources of punitive ostracism were much more likely to attribute responsibility to the targets (69%) rather than to the self (18%) or to the situation (13%). Not ostracism and role-prescribed incidents, on the other hand, were attributed more often to the situation (47% and 53%, respectively) than to the target (9% and 14%, respectively).

Impact of Ostracism on Sources

Two reactions were most apparent in our sources. When ostracism resulted in changed feelings, sources were more likely to feel increased control (39% compared with 22% decreased) and decreased belonging (39% compared with 12% increased). Self-esteem increased (24%) about as often as it decreased (25%), as was the case for meaningful existence (18% increased, 17% decreased).

Feelings of belonging were significantly reduced as a function of all recorded motives except for role-prescribed. Feelings of control were increased when using ostracism for all motives, except defensive and not ostracism. Self-esteem was increased only when the motive was punitive. Participants' reports of meaningful existence were unaffected by motives.

The sources reported that their anger decreased when they decided their act was not an instance of ostracism (i.e., not ostracism), but increased for defensive and punitive motives. Sources felt more obligated to apologize when they reported that the incident was not ostracism (perhaps to clarify a potential misinterpretation), but did not feel obliged to apologize when their motive was punitive.

Sources felt angrier, less repentant, and at the same time better about themselves after ostracizing someone to punish them than when they defensively ostracized in order to deflect some form of ego threat against themselves. Participants also reported diminished feelings of belonging and increased anger after engaging in punitive, as opposed to oblivious, ostracism. Our finding that sources' self-esteem increases when they punitively ostracize appears to contradict the role-play findings in our train-ride studies (discussed in Chapter 7). With that paradigm, we find punitive sources indicating they experience a loss in self-esteem. In these data, participants chose to ostracize, whereas with the train-ride studies, they were instructed to ostracize. It is likely these differences in self-esteem may reflect this difference. When people ostracize others, particularly as a punishment, they are probably much less likely to feel badly about their behavior.

Compared to role-prescribed ostracism, behaviors subsequently regarded as "not ostracism" resulted in lower feelings of control and self-esteem, and an increased need to apologize. This result may be an arti-fact of the method, which undoubtedly made salient the potential impact of ostracism on targets.

THE SOR-T STUDY

Forty-four individuals recruited from advertisements participated in this study. Once again, the 13 males and 31 females were paid for their ex-penses during a 2-week study. This time, as shown in Figure 10.2, they recorded episodes in which they felt ostracized by others.

Diversity of Episodes

As with the source records, there was an incredible diversity of entries. Some seemed relatively innocuous, as was the case with this entry: "I was in the grocery store and the shop assistant knew I was coming to pay because I had received eye contact, but she still turned away and car-ried on reading her newspaper." Others were much more personal (and embarrassing), as with this young man: "I was sharing a romantic eve-ning with my partner and I broke wind unexpectedly—she left the room saying that I had spoilt the mood and atmosphere and that she had lost her image of what the perfect night would be." Some took place over the Internet, as in this example: "I went in to a chat room on the Internet in which I hadn't been before, I said hi and no one responded." One entry was particularly noteworthy because the diary itself was instrumental in the subsequent ostracism: "When I was having a look at what I wrote in the diaries for SOR, he looked in to what I had written. I just finished reading then, so I closed them, he said I was hiding them from him. He got upset because I share this personal account with a stranger but not with him. Since then he's been ignoring me by not responding and re-moving himself from me physically."

Frequency and Categories of Targets' Reports of Ostracism

There were a total of 737 ostracism episodes entered over the 2-week period, which averaged out to being almost 17 episodes per person, a little more than one per day. This figure is remarkably similar to the number of source-generated entries.

The average duration of each episode was a half hour, but—as might be expected—the range was quite large (from 1 minute to 36 hours). Our targets felt they had been ostracized mostly by acquain-tances (31%) and strangers (30%), followed by ordinary friends (16%),

Date _____   Your code # _____

1. What time did the ostracism occur? Start _____ End _____

2. Who ostracized you (gender and initials)? M, F____ M, F____ M, F_____
   or groups greater than three: # Males____ # Females____

3. What was your relationship to the person(s) who ostracized you? (Place the initials of the individual(s) in the space provided. If initials unknown, place a tick.)
   Stranger ___ Acquaintance ___ Ordinary friend ___ Close friend ___
   Relationship partner ___ Relative___

4. Was the person(s) who ostracized you inferior in status to you ___
   your equal ___ or superior in status ___?

5. Were you the only one being ostracized? Yes___ (go to #7)   No___
   If No, how many others? _____
   Were you all part of a group/team ___ or strangers to one another ___?

6. What was your relationship to the other person(s) who were also being ostracized? (Place the initials of the individual(s) in space provided. If initials unknown, place a tick.)
   Stranger ___ Acquaintance ___ Ordinary friend ___ Close friend ___
   Relationship partner ___ Relative___

7. What kind of ostracism was it? (Tick one option on each line.)

V	Social ___	Cyber ___	Physical ___		
M	Not ostracism ___	Role-prescribed ___	Punitive ___	Defensive ___	Oblivious ___
Q	Barely ___	Slight ___	Moderate ___	Substantial ___	Complete ___
C	Totally unclear ___	Pretty unclear ___	Moderate ___	Pretty clear ___	Totally clear___

8. The reason ostracism occurred was primarily because of:
   Me___ Them___ Situation___

9. Compared to how you were prior to the ostracism, how did your feelings change as a result of the ostracism?

Lower on belonging	−3 −2 −1 0 +1 +2 +3	Higher on belonging
Lower on control	−3 −2 −1 0 +1 +2 +3	Higher on control
Lower on self-esteem	−3 −2 −1 0 +1 +2 +3	Higher on self–esteem
Lower on meaningful existence	−3 −2 −1 0 +1 +2 +3	Higher on meaningful existence
Less angry	−3 −2 −1 0 +1 +2 +3	More angry
Less apologetic	−3 −2 −1 0 +1 +2 +3	More apologetic

10. What happened? (*Write on back of page.*) Please describe the event. Where did it take place? If it is related to a previous ostracism or to ongoing ostracism, tell us about it. Current date/time _____

FIGURE 10.2. Sydney Ostracism Record for targets of ostracism (SOR-T).

close friends (12%), relatives (6%), and relationship partners (5%). They recorded more instances of being ostracized by sources who were of equal status (76%), with only 15% of the episodes of ostracism by sources who were superior and 8% by sources who were inferior in status.

Targets recorded more instances of social ostracism (70%) than any other type. This was followed by 18.5% of cyberostracism episodes, and by 10.5% involving physical ostracism. The motives were spread out more across the various options: the highest percentage of motives were attributed to role-prescribed episodes of ostracism (26%), then not ostracism (25%), oblivious ostracism (20%), punitive ostracism (17%), and finally defensive ostracism (12%).

Their judgments as to the quantity of ostracism that occurred in each episode also ranged across all points on the continuum, roughly resembling a bell-shaped distribution: barely (16%), slight (25%), moderate (27%), substantial (18%), and complete (13%). The same sort of bell-shaped distribution emerged for our targets' recordings of the episodes' causal clarity: 13.5% totally unclear, 19% pretty unclear, 27% moderately clear, 25% pretty clear, and 14% totally clear.

When asked to place blame or responsibility for the episode with themselves, the source, or the situation, they blamed 41% of the episodes on the source, 37% on the situation, and only 12% of the ostracism episodes on themselves (almost 10% of the episodes had no option checked on this question).

Impact of Being Ostracized

Overall, if any change was noticed, participants recorded decreased levels in each of the four fundamental needs. Fifty-six percent of the episodes resulted in decreased feelings of belonging compared to only 2% that increased belonging. Similarly, 52% of the episodes decreased control, compared to only 4% that increased it. Almost half (46%) the episodes resulted in decreased self-esteem, with only 3% increasing it. And 25% of the episodes resulted in diminished feelings of meaningful existence, whereas only 2% of the episodes increased these feelings. Anger was more likely to be increased (43%) than decreased (7%), whereas the felt obligation to apologize was more likely to decrease (32%) than to increase (13%).

The motive attributed to the ostracism had an important impact on the needs. Punitive (70%) and oblivious ostracism (69%) resulted in the highest percentage of a lost sense of belonging, followed by defensive (57%), not ostracism (51%), and role-prescribed (40%). The same pattern emerged for self-esteem (60%, 60%, 46%, 39%, and 32%, respectively), and meaningful existence (37%, 34%, 26%, 16%, and 16%, respectively). The impact on control followed a slightly different pattern. Highest loss of control again was for punitive (66%) and oblivious (67%), but then the other three motives were about equal in their threat to control (44% for defensive, 45% for not ostracism, and 41% for role-prescribed).

SUMMARY OF DIARY FINDINGS

The results thus far of both diary studies are informative and provocative. The event-contingent self-report method provides us with information about the frequencies and consequences of ostracism in peoples' everyday lives. On average, ostracism was experienced daily by sources and by targets. If our results held true for the world's population, we could estimate that we ostracize others over 25,000 times in our lives, and others ostracize us another 25,000 times.

The effects of ostracizing and of being ostracized converge with the evidence gained in our other studies. For targets, all four needs are threatened, whereas none are fortified. Targets feel lowered levels of belonging, control, self-esteem, and, to a lesser extent, meaningful existence. They also feel angry. Sources, on the other hand, feel increased levels of control as a result of using ostracism. But they also suffered threats to belonging. Self-esteem appeared to be affected, but in some instances it was threatened and in others it was fortified. Clearly, more analyses are needed to understand the particular combination of dimensions, attributions, and relationship variables that produce the specific effects observed in these studies.

It will also be useful to examine whether the duration or frequency of the ostracism, again in combination with the other factors, reveals more severe reactions. As hypothesized in the model, as the duration and exposure to ostracism increases (for targets), reactions should shift from self-repair to internalization. We now turn toward our last program of research—structured interviews of long-term targets and sources—to see if the evidence gathered from these individuals is consistent with this proposition.

STRUCTURED INTERVIEWS OF INDIVIDUALS WITH LONG-TERM EXPERIENCE WITH OSTRACISM

There are fewer methods available to uncover effects of long-term exposure to ostracism. For obvious reasons, we cannot use experiments, so we are left to rely on correlational and qualitative approaches. For several years now, we have been interviewing individuals who have long-term exposure to ostracism—either as targets, sources, or both. Initially we began with unstructured interviews that were largely exploratory. We wanted the interviews to be in the control of the interviewees. To this end, Sonja Faulkner interviewed 32 people (22 females and 10 males), 17 of whom were long-term targets, nine of whom were sources, and six of whom said they were both. These people came to us in response to a newspaper ad we placed asking for the participation of individuals who had had long-term experience with the silent treatment (Faulkner & Williams, 1995).[1]

The results of these interviews were eye-opening. One woman had been given the silent treatment by her husband for the last 40 years of his life. She said her life was worthless—that she would have rather have been beaten. Another woman claimed she became promiscuous after her father refused to talk to her for several months. Still others claimed that the silent treatment drove them to various maladaptive responses, from anorexia to attempted suicide. Most of our sources themselves used the silent treatment in relationships as their first line of defense. They felt it was powerful and effective. Some used it because they could not achieve control or power in the relationship with any other tactic, but others used it on everyone they had relationships with, simply because it worked so well. One 65-year-old woman said, "I use the silent treatment whenever there may be a fight or confrontation. The silent treatment accomplishes for me all the things that fighting does for other people: control, power, and punishment. It gives me pleasure, and I'm in control. I also think it is funny how people grovel. I never feel guilty or ashamed; because it's always justifiable. . . . The Rolling Stones talk about satisfaction. This is how I get mine." We observed that long-term sources, like our laboratory sources, were rewarded with increased control. It is important to acknowledge, however, that both target and source accounts are post-hoc naïve theories used to understand (and possibly justify) one's own problematic behavior.

The information we gleaned from these interviews was certainly consistent with the notion that after a while coping mechanisms that attempt to repair threatened needs begin to fail, resulting in lowered senses of belonging, control, self-esteem, and meaningful existence. When this happens, it appeared that our targets felt isolated and alienated, helpless, worthless, and depressed. But because we let the interviewees direct the course of the interviews, we had a very uneven set of data for each person. Some discussed their health, others did not. Some concentrated on what led up to their ostracism, while others focused on how they dealt with it.

The information from these interviews was disturbing, but was certainly consistent with our predictions regarding long-term exposure to ostracism. Therefore, Lisa Zadro and I developed a structured interview that first allowed for the interviewee to give us whatever information he or she wanted without our interference. Then we proceeded to ask specific questions that we derived from the model. Once again, individuals in the community responded to newspaper or magazine advertisements asking for participation in interviews by people who had long-term experience with ostracism or the silent treatment. Additionally, because I had been requested to give several media interviews on ostracism, listeners, readers, and viewers of these interviews sometimes contacted me directly asking to be involved in the research.

Because of this method of procurement, the people we have interviewed so far represent a self-selected convenience sample. The experiences these people reveal to us may be related to the ostracism they endured, or it may be related to any number of other factors. Thus, our findings based on these interviews must be regarded with caution. Nevertheless, we think the information we are accumulating is worthy of attention because it represents the only programmatic research with long-term ostracism.

The structured interview was patterned after Yuille's (1988) suggestions for aiding recall for children's eyewitness testimony. It consists of seven sections: free recall; specific questions derived from the model (e.g., visibility, motive, quantity, causal clarity); thoughts, feelings, and actions of the interviewee as they pertained to instances of ostracism; consequences of ostracism (e.g., social life, their relationship with others, and health); propensity for and methods used to ostracize or to respond to being ostracized; possible means of terminating ostracism; and needs threat (e.g., agreement with statements such as "My life is meaningless" or "My self-esteem is low").

Some interviews were conducted in person but most of them were done over the telephone. Participants agreed to have the interviews audiotaped in all instances, and these tapes were later transcribed verbatim. Participants were assured of confidentiality and anonymity, and so all identifying information was removed.

The interviews usually lasted about 2 hours. So far, we have had over 90 letters, faxes, or e-mails and 112 phone calls in response to the advertisements or the interviews, from every state in Australia; we have even had two contacts from Tahiti and Hawaii. About three times as many targets as sources have responded, and about four times as many women as men have responded. The ages of our respondents ranged from 23 to 68 years old. They represent the full socioeconomic spectrum. From this group, we have just finished our 38th interview, 30 of which were with females (6 sources and 24 targets) and eight of which were with males (4 sources, 4 targets).

Target Interviews

For many of our interviewees, this was an extremely emotional experience. Often, it was their first chance to speak to someone about their experiences. On many occasions, we were told, "I thought I was the only one. . . . I thought I had made up the term [the silent treatment]." In fact, there were many labels for the treatment they received: "no speaks," "the pout, " and "silent hell, " to name a few.

Most of our interviewees were given the silent treatment by one person (52% of them by their relationship partner); the others were targets of group ostracism (e.g., several family members, work colleagues, school peers). Many were extremely worried about anonymity, concerned that the sources of the ostracism would find out and punish them further.

There were two general categories of long-term ostracism targets: those who were subjected to long and *continuous* ostracism over months and years, and those who experienced frequent yet *episodic* occurrences. For example, a 55-year-old woman told us that as a child she had been a target of mental and physical abuse by her stepfather, who was a champion boxer. One day her mother came into her room and announced, "Dad thinks it would be easier not to speak to you." So, from then on, her father ignored her. She said, "At first it was a relief . . . but then I kept thinking how bizarre this was. I longed to be able to put it right. I began to think that this was all I was worth. I thought that I was a horrible person, that I was not worth speaking to." Her father gave her the silent treatment for 6 years before she ran away from home. A 40-year-old mother of two was an example of an episodic target. Her parents had ostracized her throughout her life, usually for 3 to 6 months at a time. Even during the time of the interview, her parents had not spoken to her for 6 months because they blamed her for the breakdown of her marriage. She said, "My father has given me the silent treatment whenever he's been upset with me ever since I was 12 years old. Now I'm 40 years old and my father hasn't talked to me for the last 6 months. Recently, he was in hospital and I was told he might die. I decided I had to go see him, even if he wasn't talking to me. I walked up to him and held his hand and said 'Oh Daddy, please don't leave me.' He looked at me, his eyes were welled up with tears, then turned his head away from me. He still wouldn't talk to me . . . his death would be the final silence."

We asked our targets if they knew when they were about to get the silent treatment, and whether there was a period of time when they might be able to somehow avoid getting it. Many indicated they became expertly "attuned" to nonverbal signals made by their sources. One middle-aged woman was given the silent treatment repeatedly throughout her life by her mother. She said, "There was certain ways that she would look. That was the first hint—the way she would twist her mouth or something. I'd know something's happening here. . . . " Another woman was a target of episodic cyberostracism from a lover she had met through a chat room (see Chapter 8). She picked up on text cues, the use of monosyllabic or one-word answers (e.g., "k" instead of "okay") without reciprocated questions.

Some of our targets were what we might refer to as "perpetual targets," perhaps creating the behaviors in others that they hate the most, resulting in being targets of ostracism from several independent sources. For instance, one woman said to us "[people not talking to me] was what I hated more than anything really. And so . . . I told my husband that [the silent treatment] was one of my mother's methods and so he started to use it too. . . . I must be the sort of person that it works with."

Even in the first stages of the interviews, when our interviewees were free to say anything they wished without direction, we noted instances of internalized need loss. For example, one woman said, "You didn't belong. You thought 'I'm a mistake, I shouldn't be here, I'm not wanted here.' That's what you felt." Another target said, "I'm just no good at anything . . . failure, failure, failure." Still another told us, "I felt helpless in so many areas of my life." A middle-aged woman said, "It [the silent treatment] made me question 'What's it all for? . . . Why am I still here?' . . . whereas before I never questioned that. I knew why I was there and I knew what it was all for."

Some engaged in self-destructive behaviors. One young woman, speaking about when her schoolmates ostracized her in grade school, said, "At one stage they refused to speak to me for 153 days, not one word at all, doctor. That was a very low point for me in my life and on the 153rd day, I swallowed 29 Valium pills." Another showed signs of self-isolation. One woman avoids social situations in general because, in her words, "I am [now] overly receptive to any other signs of rejection by others." Because of this, she has little opportunity to regain a sense of belonging, self-esteem, or meaningful existence. Of course, it could be said that she has maintained a sense of control, because she controls and prevents future rejection. One woman became oversensitized to silence, saying, "I think one of the worst things in life would be to be deaf. . . . I cannot bear silence. . . . I have to sleep with the radio on at night."

We noted that with many of our targets, the silent treatment often went hand-in-hand with verbal and/or physical abuse. First they would be yelled at or hit, then they would be subjected to lengthy bouts of the silent treatment by the source. Perhaps the silent treatment was used defensively for these sources, as a way to avoid confronting their objective forms of abuse. But, surprisingly, many targets stated that they preferred to be hit than given the silent treatment. A young woman who was in a position to make the comparison received silent treatment (which she referred to as "mental cruelty") from her third husband for 10 years. She said, "My second husband, who was an alcoholic, used to physically abuse me, but the bruises and scars healed very quickly and I believe that mental cruelty is far more damaging than a black eye."

In the free recall section, 80% of targets revealed that they had health problems that they attributed to being targets of ostracism. These ailments ranged from those that could be considered stress-related (e.g., migraines, heart palpitations), to others that might be related to suppressed immune functioning (e.g., recurring colds, bronchial problems, chronic fatigue syndrome, high blood pressure).

How did individuals who received long-term ostracism perceive the people who ostracized them? A large number stated that they did not know why they were ostracized: one moment things were fine, then suddenly they were being ignored. Many regarded the ostracizers as being stubborn—so many in fact that we are looking for validated stubbornness scales to test their hypothesis. Silence was sometimes a general characteristic of sources. For instance, many husband sources were described as "the strong, silent type." But there were just as many who had no clue about their husband's propensity for silence, calling their shifts to silence as a kind of "Jekyll and Hyde" change.

How do targets get the sources to stop? They had very few answers to this question, which may account for their predicament of being ostracized repeatedly throughout their lives. Almost none of the targets suggested strategies or had advice as to how to stop being ostracized while it was ongoing. They tried many countertactics. They reciprocated the silent treatment, but usually found that eventually they were the ones to try to mend the rift. They yelled, hurled insults, or even resorted to physical violence. But this only exacerbated the problem, making it more likely that they would have to apologize. The most common suggestion for ending the ostracism was to end the relationship. Only one individual felt she had successfully dealt with her husband's repeated use of episodic ostracism without resorting to resignation or divorce. She said she realized that her husband gave her the silent treatment whenever he needed to be alone. She also realized that this was a temporary state, and that his use of the silent treatment did not signify lack of love or a desire to disengage permanently. So, in her words, "I said to myself 'Well, why talk to him when I can just be with him? And when he feels like talking, he'll talk.'" She said that when he gives her the silent treatment, she carries on as if things are normal. Instead of asking him to go out of the house to do something, she simply grasps his arm and takes him with her. She gets the company; he gets to continue not talking. For them, this seems to work.

Source Interviews

Although fewer in number, the sources who answered our advertisements were very open and forthcoming. Some were looking for advice about how to quit; others had no intention of quitting. In fact, we came up with two descriptions that fit most of our sources: the *proud* and the *penitent*. The proud enjoyed the power that came from using the silent treatment. A young woman who had used the silent treatment on loved ones since she was 13 years old said, "I'm gonna use the silent treatment till the day I die. I have often given the silent treatment to my husband, as I believed it was my best weapon. . . . It can make a grown man cry, without having to hit him over the head." The penitent were remorseful and wished they could stop giving the silent treatment to others. One said, "I am not proud of giving this treatment, and often feel I have let myself down by doing it."

Regardless of being proud or penitent, in agreement with many targets, almost all sources described themselves as "stubborn." One woman said, "I'll hold a grudge till the day I die. I've still got a grudge against a 6-year-old boy who got me into trouble for playing 'I'll show you mine if you show me yours' behind the bike shed when we were in kindergarten." One woman got angry at her grocery clerk with whom she used to have friendly conversations. Ten years later, she saw him and he her, and she still felt compelled to turn away, even though it was clear to her that he wanted to talk.

Sources always had a reason for ostracism. Several sources mentioned using the silent treatment to "level the playing field." One woman regularly gave her husband the silent treatment "because I can't match his quick-wittedness and retorts. I get too confused and too tongue-tied. I get tongue-tied and can't think straight so I just shut up because I don't want to put my foot in my mouth any further." Others use it because they know it is powerful and makes it difficult for their targets to regain the upper hand.

All sources seemed to have their own silent treatment technique, but we found a convenient duality: some are what we call *quiet* ostracizers and others are *noisy*. The quiet ones do not draw attention to their use of the tactic. As one said, "I wipe them completely off the face of the earth. That means that I don't acknowledge them, I don't speak to them." The noisy ones are rather demonstrative in their use of ostracism. One source had a rather long list of behavioral requirements accompanying her use of the silent treatment: "Sometimes 'the glare' goes with the silence, but most of the time it's the silence and the stiff jaw. Stiff jaw, nose up . . . and give 'em the half-shut eye. Sort of dismissive glare, turn your head away." Other examples involved stomping around the same room, slamming drawers and doors, and in other ways making a noisy show of silence.

From our impressions, quiet ostracism appeared to be less effortful and lasted for longer periods of time, usually falling into the category of continuous. Noisy ostracism was effortful and usually episodic. It seemed to us that the quiet type was a genuine indicator of social death—a total divorce from and disengagement of interest with the target. Noisy users tended to regard their use of the silent treatment as a temporary tactic, aimed at showing their displeasure and used to get the target back into the fold by apologizing or begging for attention. One noisy user said to us, "Realistically, trying not to talk or doing the silent treatment for 5 days was bloody hard. . . . Usually by the fifth day if he'd come home with a bunch of flowers I'd think 'Oh thank God.' "

But ostracism did not always have its intended outcome. One woman said, "One day . . . I decided that I wouldn't bother to speak to [my husband] at all, apart from answering him as briefly as possible if he spoke to me. I managed to keep this up for some days, possibly a week or so, but finally he did something which really annoyed me so I spoke. . . . He was taken aback and I was disturbed by his response which was 'But you've been so happy lately!' "

As indicated in our other studies, sources report having needs threat and fortification. Most consistently, they reported an increase in control over the target and over the situation, but sometimes they felt they ended up losing this control to the tactic itself. As one father said, "To terminate the ostracism, however, was an extremely difficult process. I could only begin with grudging, monosyllabic responses to his indirect overtures. I was only able to expand on these responses with the passing of time. . . . Ostracism can be like a whirlpool, or quicksand, if you, the user, don't extract yourself from it as soon as possible, it is likely to become impossible to terminate regardless of the emergence of any subsequent will to do so."

Why is it so difficult to discontinue? One reason appears to be that sources fear losing face. In order for them to cease using the silent treatment, the target must show sufficient contrition or effort so as to make the source appear generous in his or her willingness to once again regard the target's existence. We also heard considerable agreement by long-term sources that each time they used ostracism it became easier and easier to do. As one man said, "I got stronger and felt more comfortable. . . . I would see [the target] in the early days and I'd get an adrenalin rush. I'd think, 'I don't want to be in the room with you, I want out of here' . . . but as time goes on I don't feel like that." Thus, with continued use, perhaps ostracism becomes less effortful and is less likely to deplete one's cognitive resources. Thus, continuing with it becomes easier because there is little cost associated with its use.

Another consistent tendency was for sources to mention that they themselves had been subjected to the silent treatment when they were children. Targets, too, mentioned that their partners' parents were likely to use the silent treatment. Thus, although we find that most people use some form of ostracism in their day-to-day lives, for some people it becomes their dominant method of coping with interpersonal problems. For these people, it seems as though they have learned to use ostracism, particularly the silent treatment, from their upbringing. This sentiment is best expressed by the mother who said, "I'm probably passing it on to my 4-year-old because when he gets angry, he storms off. He'll tell my youngest son 'Don't talk to Mum, I'm angry at her!' " It is, of course, possible that the use of ostracism as the first line of defense runs in families, as suggested by what a man told us: "At the present moment, my sister aged 58 in the United States won't talk to either my father or myself—for supposedly differing reasons. My father's sister has not spoken to him for over 30 years. My mother's brother once refused to talk to his wife for 6 months. My mother regularly refused to talk to me or my sister for days at a time. It seems like ostracism is a congenital condition in my family."

What advice do sources have as to how to get them to stop using the silent treatment? According to our sources so far, the worst thing to ask is "What's wrong?" or "What have I done wrong?" As one woman said, "I get really mad when they go 'I don't know what I've done wrong.' Then I get even quieter. . . . I think that if they do something that bad and they don't know what they've done wrong, they are really stupid." Instead, our sources say the best thing is to leave them alone. Then, after some period of time elapses, apologize (or, as one source said, "And give me presents"). Of course, this sort of response by targets would simply reinforce the sources' use of the silent treatment. Not only can sources deprive their partners of fundamental needs, but if they are able to extract an apology (or presents) from the targets, they can completely exonerate themselves of any wrongdoing. What could be better?

Summary

Most of our observations at this point are impressionistic. We need to accumulate a larger number of interviewees, and subject these data to more rigorous forms of qualitative analysis. Nevertheless, the observations I have noted represent dominant themes in our interviews. We hear the same things over and over again. Still, our sample is self-selected. The targets may be individuals who bring the ostracism upon themselves. They may react to any form of disagreement with such ferocity that their significant others are left with nothing else to counter with except silence. Also, except for one instance in which both the husband (source) and the wife (target) agreed to interview with us, we are only getting one side of the story. As Baumeister and Catanese (2001) observed, there are very typical patterns in victims' stories and perpetrators' stories. Victims see themselves as blameless, and view the consequences of the acts as overly hurtful and long lasting. Perpetrators believe their behavior is precipitated by the victims, and contextualize the incidents in shorter time frames with less harmful consequences. Our impressions, therefore, must take into account these standard cognitive and motivational biases that characterize victim and perpetrator accounts.

CONCLUSIONS

The results of both paradigms, event-contingent diaries and structured interviews, provide insight into the experience of long-term ostracism. People encounter episodes of ostracism daily. Many of these episodes are misinterpretations of events, and are quickly reinterpreted as not being instances of ostracism. Others are role-prescribed episodes of ostracism that we, as societies, adhere to because of our customs. Many of us, in fact, would probably prefer not to talk to strangers in the elevator, or wait staff in restaurants, or seatmates on buses. The acceptance of this mild form of ostracism allows us to maintain our personal space and privacy. In these cases, it is quite likely that ostracism is harmless, having little negative influence on targets, nor any benefits for sources.

Other episodes are not so benign. When ostracism is used to punish or to preempt harmful encounters, and is experienced repeatedly or for long periods of time, then targets seem to lack sufficient resources to cope. Consequently, they begin to internalize the message that ostracism inherently delivers: they are no longer a part of the other person or group, they have no control over their situation, they are bad, and their existence is meaningless. Long-term sources of ostracism either feel empowered and almost gleeful in their discovery of such a powerful form of social influence, or they recognize the damage its use has caused and wish desperately to abandon what appears to be a habitual response to unpleasant social circumstances.

We have fewer observations with individuals who report long-term exposure to what they considered to be oblivious ostracism. We suspect that sources of this behavior will be, as the term implies, oblivious to their behaviors, and will not suffer or benefit greatly from its use. Of course, others who are on the receiving end of oblivious ostracism may join forces and react against what they perceive to be arrogant and unfair treatment. But if individuals experience long-term oblivious ostracism by others, I suspect they will be resigned to an utterly powerless sense of meaningless existence. They will have been cut dead.

NOTE

1. See also Chapter 2, where material and a number of quotations from these interviews were first introduced and discussed.

Reflections and Future Aims

This book reports research accomplished and work in progress. There is still much work to be done. This last chapter summarizes what we now know about ostracism, integrates these findings with recent results found in other laboratories, and identifies important questions for future research.

In Chapter 3, I presented a working model of ostracism. I formulated the model after reviewing the literature from a variety of disciplines, and after I conducted a few exploratory studies. I intended the model to act as a guide, a map of "the big picture" of ostracism. I figured that in some ways the model would be overinclusive, but that it would not surprise me that it was insufficient to allow a full understanding of ostracism. For instance, I knew that although we could describe ostracism as an act of ignoring and excluding, that all such acts would not have the same impact, or even be regarded as ostracism by most people. And, although I included a box in the model aimed at listing the antecedents of ostracism, it is now clear to me that the model needs to be extended considerably to direct our attention to the impact that ostracism has on the people who use it: the sources. Thus, the model still remains as it was intended: a working model that will both guide research and accommodate modifications with new discoveries.

SUPPORT FOR THE MODEL

Although the model can be considered as a map, there is no single starting point. Our choices of what to examine first reflect our own biases and interests, and also probably reflect those questions that can be attacked more easily. Thus, we have tested some aspects of the model more than others.

For example, the top right box of the model (see Figure 3.1), antecedents, has been barely scratched. We have little information on what triggers ostracism rather than some other aversive interpersonal behavior. A few of our studies suggest that certain types of people (or, more correctly, people with certain traits) are more prone to use ostracism. We have some evidence that people with low self-esteem (Sommer et al., in press) and those with insecure attachment styles (Boeckman, 2000; Williams & Zadro, 1999) are associated with greater use of the silent treatment. Undoubtedly, this information is incomplete, and more research is needed to examine individual differences that predict a preference for using ostracism. More likely, because we find that most people admit to using various forms of ostracism in their lives, even with their loved ones, ostracism is triggered by social-situational events. These can include behaviors emitted by the potential targets that would cause most anyone to ostracize them, or factors present in the social situation that make ostracism the preferred tactic over argument or physical confrontation. We are currently testing methods to induce ostracism, to see if, in a laboratory setting, we can find variables that increase the likelihood of its use. But the laboratory may not be the best place to look for this answer, and we may have to look to other methods.

Another relatively undertested aspect of the model concerns "moderators." I reasoned that the same act of ostracism could have wildly different consequences on a target depending upon that target's personality and interpretation of the event. I still find this to be a compelling proposition, but we haven't yet directed much of our attention to it. Examinations of narratives suggest that people with higher levels of self-esteem are less likely to make the negative assessments the silent treatment often causes, and are more likely to simply avoid interpersonal relations that involve it. In an undergraduate honors thesis, Chris Nadasi (1992) found that whereas introverts' self-reports showed less negative influence from ostracism (using the ball-tossing paradigm), their nonverbal behavior suggested otherwise. In his PhD thesis, Barth Reilly (1996) found that people scoring higher in loneliness were more likely to react negatively to ostracism than those who were not lonely, when involved in a conversation paradigm. On the other hand, we found that self-esteem was unrelated to short-term manipulations of cyberostracism (Williams et al., 2000). Clearly, more work needs to be done to determine the conditions under which self-esteem moderates reactions to ostracism and rejection.

It seems very reasonable that an individual's attributional style also moderates the impact of ostracism. Targets of ostracism who are more inclined to make dispositional attributions of others' behaviors, that is, to believe that aspects of their characters cause them to act as they do, should be less threatened by ostracism; those who are more prone to believe that they themselves are responsible for others' behaviors should be more threatened. However, Zadro, Walker, Williams, and Richardson (2000) found that individuals who scored higher on external locus of interpersonal control (thinking that what happened in their social relations had more to do with the desires and behaviors of the others than themselves) reacted more negatively to ostracism (physiologically, but not with self-reports) than those high in internal locus of interpersonal control. External locus of interpersonal control targets could still have surmised that the sources chose to ostracize them because they (targets) were in some way to blame.

Finally, there is some evidence that attachment style affects peoples' perception of the frequency with which they are ostracized and their reaction to it. Boeckman (2000) recently found that people with less secure styles of attachment reported more incidence of being ostracized. Likewise, in our questionnaire studies (Williams & Zadro, 1999), we find that those with insecure attachment styles are more likely to report being given the silent treatment, that they react more negatively to it, and that they are more likely to use it.

Taxonomic Dimensions

I argued at the outset that it might be useful to distinguish between different types of ostracism, because it seemed unreasonable to assume that all forms of being ignored and being included were similarly consequential. We have examined the justification for partitioning ostracism into different types, varying along four dimensions: visibility, motive, quantity, and causal clarity.

Visibility

We have investigated through various methods all three types of ostracism that vary across visibility; these include physical, social, and cyberostracism. Through our examinations of narratives and structured interviews, we conclude that physical ostracism can be quite unpleasant and distressing, but that it can also afford both parties the opportunity to cool down and gather their thoughts so that further discord is not amplified once sources and targets are reunited. Another distinctive and potential positive feature of physical ostracism is that it comes with its own endpoint. A reunion between source and target provides a clear marker that can be interpreted as a green light to resume social interaction. In social and cyberostracism, no clear markers exist, putting the onus on either the source or the target to make a reconciliation attempt. Because of this, either the source or the target risks losing face if his or her attempt is spurned. Social ostracism, however, appears not only to be highly frustrating but often can ignite rage and retribution. Even in some of our role-play studies, we observed attempts to gain recognition taking precedence over rehabilitating sense of belonging or self-esteem. In many of our laboratory studies, however, targets do not take control and force sources to recognize them; instead, they sit slumped in their seats with resignation. When do we expect to see one reaction or the other? Once the episode ends, they attempt to regain or repair their threatened needs. Cyberostracism, however (in our chat-room studies in particular), is met not with resignation but with demands for clarification and confrontation. Although we can only speculate at present, it would appear that these different forms of ostracism result in different behavioral, emotional, and cognitive consequences for targets. Thus, again it seems useful to distinguish the mode by which ostracism occurs.

Motive

I have proposed that the simple act of being ignored and excluded is not sufficient to threaten fundamental needs; it depends upon the perceived or intended motive behind such acts. After such an act, an individual may decide that he or she is not being ostracized after all (i.e., not ostracism). Role-prescribed ostracism occurs when people ignore others because the norms within that culture allow or even encourage this form of ignoring. People routinely ignore their fellow passengers on elevators, trains, buses, and planes (see Goffman's "norm of civil inattention," 1963). Through diary studies and informal discussions, we know that people recognize this behavioral pattern in themselves and others. But we also know that the impact of this sort of ostracism is negligible. Whether we manipulate the situation or the scenario to be role-prescribed or we ask people to report instances in which it occurs, we find that targets of this sort of ostracism indicate no change in feelings or cognitions when compared to how they were feeling prior to the ostracism. When people find themselves engaging in role-prescribed ostracism, they also report no impact on their feelings or thoughts. Targets of punitive, defensive, or oblivious ostracism, however, show signs of emotional distress and report lower levels of belonging, control, self-esteem, and meaningful existence. Sources, however, report that engaging in these types of ostracism increases their sense of control and power. Thus, it appears to be useful to distinguish between different motives of ostracism. More research is needed to distinguish between oblivious ostracism and punitive ostracism. It is my feeling that whereas both are certainly aversive and unpleasant, oblivious ostracism is more threatening. Punitive ostracism, when perceived as such, should at least provide targets with the comfort of knowing they are "objects of inattention." That is, they know that they are worthy of others' *intentional* acts of ostracism. If instead, individuals conclude that others don't even notice them in the first place, then there seems to be nothing in which targets of ostracism can take solace.

Quantity

Quantity of ostracism refers to the observation that ostracism varies in how much ignoring and exclusion is occurring. In anthropological accounts, in narratives, and from our interviews, we know that ostracism is sometimes indicated through subtle shades of inattention, which we call *low quantity* (e.g., less eye contact, monosyllabic responses, answering questions but not initiating conversation), and at other times with full-blown ignoring and exclusion, what we call *high quantity*. I had thought initially that moderate quantities of ostracism might be more aversive than high quantities simply because ambiguity would be greater. Targets of moderate quantities of ostracism might be less certain that they are being ostracized and consequently might question their own perceptions and paranoia. On the other hand, a great deal of social psychological research demonstrates that if individuals can possibly interpret events in a self-serving protective manner, they will. Thus, targets of moderate amounts of ostracism might be more easily able to dismiss, reinterpret, or deny any evidence that they are being ignored and excluded. In our only study to date that manipulated quantity, we found support for the self-protective hypothesis: increasing the quantity of (cyber) ostracism resulted in reports of lower mood and higher perceptions of exclusion (Williams et al., 2000). It remains to be seen if there are conditions under which the ambiguity that accompanies moderate quantities of ostracism makes matters worse for targets.

For sources, choosing to engage in moderate quantities of ostracism rather than high quantities could provide them with the ability to deny any accusations the targets might make with reference to being ostracized: such sources could easily refer to instances in which they gave answers or attended to targets.

Causal Clarity

Sometimes ostracism is given without explanation and targets are left bewildered and searching for explanations about whether they are being ostracized and, if so, why? Other times, clear pronouncements of ostracism are given, as in the Amish proclamation of Meidung, or even within close interpersonal relationships, as when a partner says, "I'm not going to talk to you." Again, my thinking was that low causal clarity was more ambiguous, and therefore would cause more consternation, rumination, and potentially negative self-thoughts. A target of ostracism in which there was low causal clarity would not only have to grapple with whether his or her perceptions of ostracism were accurate, but would also have to generate plausible justifications for the ostracism. This might involve a rather extensive list of wrongdoings which, when contemplated, would result in higher levels of self-blame and self-derision. When the cause for the ostracism is clear, the target can at least focus on the transgression that is alleged, and has more opportunity to dismiss it, correct his or her behavior, or apologize. In one study (Ezrakhovich et al., 1998), we have found marginal tendencies showing that when targets could clearly attribute their ostracism to the fact that they were late for the experiment, they contributed less effort to the group task than when it was not clear why they were being ostracized. Assuming that contributing to the group's effort is a means to cope with higher levels of needs threat, these results are consistent with the notion that targets need to cope less with causally clear than with causally unclear ostracism.

Impact on Four Needs

The psychological literature provides considerable support for propositions that there are at least four fundamental human needs: (1) the need to belong (Baumeister & Leary, 1995), (2) the need to control (Seligman, 1975; Skinner, 1996), (3) the need to maintain high self-esteem (Steele, 1988; Tesser, 1988), and (4) the need to buffer against the realization of one's mortality and meaningless existence (Greenberg et al., 1986). I have not tried to determine whether any of these needs supersedes or is encapsulated by the other needs (but, for such an attempt to distinguish between self-esteem and belonging, see a study by Rudich and Vallacher [1999]). For my purposes, there seems to be sufficient evidence to regard each need as important and, although potentially overlapping, distinct.

I consider ostracism to be unique in its potential ability to pose a threat to all four needs. Ostracism serves to severe bonds, withdraw control, derogate, and render invisible and insignificant its targets. Furthermore, I proposed that these needs could be threatened within moments of when targets perceive the ostracism. The power of ostracism lies in these two propositions: it can simultaneously diminish four fundamental human needs, and it can do so quite quickly. The additional feature that explains ostracism's apparent ubiquity and frequency it that sources can employ it without a great deal of effort and in such a way that they can deny that they are doing it.

The research reported in this book provides strong support for the first two propositions. Whether we rely on self-reports or make inferences based on behaviors, whether we employ role play, simulations, diaries, interviews, or experimental manipulations, we observe repeatedly that for targets of ostracism all four needs are threatened. It is, of course, not always the case that all four needs are simultaneously and equally diminished. In some cases, in particular, we are unable to detect effects on our measures for meaningful existence. In some respects, this may simply reflect our inability to measure this concept in an appropriate fashion. Or it may reflect the difference between short-term and clearly temporary manipulations of ostracism, where we are less able to detect an impact on meaningful existence, and longer, more permanent exposures to ostracism, where we do see its impact.

Finally, although not initially part of the model, we have found that two of these needs, belonging and control, are often fortified in individuals or groups who employ ostracism on others. We will return to this finding shortly.

Short-Term versus Long-Term Reactions

Individuals will generally react to ostracism differently depending upon whether they have been exposed to the ostracism briefly or they have had to endure it on a more continuous basis. Specifically, targets of short-term ostracism will attempt to regain or repair the needs that were threatened; targets of long-term ostracism will essentially internalize or adapt to lower need levels. The latter will either not expect or will not attempt to enhance basic levels of belonging, control, self-esteem, or meaningful existence, or, worse, they will show the pathologies that would be expected in the absence of satisfying these needs: mental and physical ill health, alienation, marginalization, helplessness, depression, despondency, and worthlessness. The basic premise behind this temporally distinct reaction is that individuals have at their disposal a finite amount of psychological resources to cope with threats to fundamental needs. These resources are called up and expended when needs threat is initially encountered, and, if successful, can serve to replenish the diminished needs. If, however, they are unsuccessful in fortifying the threatened needs, or if the ostracism persists regardless of these stopgap measures, then the psychological resources are depleted, and resistance is low or absent. Considerable evidence by other researchers supports such a temporal shift for each of the fundamental needs.

Most of the studies reported in this book examine the consequences of short-term ostracism. The results have been largely supportive of the needs threat–repair prediction. Targets of short-term ostracism are more likely to work harder in group settings (Ezrakhovich, et al, 1998; Williams & Sommer, 1997), employ cognitive strategies that enhance self-esteem and commonality with others (Gardner, Pickett, & Brewer, 2000; Ko, 1994; Zadro & Williams, 1998b), desire and exert greater control over others (Lawson Williams & Williams, 1998), and conform more to others' unanimous (yet incorrect) perceptual judgments (Williams et al., 2000).

Evidence for long-term consequences is, of course, more difficult to obtain. Ethical concerns would obviously prohibit any attempt at assigning individuals to long-term ostracism for experimental purposes. What we must turn to, instead, are methods that tap into the impressions of individuals who have endured long-term episodes of ostracism. As a consequence, cause and effect becomes less clear. Nevertheless, in our interviews with targets of long-term ostracism, who in most cases have been receiving the silent treatment from significant others, we have repeatedly heard reports of the misery that followed such treatment. Physical ailments were unanimously reported, even without prompting. Depression, seeking therapy, eating disorders, unwillingness to leave abusive relationships, promiscuity, and suicidal ideation and actual attempts were commonly reported.

Although no temporal shift was hypothesized for sources of ostracism, the evidence we have accumulated allows for some speculation that something similar might be happening for sources as they persist in using ostracism over a long period of time. Sources of ostracism in our laboratory and role-play studies show need fortification, particularly for control and sometimes belonging (if there is another cosource of ostracism). Regarding desires for control and belonging, they may feel sated or even oversatisfied. An obvious hypothesis that has not yet been tested is that ostracism sources, compared to sources of inclusion or argument, should be less likely to engage in need repair. But, for some of our long-term users of ostracism, we detect that while they enjoy an immediate feeling of power and control over the target, the obligation to maintain the silent treatment in the absence (or even sometimes in the presence) of total capitulation by the targets commits them, indeed controls them, to continue using the silent treatment beyond what they ever would have imagined they would have done.

What Alterations Need to Be Made to the Model?

As I have indicated, a good deal of information has surfaced from our research on the effects of ostracism on those who use the tactic. The model was not developed to explain the consequences of ostracizing on the ostracizers. The antecedents portion of the model focuses on what causes people to ostracize others, which pertains to sources as well as targets. The model needs to be expanded to accommodate the impact, costs, and benefits to people who engage in ostracism. We have observed in several studies now that sources of ostracism, at least in the short term, are rewarded with increased feelings of control and power. If there are two or more cosources, they report feeling a stronger bond with each other, when compared to cosources who engage in verbal argument with a target. In this sense, we observe the opposite impact on two of the four fundamental needs, belonging and control. It is certainly tempting, if only because of the theoretical symmetry, to propose that the same needs that are threatened in targets are fortified in sources. However, so far there is no evidence that engaging in ostracism increases sources' sense of self-esteem or meaningful existence. Currently, my PhD student Lisa Zadro is working on such a task, trying to develop a model that predicts when people will ostracize and how it will affect them in the short and long term.

RECENT RESEARCH BY OTHER INVESTIGATORS

Two recently published studies are particularly relevant to ostracism and to my theory. The first is a set of studies by Gardner et al. (2000) that demonstrates that targets of exclusion are more likely to attend to and remember social information. The second, a set of six experiments by Tice, Twenge, and Schmeichel (in press), demonstrates that exclusion can lead to antisocial behavior. Both of these sets of findings deserves closer attention.

Effects of Social Exclusion on Selective Memory

Gardner et al. (2000) reasoned that if the need to belong was similar to other needs, like hunger, then depriving individuals of a sense of belonging should have similar effects on attention and memory. When people are hungry, they are more likely to attend to food-related information and stimuli, and are more likely to recall information about food, than when they are not hungry. Therefore, socially excluded individuals should be more likely to attend to and recall social information than socially included individuals. These researchers used a chat-room paradigm to manipulate social exclusion and inclusion. After a brief get-acquainted chat, participants were either excluded from engaging in further discussion with two others or continued to be included.

The results of both studies show clear support for the idea that social exclusion deprives its targets of the need to belong, and that the response to this deprivation is similar to other types of need deprivation: individuals behave in ways that would increase their likelihood of need fulfillment. If hungry, the adaptive response would be to be especially attentive to food stimuli in order to increase chances for food acquisition. Similarly, if through social exclusion one has a stronger need to belong, then it would be adaptive to attend to and recall socially relevant information. This directed attention could increase the likelihood that social-deprived individuals could reacquire the desired social bonds.

Effects of Social Exclusion on Antisocial Behavior

In many of my studies, a frequent behavioral reaction for ostracism targets is to display signs of despondent resignation. In the ball-tossing and conversation paradigms, after maintaining eye contact and a hopeful expression, targets routinely slump back in their chairs and stare at the wall or the floor. However, this is not the only behavioral reaction. Indeed, in the 5-day Scarlet Letter Study (Chapter 5), the chat-room paradigm (Chapter 8), and from our structured interviews (Chapter 10), we observed offensive proactive reactions. In these studies, targets of ostracism engaged in all sorts of attention-getting behaviors that demanded recognition and reaction from others.

In the Scarlet Letter Study, this motive for recognition and reaction was paramount. Rather than being obsequious and overly pleasant, and instead of responding with despondent resignation, these targets went out of their way to provoke responses from the sources. One target plastered an "O" on his head simply to get a laugh (and when he got an angry response from one of the sources he felt exhilarated!). Our chat-room participants often fill their screens with questions and sarcastic provocative remarks, forcing the other chatters to notice their virtual presence. And, in our interviews with long-term targets, we have noted several who at some point in the ostracism process tried to provoke a response even if it was an angry response. They insulted, yelled at, and sometimes threw objects at the source just so they would be recognized—just to get a reaction, any reaction. Thus, rather than always expecting that targets will attempt to behave in ways that will facilitate their readmission into groups, under some circumstances or with certain people, we might expect behaviors that, instead, demand recognition of any sort.

James (1890) said it was important to be recognized, and to be recognized favorably. I suggest that at some point, it becomes sufficient to be recognized, favorably or not. This sort of reaction is consistent with what would be expected from experiencing diminished control and loss of meaningful existence. To regain control and to reaffirm that one's existence has meaning and consequence simply requires obtaining recognition from others and forcing them to change their behavior. If regaining control and meaningful existence takes precedence over belonging and self-esteem, then rather than trying to improve one's appeal to others in order to be accepted (belonging) and appreciated (self-esteem), we might expect that any type of provocative behavior will surface, even if it can be characterized as antisocial. To provoke recognition and reaction from others, even (or especially) antisocial acts are likely candidates.

Recently, Tice et al. (in press) conducted a series of experiments on reactions to social exclusion. All led to reactions that could not be considered to enhance the belongingness status of the target, but instead were indicative of provocative, even antisocial, behavior. After being actively rejected by others, or even when simply primed with rejection cues, their participants (compared to others who were included or who received alternative aversive consequences) gave negative and damaging assessments to a job applicant, cheated on tests, helped less, thought others to be less attractive, and competed more in a game in which cooperation would be most mutually beneficial. Although the authors found that exclusion and rejection leads to antisocial behaviors, I think it is just as plausible to suggest that their participants were merely attempting to regain a sense of control or recognition. Participants may have felt that their negative evaluations of the job applicant would have a tangible consequence, thus giving them a sense of control. Participants who disobeyed examination instructions took control. Saying no to a requested favor demonstrates taking control. Perceiving others as unattractive and not wanting to form bonds with them allows the target to control the social situation rather than putting themselves in the situation in which someone else can (once again) reject them. And, by competing in a zero-sum game, participants can effectively determine (control) the outcome for both participants (even though it is a negative outcome). If they chose to cooperate, their outcomes would depend upon what their partner chose to do.

Clearly, reactions to ostracism or other forms of rejection can vary widely, from increasing attempts to contribute to groups (Ezrakhovich et al., 1998; Williams & Sommer, 1997), to conforming to others (Williams et al., 2000), to behaving in such ways that practically assure future rejection (Tice et al., in press). Two students at Columbine High School in Colorado claimed that their peers ostracized them. Their reaction to this ostracism was not to conform to the larger group so that they could achieve acceptance and inclusion, but instead to lash back at these students with bombs and guns. The key question is, Under what conditions will targets attempt to improve their image and strengthen their need to belong, and under what conditions will they choose to take control, even to the extent that their behaviors become antisocial and violent?

FUTURE RESEARCH

In this section, I briefly consider several questions that merit future attention.

Is Ostracism Ever Positive?

Paul Tillich is widely attributed for saying, "Our language has wisely sensed the two sides of man's being alone. It has created the word 'loneliness' to express the pain of being alone, and it has created the word 'solitude' to express the glory of being alone." When I discuss the silent treatment on a radio program, someone from the audience invariably calls in saying, "I wish my wife [or husband] would give me the silent treatment!" My former colleague told me he longed for just one day in which students would ostracize him. Celebrities often resort to disguise so that they will not be recognized in public. Are these desires to be ignored and excluded genuine? My guess is that for people who are overstimulated by inclusion and conspicuity, ostracism might just provide the haven they seek. Whether they would enjoy being unseen and unheard for long periods of time is another matter. I would venture to say they would not. Indeed, there may be an optimum amount of social stimulation and recognition that people desire, and this level can be overachieved as well as underachieved. Although my focus so far has assumed that withdrawal of attention and inclusion is threatening, it would be worthwhile to investigate if and when such withdrawal was preferred or enjoyed, and for how long it is appreciated.

Time-Out as a Disciplinary Method

It is common practice in most school systems and in many homes to discipline children using some form of "time-out" procedure. Though considered socially acceptable, time-out is, strictly speaking, a form of ostracism. As we have seen, many forms of ostracism have deleterious psychological and physiological effects on its targets. A perusal of the time-out literature suggests a primarily atheoretical approach that relies heavily on case studies. The interesting thing about these case studies is that there does not appear to be a uniform agreement on what exactly constitutes time-out. Sometimes students are sent to detention rooms to sit alone for an unspecified duration. Sometimes students remain in class, sitting in their seats, but are designated either verbally or by donning an armband or some other symbolic article that they are not to be spoken to or given any attention by anyone in the classroom. There are myriad variations between these two extremes. Which of these is most effective for obtaining discipline, and which might provoke unwanted side effects, does not seem to be known.

There appears to be no substantive review article or meta-analysis of this literature that speaks to the overall effectiveness of time-out, or even to which forms of time-out are more effective than others. Using the dimensions listed within the model, it would be worthwhile to conduct a meta-analysis of the time-out literature, testing theory-derived hypotheses that certain types of time-out will be effective behaviorally and emotionally, whereas others may have unintended behavioral and/or emotional side effects. With such an analysis, precise predictions using experimental research in the laboratory and in the field could instruct us as to if, and how, time-out could be best implemented. Take, for example, a student who is socially ostracized within the classroom for an unspecified period of time. If the primary threat is to belonging, then some students may improve their behavior so that they will be more accepted by others in the class. However, if students are repeatedly given time-out, they may accept the label of deviant and outsider, thus becoming *more* alienated from the class. Likewise, if control is primarily threatened, then one way to regain control is to become more disruptive. If recognition is most desired, then it may be more important for students to provoke responses, even negative ones, rather than feeling invisible.

Physiological Effects of Ostracism

In Chapter 1, I reported that others found that ostracism may have detrimental physiological and health-related consequences (McGuire & Raleigh, 1986). However, this research comes primarily from observing nonhuman primates who have been separated from their peers. Similarly, studies examining the health-related consequences of ostracism-like circumstances in humans (e.g., Kiecolt-Glaser, Cacioppo, Malarkey, & Glaser, 1992) have focused on individuals who have been isolated from social contact. Thus only physical ostracism has been examined, and only in a few studies. Likewise, questions regarding health-related consequences of ostracism in humans have tended to focus only on the targets. To understand the nature of ostracism further, there is a need to assess the physiological and health-related effects for both targets and sources of ostracism. Currently, Lisa Zadro and I are investigating the physiological impact on targets of short-term ostracism. We have found some evidence of physiological challenge and stress even for 4 minutes of cyberostracism. Studies are now being conducted in our laboratory that further test the short-term physiological consequences of ostracism. We are also accumulating self-report data on stress and physical symptoms following short- and long-term episodes of ostracism. Finally, Ciarocco et al. (2001) have reported that engaging in exclusionary behavior, such as ignoring someone, depletes cognitive resources. Might it also impact negatively on sources' physiological and health-related responses? One aim of Lisa Zadro's dissertation research is to assess the short- and long-term physiological and health-related consequences of social ostracism in terms of the effect on specific physiological structures (such as the cardiovascular system) and general overall health. She plans to examine the responses of both targets and sources to social ostracism.

Being Disowned

Another topic we hope to examine is the phenomenon of being disowned or disinherited. How do people react after their parents say to them, "You are no longer my child" or "You are not a member of our family"? Only a few articles have been written on this potentially devastating form of ostracism, so we hope to conduct structured interviews with both targets and sources. This may not only provide us with more information about long-term ostracism, but might go beyond the effects of the silent treatment. Being disowned, perhaps more than any other form of ostracism, deprives individuals of their strongest, most permanent bonds, and the roots to which their existence is tied.

Ostracizing Groups

So far, our research has concentrated on ostracism of individuals. What happens when small groups are ostracized? The significance of this question is apparent when we observe recent news reports of violent behavior by *small groups* of individuals who claim to be ostracized and marginalized by larger groups. The two students from Columbine High School mentioned earlier turned to guns and bombs to exact revenge for being ostracized by the other students in the school. Perhaps ostracized groups are more likely than ostracized individuals to act aggressively. Such incidences demand that we understand how groups of individuals who are ostracized feel and behave. Using our ball-tossing or cyberball paradigms, we could investigate how individuals react toward and with others who are also ostracized. My hunch is that targets of ostracism will form strong bonds with one another, and that they will feel empowered and motivated to act out in ways that will regain their sense of control and command recognition.

Another important line of research would be to examine the preexisting relationship between the target and other group members. Considerable research and theory has been devoted recently toward understanding how individuals define themselves in relation to groups, and how one's in-group, compared to one's out-group, differentially affects cognition, emotion, and behavior (for a review, see Hogg & Williams, 2000). Already in our cyberostracism studies (Williams et al., 2000) we have observed tendencies for targets to be less affected when out-group members, compared to in-group or mixed-group members, ostracized them. Undoubtedly, additional research will uncover other important aspects of the relation of others to self with respect to being ostracized and to ostracizing.

Coping with Ostracism

Probably the most frequent question I get from people and the media is, "If a person is being ostracized, how does he or she stop it?" The answer to this question is particularly important to individuals who are on the receiving end of continuous or repeated bouts of the silent treatment given to them by a significant other. Interestingly, we also get this question from chronic users of the silent treatment. They feel that the tactic has become so second nature to them that they don't know how to stop. They also realize that it usually works to their advantage, which also makes it hard to stop. It is perhaps because this is such a difficult question to answer, both intuitively and from research, that ostracism, particularly the silent treatment, is so pervasive. If it were easy to deal with, its power and effectiveness would be severely limited, and consequently it would be used less frequently.

Nevertheless, based in part on the various dimensions of ostracism that I lay out in the model, and in part from suggestions offered from long-term targets of ostracism, some courses of action appear more promising than others. I will first make some suggestions to chronic sources of the silent treatment. If you really want to stop using it, shift from employing social ostracism to physical ostracism. That is, instead of pretending your partner, relative, or friend doesn't exist while maintaining a physical presence with him or her, simply leave his or her presence. Go out for a walk or take in a movie. Getting away will allow you to think through whatever it was that made you angry, and will not simultaneously escalate your and your target's emotional reactions. Having to maintain such a pretense depletes your cognitive resources, preventing you from thinking rationally about the problem.

Also, committing oneself to a public stance of ignoring makes it difficult to reverse that commitment. With social ostracism there is no clear stopping point for your behavior. In order to save face and not look foolish, you not only continue it, but you may justify your behavior by manufacturing additional reasons for its use. Thus, your anger grows instead of diminishing. With physical ostracism, your eventual reunion with the target can be used as a temporal marker for change. Once you are again with your target, you can take the opportunity, without losing face, to say, "Okay, let's talk about it." Doing so seems more natural than having to pick an arbitrary point during social ostracism to move toward discussion. Even better, before exiting, if you said something like, "I need some time alone; I'll be back in 2 hours," then one aspect of ostracism's ambiguity would be removed, making it easier for your target to deal with his or her own behavior that may have triggered your anger, rather than forcing him or her to worry about *whether* you would return.

As for targets, what is the best course of action if you suddenly find yourself being given the silent treatment? Clearly, from laboratory, role plays, and interviews, we are aware of many common responses. One is to provoke a reaction from the source. This, of course, can be quite risky and self-defeating if the provocation is such that you are saying or doing harmful things to the source. Throwing a marble ashtray at his or her head may get a response, but it certainly won't be the sort of response that will improve the situation. Neither would hurling insults or bringing up more fodder from past disagreements. Even trying to provoke laughter may be unhelpful if it sends a message to the source that his or her anger is trivial and unimportant. Another common response is to retaliate with silence. If he or she pretends you don't exist, then you can pretend he or she doesn't exist too. Such reciprocity hardly seems helpful. It creates a contest of wills and makes it a certainty that the ostracism will last longer. Neither person wants to be the first to break down, so the silence goes on and on and on. Both provocation and retaliation, of course, give targets an immediate sense of control, which is probably why these responses are so common. But control is illusory and may eventually result in less control. Soon the commitment to silence will control you. As the father who wrote about his use of ostracism on his son said, "Ostracism can be like a whirlpool, or quicksand, if you, the user, don't extract yourself from it as soon as possible, it is likely to become impossible to terminate regardless of the emergence of any subsequent will to do so."

So, what is left to do? Because social ostracism is a continual reminder of being ignored, of being a nonentity, perhaps the best course of action would be to remove yourself from the "social death" to which you are being subjected. Leaving the social presence of the source will permit you and the source to reflect on the problem without having to maintain and be subjected to the pretense. As I suggested for sources, it may even be better if before leaving, you say something like, "I'm going to go out for a walk; let's try talking about this when I get back." And then, when you return, be willing to make the suggestion that you now discuss the problem. Of course, there is no guarantee that the source, particularly if he or she is stubborn, will now stop the silence. Targets must not allow themselves to be controlled by it. Once it is clear to the source that the silence is effective, he or she is reinforced for engaging in this tactic, and will use it again and again.

One of our targets of continuous silent treatments from her husband said that initially, she was devastated by his use of this tactic. She tried various counterattacks, like provocation and retaliation, but these reactions only seemed to make things worse. Finally she had a revelation: this is what her husband does, and he eventually gets over it. She accepted it and didn't let it bother her. Rather than resigning herself to its use on her, she continued as though it wasn't happening. She persisted in having a conversation, albeit one-sided, with her husband and acted as though he were answering. She'd include him in her thoughts and in her activities. She would even grab his arm and take him on walks or shopping. She found that he would begin interacting with her sooner this way. Whether or not her method of reacting would work similarly well for others is open to question, but she may be on to something. She appears to maintain her sense of belonging, control, self-esteem, and meaningful existence without making things worse in the process.

I have been discussing chronic ostracism as though it was something inherent in the source, which sometimes it appears to be. But what if one finds him- or herself on the receiving end of ostracism and the silent treatment from a variety of independent sources? Blame cannot always be shouldered by the source. This may mean that there is something in the target's behavior that elicits ostracism from others. If so, thoughtful self-analysis would seem to be in order. If individuals outshout their partners, or refuse to listen and consider what others are saying, then the other people may feel their only alternative is simply to go silent.

The most extreme response would be to extricate oneself permanently from such treatment. Indeed, our analysis of narratives that people wrote about their experience with the silent treatment suggested that individuals high in self-esteem were more likely to exit relationships in which they were targets of the silent treatment. Because these individuals had high self-esteem, they knew there were better alternatives waiting for them outside the relationship. This is a big and permanent response, and should give pause to people who chronically use it as a tactic of social influence. It may result in the complete loss of a relationship.

Future research could experimentally test remedies to the impact of ostracism. Guided by the propositions of my model, inoculation may be one way to guard against its impact. If the needs (i.e., belonging, control, self-esteem, and meaningful existence) were fortified prior to ostracism, would targets be shielded against its effects? For example, would it be sufficient simply to ask people to write down important groups to which they belong prior to being ostracized? Others (Sommer et al., in press; Tice et al., in press) have found that exposing individuals to subconscious primes of rejection and exclusion concepts results in negative consequences that are similar to more dramatic forms of ostracism. If targets are primed with inclusion and social recognition primes, might they be more resistant to acts of ostracism?

Advice to Those in Relationships in Which the Silent Treatment Is Used

It is, of course, too early in the course of our investigations to be confident in dispensing advice. Nonetheless, I am always asked for advice when I talk about the silent treatment. I cautiously suggest the following advice to sources:

- Refrain from using the silent treatment; its effects are far more damaging to the relationship than you probably imagine.
- If you must give it, say that you are upset, that you don't wish to talk because you need some time to yourself; and that you will come back and discuss the matter in a specified amount of time (preferably, no longer than a few hours). That way, the target is aware that it is occurring, why it is occurring, and that it will end.
- It is probably better to remove yourself physically from the situation for a while than to maintain the silent treatment in the presence of the target. Cooling off and giving oneself the necessary time-out are easier if one is not engaged in constant effortful attempts to pretend that the target does not exist.
- I am not so willing to give any advice at this time to targets. It is much easier to suggest that the silent treatment not be used, or if it is, how it should be done, than to say how someone should deal with it. The best I can suggest at this point is to be aware of signs that you are shifting from coping with acts of ostracism by attempting to regain the needs that have been threatened, to accepting the insidious message that ostracism delivers (that one is cut

off, helpless, bad, and meaningless). When these signs surface, exiting the group or the relationship may be the best option.

CONCLUSIONS

Ostracism is ubiquitous and powerful. Fear of rejection and exclusion has for years been assumed to explain the power of groups to influence individuals. In order to belong and be included, we conform, comply, obey, engage in groupthink, stereotype out-groups, and inhibit prosocial tendencies. If we persist in resisting the group, we risk being excluded, ignored, and rejected; we risk being ostracized. Within minutes, ostracism chips away at our senses of belonging, control, self-esteem, and meaningful existence. As a consequence, we grasp for opportunities to rebuild what ostracism removed. If we fail to do so, repeated exposure to ostracism may leave us defenseless. We may accept our fate; we may feel alienated and marginalized, helpless, depressed, and worthy of no better treatment.

We need to devote our attention to understanding why ostracism is used, when it is used, how it affects those who use it, and, perhaps most importantly, how it affects those who are subjected to it. The model presented in this book offers a framework to guide such investigations. The results of the research thus far provides initial support to several of its propositions. We have just scratched the surface, asking more questions than we have answered. It is my hope that by turning our attention to what happens during ostracism, rather than on why we avoid it, we will gain a better understanding of this fundamental social process.

References

Abbott, E. (1911). *A history of Greece: Part II*. New York: Longmans, Green.

Abrams, D., & Hogg, M. (1990). *Social identity theory: Constructive and critical advances*. New York: Springer-Verlag.

Ainsworth, M. S. (1989). Attachments beyond infancy. *American Psychologist, 44*, 709–716.

Alexander, R. D. (1986). Ostracism and indirect reciprocity: The reproductive significance of humor. *Ethology and Sociobiology, 7*, 253–270.

Allerton, M. (1998, May–June). Time's up for exclusionary time out. *PsychDD Newsletter, 36*, 5–9.

Asch, S. E. (1956). Studies of independence and conformity: A minority of one against a unanimous majority. *Psychological Monographs, 70*(9, Whole No. 416).

Asher, S. R., & Coie, J. D. (Eds.). (1990). *Peer rejection in childhood*. New York: Cambridge University Press.

Asher, S. R., & Parker, J. G. (1989). Significance of peer relationship problems in childhood. In B. H. Schneider, G. Attili, J. Nadel, & R. P. Weissberg (Eds.), *Social competence in developmental perspective* (pp. 5–23). Amsterdam: Kluwer Academic.

Australian Bureau of Statistics. (1997). *Part time, casual and temporary employment*. Canberra: Australian Government Publishing.

Baldwin, M. W., & Sinclair, L. (1996). Self-esteem and "If . . . then" contingencies of interpersonal acceptance. *Journal of Personality and Social Psychology, 71*, 1130–1141.

Bandura, A. (1997). *Self-efficacy: The exercise of control*. New York: Freeman.

Barner-Barry, C. (1986). Rob: Children's tacit use of peer ostracism to control aggressive behavior. *Ethology and Sociobiology, 7*, 281–293.

Barnett, P. A., & Gotlib, I. H. (1988). Dysfunctional attitudes and psychosocial stress: The differential prediction of future psychological symptomatology. *Motivation and Emotion, 12*, 251–270.

Bartholomew, K., & Horowitz, L. M. (1991). Attachment styles among young adults: A test of a four-category model. *Journal of Personality and Social Psychology, 61*, 226–244.

Basso, K. H. (1972). "To give up on words": Silence in Western Apache culture.

In P. P. Giglioli (Ed.), *Language and social context* (pp. 67–86). Baltimore: Penguin Books.

Baumeister, R. F. (1994). Self-esteem. In V. S. Ramachandram (Ed.) *Encyclopedia of human behavior* (pp. 83–87). San Diego, CA: Academic Press.

Baumeister, R. F., & Catanese, K. (2001). Victims and perpetrators provide discrepant accounts: Motivated cognitive distortions about interpersonal transgressions. In J. P. Forgas, K. D. Williams, & L. Wheeler (Eds.), *The social mind: Cognitive and motivational aspects of interpersonal behavior* (pp. 274–293). London: Cambridge University Press.

Baumeister, R. F., & Leary, M. R. (1995). The need to belong: Desire for interpersonal attachments as a fundamental human motivation. *Psychological Bulletin, 117,* 497–529.

Baumeister, R. F., Stillwell, A., & Wotman, S. R. (1990). Victim and perpetrator accounts of interpersonal conflict: Autobiographical narratives about anger. *Journal of Personality and Social Psychology, 59,* 994–1005.

Baumeister, R. F., & Tice, D. M. (1990). Anxiety and social exclusion. *Journal of Social and Clinical Psychology, 9,* 165–195.

Baumeister, R. F., Wotman, S. R., & Stillwell, A. (1993). Unrequited love: On heartbreak, anger, guilt, scriptlessness, and humiliation. *Journal of Personality and Social Psychology, 64,* 377–394.

Beehr, T., Drexler, J., & Faulkner, S. (1997). Working in small family businesses: Empirical comparisons to non-family businesses. *Journal of Organizational Behavior, 18,* 297–312.

Bettencourt, L. A. (1997). Customer voluntary performance: Customers as partners in service delivery. *Journal of Retailing, 73,* 383–406.

Blascovich, J., & Mendes, W. B. (2000). Challenge and threat appraisals: The role of affective cues. In J. P. Forgas (Ed.), *Feeling and thinking: The role of affect in social cognition* (pp. 59–82). New York: Cambridge University Press.

Boehm, C. (1986). Capital punishment in tribal Montenegro: Implications for law, biology, and theory of social control. *Ethology and Sociobiology, 7,* 305–320.

Boekmann, R. (2000, April). *Individual differences in attachment style may affect adults' propensity to be vigilant or trusting of equity/fairness in adult romantic relationships.* Paper presented at the meeting of the Society of Australasian Social Psychology, Fremantle, Australia.

Bowlby, J. (1977). The making and breaking of affectional bonds. *British Journal of Psychiatry, 130,* 201–210.

Brooks, N. C., Perry, V., & Hingerty, S. E. (1992). Modifying behavior through time out from positive reinforcement. *Vocational Evaluation and Work Adjustment Bulletin, 25,* 93–95.

Bruneau, T. J. (1973). Communicative silences: Forms and functions. *Journal of Communication, 23,* 17–46.

Burger, J. M. (1992). *Desire for control: Personality, social and clinical perspectives.* New York: Plenum Press.

Burger, J. M. (1995). Need for control and self-esteem: Two routes to a high desire for control. In M. H. Kernis (Ed.), *Efficacy, agency, and self-esteem* (pp. 217–233). New York: Plenum Press.

Buss, D. M. (1990). The evolution of anxiety and social exclusion. *Journal of Social and Clinical Psychology, 9,* 196–201.

Buss, D. M. (1992). Manipulation in close relationships: Five personality factors in interactional context. *Journal of Personality, 60,* 477–499.

Buss, D. M., Gomes, M., Higgins, D. S., & Lauterbach, K. (1987). Tactics of manipulation. *Journal of Personality and Social Psychology, 52,* 1219–1229.

Cairns, R. B., & Cairns, B. D. (1991). Social cognition and social networks: A developmental perspective. In D. J. Pepler, & K. H. Rubin (Eds.), *The development and treatment of childhood aggression* (pp. 249–278). Hillsdale, NJ: Erlbaum.

Cairns, R. B., Cairns, B. D., Neckerman, H. J., & Ferguson, L. L. (1989). Growth and aggression: 1. Childhood to early adolescence. *Developmental Psychology, 25,* 320–330.

Cannon, W. B. (1942). "Voodoo" death. *American Anthropologist, 2,* 169–181.

Cardarelli, R. (Producer), & Wertmüller, L. (Director). (1975). *Swept away . . . By an unusual destiny in the blue sea of August* [film]. (Available from Amazon.com)

Carver, C. S., & Scheier, M. F. (1978). Self-focussing effects of dispositional self-consciousness, mirror presence, and audience presence. *Journal of Personality and Social Psychology, 36,* 324–332.

Chen, M., Froehle, T., & Morran, K. (1997). Deconstructing dispositional bias in clinical inference: Two interventions. *Journal of Counseling and Development, 76,* 74–81.

Cheung, C. K. T. (1999). *Ostracizing clients on the Internet: The effects of not responding to electronic mail inquiries.* Unpublished master's thesis, University of New South Wales, Sydney, Australia.

Cialdini, R. B. (1993). *Influence: Science and practice* (3rd ed.). New York: HarperCollins.

Ciarocco, N. S., Sommer, K. L., & Baumeister, R. F. (2001). Ostracism and ego depletion: The strains of silence. *Personality and Social Psychology Bulletin, 27,* 1156–1163.

Cooley, C. H. (1902). *Human nature and the social order.* New York: Scribner's.

Cowley Internet. (1997). *Cowley small business newsletter: February 1997* [Online] Available: http://www.cowleys.com.au/public/newscsn3.htm.

Craighead, W. E., Kimball, W. H., & Rehak, P. J. (1979). Mood changes, physiological responses, and self-statements during social rejection imagery. *Journal of Consulting and Clinical Psychology, 47,* 385–396.

Crosby, L. A., Evans, K. R., & Cowles, D. (1990). Relationship quality in services selling: An interpersonal influence perspective. *Journal of Marketing, 54,* 68–81.

Curley, S. P., Yates, J. F., & Abrams, R. A. (1986). Psychological sources of ambiguity avoidance. *Organizational Behavior and Human Decision Processes, 38,* 230–256.

Davis, B. O. (1991). *Benjamin O. Davis, Jr., American: An autobiography.* Washington, DC: Smithsonian Institution Press.

Davis-Blake, A., & Uzzi, B. (1993). Determinants of employment externalization: A study of temps and independent contractors. *Administrative Science Quarterly, 38,* 195–223.

Deci, E. L., & Ryan, R. M. (1995). Human autonomy: The basis for true self-esteem. In M. H. Kernis (Ed.), *Efficacy, agency, and self-esteem* (pp. 31–49). New York: Plenum Press.

DePaulo, B. M. (1992). Nonverbal behavior and self-presentation. *Psychological Bulletin, 111,* 203–243.

DePaulo, B. M., Kashy, D. A., Kirkendol, S. E., Wyer, M. M., & Epstein, J. A. (1996). Lying in everyday life. *Journal of Personality and Social Psychology, 70,* 979–995.

de Waal, F. B. M. (1986). The brutal elimination of a rival among captive male chimpanzees. *Ethology and Sociobiology, 7,* 237–251.

Dittes, J. E. (1959). Attractiveness of group as function of self-esteem and acceptance by group. *Journal of Abnormal and Social Psychology, 59,* 77–82.

Dodge, K. A., Pettit, G. S., McClaskey, C. L., & Brown, M. M. (1986). Social competence in children. *Monographs of the Society for Research in Child Development, 51*(2, Serial No. 213).

Duck, S., Rutt, D. J., Hurst, M. H., & Strejc, H. (1991). Some evident truth about conversation in everyday relationships: All communications are not created equal. *Human Communication Research, 18,* 228–267.

Ekman, P., & Friesen, W. V. (1969). Nonverbal leakage and clues to deception. *Psychiatry, 32,* 88–106.

Ellison, R. (1952). *Invisible man.* New York: Quality Paperback Book Club.

Ewing, D. (1983). *Do it my way or you're fired!: Employee rights and the changing role of management prerogatives.* New York: Wiley.

Ezrakhovich, A., Kerr, A., Cheung, S., Elliot, K., Jerrems, A., & Williams, K. D. (1998, April). *Effects of causal clarity of ostracism on individual performance in groups.* Paper presented at the symposium on "Social Psychology on the Web," Society for Australasian Social Psychology, Christchurch, New Zealand.

Falbo, T. (1977). Multidimensional scaling of power strategies. *Journal of Personality and Social Psychology, 35,* 537–547.

Falbo, T., & Peplau, L. A. (1980). Power strategies in intimate relationships. *Journal of Personality and Social Psychology, 38,* 618–628.

Faulkner, S. J. (1998). *After the whistle is blown: The aversive impact of ostracism.* Unpublished doctoral dissertation, University of Toledo.

Faulkner, S. J., & Williams, K. D. (1995, May). *The causes and consequences of social ostracism: A qualitative analysis.* Paper presented at the 67th annual meeting of the Midwestern Psychological Association, Chicago.

Faulkner, S. J., & Williams, K. D. (1997, May). *Interviews with long-term targets and sources of the silent treatment.* Paper presented at the 69th annual meeting of the Midwestern Psychological Association, Chicago.

Faulkner, S. J., & Williams, K. D. (1999, April). *After the whistle is blown: The aversive impact of ostracism.* Paper presented at the 71st annual meeting of the Midwestern Psychological Association, Chicago.

Faulkner, S., Williams, K., Sherman, B., & Williams, E. (1997, May). *The "silent treatment": Its incidence and impact.* Paper presented at the 69th annual meeting of the Midwestern Psychological Association, Chicago.

Feldman, D. C., Doerpinghaus, H. I., & Turnley, W. H. (1994). Managing temps: A permanent HRM challenge. *Organizational Dynamics, 23*, 49–63.

Fenigstein, A. (1979). Self-consciousness, self-attention, and social interaction. *Journal of Personality and Social Psychology, 37*, 75–86.

Ferguson, O. (1944). Vocabulary for lakes, deep seas, and inland waters. *American Speech, 19*, 103–111.

Fontenot, R. J., & Wilson, E. J. (1997). Relational exchange: A review of selected models for prediction matrix of relationship activities. *Journal of Business Research, 39*, 5–12.

Friedland, N., Keinan, G., & Regev, Y. (1992). Controlling the uncontrollable: Effects of stress on illusory perceptions of controllability. *Journal of Personality and Social Psychology, 63*, 923–931.

Frone, M. R. (1990). Intolerance of ambiguity as a moderator of the occupational role stress-strain relationship: A meta-analysis. *Journal of Organizational Behavior, 11*, 309–320.

Gada-Jain, N., & Bernieri, F. (1998). *Effects of rapport synchrony on perceptions of a job interviewee.* Unpublished data. University of Toledo, Toledo, OH.

Gallimore, R., Tharp, R. G., & Kemp, B. (1969). Positive reinforcing function of "negative attention." *Journal of Experimental Child Psychology, 8*, 140–146.

Garbarino, E, & Johnson, M. S. (1999). The different roles of satisfactions, trust, and commitment in customer relationships. *Journal of Marketing, 63*, 70–87.

Gardner, W., Pickett, C. L., & Brewer, M. B. (2000). Social exclusion and selective memory: How the need to belong influences memory for social events. *Personality and Social Psychology Bulletin, 26*, 486–496.

Geller, D. M., Goodstein, L., Silver, M., & Sternberg, W. C. (1974). On being ignored: The effects of violation of implicit rules of social interaction. *Sociometry, 37*, 541–556.

Gilbert, D. T. (1995). Attribution and interpersonal perception. In A. Tesser (Ed.), *Advanced social psychology* (pp. 99–147). New York: McGraw-Hill.

Goffman, E. (1963a). *Behavior in public places: Notes on the social organization of gatherings.* New York: Free Press.

Goffman, E. (1963b). *Stigma: Notes on the management of spoiled identity.* Englewood Cliffs, NJ: Prentice-Hall; New York: Simon & Schuster, 1986.

Goodall, J. (1986). Social rejection, exclusion, and shunning among the Gombe chimpanzees. *Ethology and Sociobiology, 7*, 227–236.

Gottman, J. M. (1979). *Marital interaction: Experimental investigations.* New York: Academic Press.

Gottman, J. M. (1980). Consistency of nonverbal affect and affect reciprocity in marital interaction. *Journal of Consulting and Clinical Psychology, 48*, 711–717.

Gottman, J. M., & Krokoff, L. J. (1992). Marital interaction and satisfaction: A longitudinal view. *Journal of Consulting and Clinical Psychology, 57*, 47–52.

Graphics, Visualization, and Usability Center. (1998, December). 10th WWW

User Survey. [On-line] Available: http://www.gvu.gatech.edu/user_surveys/ survey-1998-10/

Greenberg, J., Pyszczynski, T., & Solomon, S. (1986). The causes and consequences of the need for self-esteem: A terror management theory. In R. F. Baumeister (Ed.), *Public self and private self* (pp. 189–212). New York: Springer-Verlag.

Greenberg, J., Pyszczynski, T., Solomon, S., Rosenblatt, A., Veeder, M., Kirkland, S., & Lyon, D. (1990). Evidence for terror management theory, 2: The effects of mortality salience on reactions to those who threaten or bolster the cultural worldview. *Journal of Personality and Social Psychology, 58,* 308–318.

Greenberg, J., Solomon, S., Pyszczynski, T., Rosenblatt, A., Burling, J., Lyon, D., Simon, L., & Pinel, E. (1992). Why do people need self-esteem?: Converging evidence that self-esteem serves an anxiety-buffering function. *Journal of Personality and Social Psychology, 63,* 913–922.

Greenberger, D., Miceli, M., & Cohen, D. (1987). Oppositionists and group norms: The reciprocal influence of whistleblowers and co-workers. *Journal of Social Issues, 47,* 111–128.

Greenhaus, J. H., & Beutell, N. J. (1985). Sources of conflict between work and family roles. *Academy of Management Review, 10,* 76–88.

Greenwald, A. G. (1980). The totalitarian ego: Fabrication and revision of personal history. *American Psychologist, 35,* 603–618.

Gruter, M. (1986). Ostracism on trial: The limits of individual rights. *Ethology and Sociobiology, 7,* 271–279.

Gruter, M., & Masters, R. D. (1986a). Ostracism as a social and biological phenomenon: An introduction. *Ethology and Sociobiology, 7,* 149–158.

Gruter, M., & Masters, R. D. (Eds.). (1986b). Ostracism: A social and biological phenomenon. *Ethology and Sociobiology, 7,* 149–395.

Gummesson, E. (1994). Making relationship marketing operational. *International Journal of Service Industry Management, 5,* 5–20.

Gwinner, K. P., Gremler, D. D., & Bitner, M. J. (1998). Relational benefits in service industries: The customer's perspective. *Journal of the Academy of Marketing Science, 26,* 101–114.

Haney, C., Banks, W. C., & Zimbardo, P. (1973). Interpersonal dynamics in a simulated prison. *International Journal of Criminology and Penology, 1,* 69–97.

Haney, C., & Zimbardo, P. (1998). The past and future of U.S. prison policy: Twenty-five years after the Stanford Prison Experiment. *American Psychologist, 53,* 709–727.

Harris, S. (1998, September 20). Pay-out after boy locked in cupboard. *Sydney Sunday Telegraph,* p. 35.

Harter, S. (1993). Causes and consequences of low self-esteem in children and adolescents. In R. F. Baumeister (Ed.), *Self-esteem: The puzzle of low self-regard* (pp. 87–116). New York: Plenum Press.

Hazan, C., & Shaver, P. (1987). Conceptualizing romantic love as an attachment process. *Journal of Personality and Social Psychology, 52,* 511–524.

Heider, F. (1958). *The psychology of interpersonal relations.* New York: Wiley.

Henson, K. D. (1996). *Just a temp*. Philadelphia: Temple University Press.

Herman, C. P., Polivy, J., Lank, C. N., & Heatherton, T. F. (1987). Anxiety, hunger, and eating behavior. *Journal of Abnormal Psychology, 96*, 264–269.

Heron, T. E. (1987). Timeout from positive reinforcement. In I. O. Cooper, T. E. Heron, & H. Merrill (Eds.), *Applied behavior analysis* (pp. 439–453). Columbus, OH: Merrill.

Hogg, M. A., & Abrams, D. (1988). *Social identifications: A social psychology of intergroup relations and group processes*. London: Routledge.

Hogg, M., & Williams, K. D. (2000). From "me" to "we": Social identity and the collective self. *Group Dynamics: Theory, Research and Practice, 4*, 81–97.

Insko, C. A., & Wilson, M. (1977). Interpersonal attraction as a function of social interaction. *Journal of Personality and Social Psychology, 35*, 903–911.

International Data Corporation. (1999, September). *The globalization of ecommerce* (Bulletin #NL99MR04-Giraldo, A.). http://www.idcresearch.nl/countrynetpub/moreinfo.lp?did=400437.

Jackson, J. M., & Saltzstein, H. D. (1957). The effect of person–group relationships on conformity processes. *Journal of Abnormal and Social Psychology, 57*, 17–24.

James, W. (1890). *Principles of psychology* (Vol. 1). New York: Dover.

Janoff-Bulman, R., & Wortman, C. B. (1977). Attributions of blame and coping in the "real world": Severe accident victims react to their lot. *Journal of Personality and Social Psychology, 35*, 351–363.

Jensen, J. (1987). Ethical tension points in whistleblowing. *Journal of Business Ethics, 6*, 527–542.

Jones, E. E. (1990). *Interpersonal perception*. New York: Macmillan.

Jones, E. E., & Davis, K. E. (1965). From acts to dispositions: The attribution process in person perception. In L. Berkowitz (Ed.), *Advances in experimental social psychology* (Vol. 2, pp. 219–266). New York: Academic Press.

Karau, S. J., & Williams, K. D. (1993). Social loafing: A meta-analytic review and theoretical integration. *Journal of Personality and Social Psychology, 65*, 681–706.

Karau, S. J., & Williams, K. D. (1997). The effects of group cohesion on social loafing and social compensation. *Group Dynamics: Theory, Research, and Practice, 1*, 156–168.

Keinan, G. (1994). Effects of stress and tolerance of ambiguity on magical thinking. *Journal of Personality and Social Psychology, 67*, 48–55.

Kelley, H. H., & Thibaut, J. W. (1978). *Interpersonal relations: A theory of interdependence*. New York: Wiley.

Kelley, S. W., & Davis, M. A. (1994). Antecedents to customer expectations for service recovery. *Journal of the Academy of Marketing Science, 22*, 52–61.

Kennedy, W. (1987, November 29). Military uses exam to curb whistleblowers. *Christian Science Monitor*, p. B1.

Kiecolt-Glaser, J. K., Cacioppo, J. T., Mclarkey, W. B., & Glaser, R. (1992). Acute physiological stressors and short-term immune changes: What, why, for whom, and to what extent? *Psychosomatic Medicine, 54*, 680–685.

King, M. G., Burrows, G. D., & Stanley, G. V. (1983). Measurement of stress and arousal: Validation of the stress/arousal adjective checklist. *British Journal of Psychology, 74,* 473–479.

Kipnis, D. (1984). The use of power in organizations and in interpersonal settings. In S. Oskamp (Ed.), *Applied social psychology annual* (Vol. 5, pp. 179–210). Newbury Park, CA: Sage.

Kipnis, D., Schmidt, S. M., & Wilkinson, I. (1980). Intraorganizational influence tactics: Explorations in getting one's way. *Journal of Applied Psychology, 65,* 440–452.

Kling, A. S. (1986). Neurological correlates of social behavior. *Ethology and Sociobiology, 7,* 175–186.

Ko, T. (1994). *Social ostracism and social identity.* Unpublished master's thesis, University of Toledo, Toledo, OH.

Kramer, R. M. (1994). The sinister attribution error: Paranoid cognition and collective distrust in groups and organizations. *Motivation and Emotion, 18,* 199–229.

Kraut, R., Patterson, M., Lundmark, V., Kiesler, S., Mukopahdyay, T., & Scherlis, W. (1998). Internet paradox: A social technology that reduces social involvement and psychological well-being? *American Psychologist, 53,* 1017–1031.

Ladouceur, R., Talbot, F., & Dugas, M. (1997). Behavioral expressions of intolerance of uncertainty in worry. *Behavior Modification, 21,* 355–371.

Lancaster, J. B. (1986). Primate social behavior and ostracism. *Ethology and Sociobiology, 7,* 215–225.

Latané, B. (1981). The psychology of social impact. *American Psychologist, 36,* 343–356.

Latané, B., & Darley, J. M. (1970). *The unresponsive bystander: Why doesn't he help?* New York: Appleton-Century-Crofts.

Latané, B., Williams, K. D., & Harkins, S. G. (1979). Many hands make light the work: The causes and consequences of social loafing. *Journal of Personality and Social Psychology, 37,* 822–832.

Lawson Williams, H., & Williams, K. D. (1998, April). *Effects of social ostracism on desire for control.* Paper presented at the meeting of the Society for Australasian Social Psychology, Christchurch, New Zealand.

Leary, M. R. (1990). Responses to social exclusion: Social anxiety, jealousy, loneliness, depression, and low self-esteem. *Journal of Social and Clinical Psychology, 9,* 221–229.

Leary, M. R., & Kowalski, R. M. (1995). *Social anxiety.* New York: Guilford Press.

Leary, M. R., Tambor, E. S., Terdal, S. K., & Downs, D. L. (1995). Self-esteem as an interpersonal monitor: The sociometer hypothesis. *Journal of Personality and Social Psychology, 68,* 518–530.

Lee, T. W., & Johnson, D. R. (1991). The effects of work schedule and employment status on the organizational commitment and job satisfaction of full versus part time employees. *Journal of Vocational Behavior, 38,* 208–224.

Mackay, C., Cox, T., Burrows, G., & Lazzerini, T. (1978). An inventory for the measurement of self-reported stress and arousal. *British Journal of Social and Clinical Psychology, 17,* 283–284.

Mahdi, N. Q. (1986). Pukhtunwali: Ostracism and honor among the Pathan Hill Tribes. *Ethology and Sociobiology, 7,* 295–304.

Marks, G., & Miller, N. (1987). Ten years of research on the false consensus effect: An empirical and theoretical review. *Psychological Bulletin, 102,* 72–90.

Matrix Information and Directory Services. (1997). *1997 Users and Hosts of the Internet and the Matrix* [Online]. Available: http://www.mids.org/press/pr9701.html.

McGuire, M. T., & Raleigh, M. J. (1986). Behavioral and physiological correlates of ostracism. *Ethology and Sociobiology, 7,* 187–200.

McInnes, S. (1999). *Ostracism of the invisible worker.* Unpublished master's thesis, University of New South Wales, Sydney, Australia.

McKenna, M. (1997, April 13). Worker told goodbye after "ignoring" boss. *Sydney Telegraph,* p. A7.

Mead, G. H. (1934). *Mind, self, and society.* Chicago: University of Chicago Press.

Mettee, D. R., Taylor, S. E., & Fisher, S. (1971). The effect of being shunned upon the desire to affiliate. *Psychonomic Science, 23,* 429–431.

Miceli, M. P., & Near, J. P. (1992). *Blowing the whistle: The organizational and legal implications for companies and employees.* New York: Lexington Books.

Milgram, S. (1974). *Obedience to authority: An experimental view.* New York: Harper & Row.

Morgan, R. M., & Hunt, S. D. (1994). The commitment trust theory of relationship marketing. *Journal of Marketing, 58,* 20–38.

Moscovici, S. (1980). Towards a theory of conversion behavior. In L. Berkowitz (Ed.), *Advances in Experimental Social Psychology* (Vol. 13, pp. 209–239). New York: Academic Press.

Murray, S. L., Holmes, J. G., & Griffin, D. (1996). The self-fulfilling nature of positive illusions in romantic relationships: Love is not blind, but prescient. *Journal of Personality and Social Psychology, 71,* 1155–1180.

Murray, S. L., Holmes, J. G, MacDonald, G., & Ellsworth, P. C. (1998). Through the looking glass darkly?: When self-doubts turn into relationship insecurities. *Journal of Personality and Social Psychology, 75,* 1459–1480.

Nadasi, C. (1992). *The effects of social ostracism on verbal and non-verbal behavior in introverts and extraverts.* Unpublished honors thesis, University of Toledo, Toledo, OH.

Napolitan, D. A., & Goethals, G. R. (1979). The attribution of friendliness. *Journal of Experimental Social Psychology, 15,* 105–113.

Near, J., & Miceli, M. (1987). Whistleblowers in organizations: Dissidents or reformers? In B. M. Staw & L. L. Cummings (Eds.), *Research in organizational behavior* (pp. 321–368). Greenwich, CT: JAI Press.

Nezlek, J. B., Kowalski, R. M., Leary, M. R., Blevins, T., & Holgate, S. (1997). Personality moderators of reactions to interpersonal rejection: Depression and trait self-esteem. *Personality and Social Psychology Bulletin, 23*, 1235–1244.

Ockenden, P. (1999, October). Focus on research. *Australian PC Authority, 23*, 169–170.

O'Leary, S. G., & O'Leary, K. D. (1976). Behavior modification in the school. In H. Leitenberg (Ed.), *Handbook of behavior modification and behavior therapy* (pp. 475–515). Englewood Cliffs, NJ: Prentice-Hall.

Oliver, K., Zadro, L., Huon, G., & Williams, K. (2001). The role of interpersonal stress in overeating among high and low disinhibitors. *Eating Behaviors, 2*, 19–26.

Olweus, D. (1978). *Aggression in the schools: Bullies and whipping boys.* Washington, DC: Hemisphere.

Olweus, D. (1993). *Bullying at school: What we know and what we can do.* Oxford, UK: Blackwell.

Osterman, P. (1988). *Employment futures: Reorganization, dislocation, and public policy.* Oxford, UK: Oxford University Press.

Parker, R. (1994). *Flesh peddlers and warm bodies: The temporary help industry and its workers.* New Brunswick, NJ: Rutgers University Press.

Parks, M., & Floyd, K. (1996). Making friends in cyberspace. *Journal of Communication, 46*, 80–97.

Parmerlee, M., Near, J., & Jensen, T. (1982). Correlates of whistleblowers' perceptions of organizational retaliation. *Administrative Science Quarterly, 27*, 17–34.

Pearce, J. L. (1993). Toward an organizational behavior of contract laborers: Their psychological involvement and effects on employee co-workers. *Academy of Management Journal, 36*, 1082–1096.

Pepitone, A., & Wilpizeski, C. (1960). Some consequences of experimental rejection. *Journal of Abnormal and Social Psychology, 60*, 359–364.

Peretti, P., Clark, D., & Johnson, P. (1984). Effect of parental rejection on negative attention-seeking classroom behaviors. *Education, 104*, 313–317.

Petersen, J., & Farrell, D. (1986). *Whistleblowing: Ethical and legal issues in expressing dissent.* Dubuque, IA: Kendall/Hunt.

Peterson, C., Maier, S. F., & Seligman, M. E. P. (1993). *Learned helplessness: A theory for the age of personal control.* New York: Oxford University Press.

Petty, R. E., Williams, K. D., Harkins, S. G., & Latané, B. (1977). Social inhibition of helping yourself. *Personality and Social Psychology Bulletin, 3*, 575–578.

Pfeffer, J., & Baron, J. N. (1988). Taking the workers back out: Recent trends in the structure of employment. *Research in Organisational Behavior, 10*, 257–303.

Pietromonaco, P. R., & Barrett, L. F. (1997). Working models of attachment and daily social interactions. *Journal of Personality and Social Psychology, 73*, 1409–1423.

Pittman, T. S., & D'Agostino, P. R. (1989). Motivation and cognition: Control deprivation and the nature of subsequent information processing. *Journal of Experimental Social Psychology, 25*, 465–480.

Pittman, T. S., & Pittman, N. L. (1980). Deprivation of control and the attribution process. *Journal of Personality and Social Psychology, 39*, 377–389.

Polivka, A. E. (1996). In to contingent and alternative employment: By choice. *Monthly Labor Review, 119,* 55–74.

Predmore, S. C., & Williams, K. D. (1983, May). *The effects of social ostracism on affiliation.* Paper presented at the annual meeting of the Midwestern Psychological Association, Chicago.

Pyszczynski, T., Wicklund, R. A., Floresku, S., Koch, H., Gauch, G., Solomon, S., & Greenberg, J. (1996). Whistling in the dark: Exaggerated consensus estimates in response to incidental reminders of mortality. *Psychological Science, 6,* 332–336.

Raleigh, M. J., & McGuire, M. T. (1986). Animal analogues of ostracism: Biological mechanisms and social consequences. *Ethology and Sociobiology, 7,* 201–214.

Rand, A. (1992). *Atlas shrugged.* New York: Signet. (Original work published 1957)

Rehbinder, M. (1986). Refusal of social cooperation as a legal problem: On the legal institution of ostracism and boycott. *Ethology and Sociobiology, 7,* 321–327.

Reilly, B. (1996). *Effects of loneliness on reactions to ostracism.* Unpublished dissertation, University of Toledo, Toledo, OH.

Reis, H. T., & Wheeler, L. (1991). Studying social interaction with the Rochester Interaction Record. In M. P. Zanna (Ed.), *Advances in experimental social psychology* (Vol. 24, pp. 270–312). New York: Academic Press.

Ricard, L., & Perrien, J. (1999). Explaining and evaluating the implementation of organizational relationship marketing in the banking industry: Clients' perception. *Journal of Business Research, 45,* 199–209.

Rintel, E. S., & Pittam, J. (1997a). Strangers in a strange land: Interaction management on Internet relay chat. *Human Communication Research, 23,* 507–534.

Rintel, E. S., & Pittam, J. (1997b, May). *Communicative and non-communicative silence on Internet relay chat: Management and function.* Paper presented at the 47th annual conference of the International Communication Association, Montreal, Canada.

Robbins, I., & Hunt, N. (1997). *Survey on the effects of war experience* [Online]. Available: http://salmon.psy.plym.ac.uk/intro.htm.

Roberts, L. (1997). *New Internet user survey* [On-line]. Available: http://psych.curtin.edu.au/people/roberts/newbiein.htm.

Rogers, C. (1959). A theory of therapy, personality, and interpersonal relationships, as developed in the client-centered framework. In S. Koch (Ed.), *Psychology: A study of a science* (Vol. 3, pp. 184–256). New York: McGraw-Hill.

Rosenberg, M. (1965). *Society and the adolescent self-image.* Princeton, NJ: Princeton University Press.

Rosenfeld, L. B. (1979). Self-disclosure avoidance: Why I am afraid to tell you who I am. *Communication Monographs, 46,* 63–74.

Rothbaum, F., Weisz, J. R., & Snyder, S. (1982). Changing the world and changing the self: A two process model of perceived control. *Journal of Personality and Social Psychology, 42,* 5–37.

Rudich, E. A., & Vallacher, R. R. (1999). To belong or to self-enhance? Motivational bases for choosing interaction partners. *Personality and Social Psychology Bulletin, 25,* 1387–1404.

Rusbult, C. E. (1993). Understanding responses to dissatisfaction in close relationships: The exit–voice–loyalty–neglect model. In S. Worchel, & J. A. Simpson (Eds.), *Conflict between people and groups: Causes, processes, and resolutions* (pp. 30–59). Chicago: Nelson-Hall.

Rusbult, C. E., Johnson, D. J., & Morrow, G. D. (1986). Impact of couple patterns of problem solving on distress and nondistress in dating relationships. *Journal of Personality and Social Psychology, 50,* 744–753.

Rusbult, C. E., Morrow, G. D., & Johnson, D. J. (1987). Self-esteem and problem solving behavior in close relationships. *British Journal of Social Psychology, 26,* 293–303.

Rusbult, C., Verette, J., Whitney, G., Slovik, L., & Lipkus, I. (1991). Accommodation processes in close relationships: Theory and preliminary empirical evidence. *Journal of Personality and Social Psychology, 60,* 53–78.

Saxena, V. (1992). Perceived maternal rejection as related to negative attention-seeking classroom behaviour among primary school children. *Journal of Personality and Clinical Studies, 8,* 129–135.

Schachter, S. (1951). Deviation, rejection, and communication. *Journal of Abnormal and Social Psychology, 46,* 190–207.

Schachter, S. (1959). *The psychology of affiliation.* Stanford, CA: Stanford University Press.

Schein, E. (1965). *Organizational psychology.* Englewood Cliffs, NJ: Prentice-Hall.

Schlack, M. (1995). Facing the future with Windows95. *Datamation, 41,* 43–44.

Schneider, D. J., & Turkat, D. (1975). Self-presentation following success or failure: Defensive self-esteem models. *Journal of Personality, 43*(1), 127–135.

Schuster, B. (1996). Rejection, exclusion, and harassment at work and in schools: An integration of results from research on mobbing, bullying, and peer rejection. *European Psychologist, 1,* 293–317.

Seligman, M. E. P. (1975). *Helplessness: On depression, development, and death.* San Francisco: Freeman.

Service, E. R. (1975). *Origins of the state and civilization.* New York: Norton.

Shaftel, F. R., & Shaftel, G. (1976). *Role-playing for social values: Decision-making in the social studies.* Englewood Cliffs, NJ: Prentice-Hall.

Sheler, J. (1981, November 16). When employees squeal on fellow workers. *U.S. News & World Report,* pp. 81–82.

Sherif, M., Harvey, O. J., White, B. J., Hood, W. E., & Sherif, C. W. (1961). *The robber's cave experiment: Intergroup conflict and cooperation.* Norman, OK: Institute of Group Relations.

Skinner, E. A. (1996). A guide to constructs of control. *Journal of Personality and Social Psychology, 71,* 549–570.

Smith, E. R., & Mackie, D. M. (1995). *Social psychology.* New York: Worth.

Snell, W. (1997). *Survey on romantic relationships* [On-line]. Available: http://www2.semo.edu/snell/study2.html.

Snoek, J. D. (1962). Some effects of rejection upon attraction to a group. *Journal of Abnormal and Social Psychology, 64,* 175–182.

Solomon, S., Greenberg, J., & Pyszczynski, T. (1991). A terror management theory of self-esteem and its role in social behavior. In M. Zanna (Ed.), *Advances in experimental social psychology* (pp. 93–159), New York: Academic Press.

Sommer, K. L., Ciarocco, N. J., & Baumeister, R. F. (1999, April). *Ignoring others causes a subsequent breakdown in self-control*. Paper presented at the meeting of the British Psychological Society, Belfast, Northern Ireland.

Sommer, K. L., Williams, K. D., Ciarocco, N. J., & Baumeister, R. F. (in press). When silence speaks louder than words: Explorations into the interpersonal and intrapsychic consequences of social ostracism. *Basic and Applied Social Psychology.*

Spielberger, C. D. (1983). *Manual for the State–Trait Anxiety Inventory for Adults*. Palo Alto, CA: Consulting Psychologists Press.

Steele, C. M. (1988). The psychology of self-affirmation: Sustaining the integrity of the self. In L. Berkowitz (Ed.), *Advances in experimental social psychology* (Vol. 21, pp. 261–302). San Diego: Academic Press.

Steinberg, R. (1975). *Man and the organization*. New York: Time Life Books.

Stroud, L. R., Tanofsky-Kraff, M., Wilfley, D. E., & Salovey, P. (2000). The Yale Interpersonal Stressor (YIPS): Affective, physiological, and behavioral responses to a novel interpersonal rejection paradigm. *Annals of Behavioral Medicine, 22,* 204–213.

Tajfel, H. (1970). Experiments in intergroup discrimination. *Scientific American, 223,* 96–102.

Tajfel, H., & Turner, J. (1986). The social identity theory of intergroup behavior. In S. Worchel & W. Austin (Eds.), *Psychology of intergroup relations* (pp. 33–48). Chicago: Nelson-Hall.

Tansky, J. W., Gallagher, D. G., & Wetzel, K. W. (1997). The effect of demographics, work status, and relative equity on organizational commitment: Looking among part-time workers. *Canadian Journal of Administrative Sciences, 14,* 315–326.

Taylor, S. E., & Brown, J. D. (1988). Illusion and well-being: A social psychological perspective on mental health. *Psychological Bulletin, 103,* 193–210.

Taylor, S. E., Kemeny, M. E., Aspinwall, L. G., Schneider, S. G., Rodriguez, R., & Herber, M. (1992). Optimism, coping, psychological distress, and high-risk sexual behavior among men at risk for acquired immunodeficiency syndrome (AIDS). *Journal of Personality and Social Psychology, 63,* 460–473.

Tesser, A. (1988). Toward a self-evaluation maintenance model of social behavior. In L. Berkowitz (Ed.), *Advances in experimental social psychology* (Vol. 21, pp. 181–227). San Diego, CA: Academic Press.

Tice, D. M., Twenge, J. M., & Schmeichel, B. (in press). Social exclusion and prosocial and antisocial behavior. In J. P. Forgas & K. D. Williams (Eds.), *The social self: Cognitive, interpersonal, and intergroup perspectives*. Philadelphia: Psychology Press.

Trope, Y. (1986). Identification and inferential processes in dispositional attribution. *Psychological Review, 93,* 239–257.

Turner, J. C. (1984). Social identification and psychological group formation. In

H. Tajfel (Ed.), *The social dimension: European developments in social psychology* (Vol. 2., pp. 518–538). London: Cambridge University Press/Paris: Editions de la Maison des Sciences de l'Homme.

Turner, J. C., Hogg, M. A., Oakes, P. J., Reicher, S. D., & Wetherell, M. S. (1987). *Rediscovering the social group: A self-categorization theory*. Oxford, UK: Blackwell.

Van Ments, M. (1983). *The effective use of role play: A handbook for teachers and trainers*. London: NP Kogan Page.

Veenstra, G. J., & Scott, C. G. (1993). A model for using time out as an intervention technique with families. *Journal of Family Violence, 8*, 71–87.

Von Hippel, C., Mangum, S. L., Greenberger, D. B., Skoglind, J. D., & Henemen, R. L. (1997). Temporary employment: Can organizations and employees both win? *Academy of Management Executive, 11*, 93–104.

Von Hippel, C., Mangum, S. L., Greenberger, D. B., Skoglind, J. D., & Henemen, R. L. (1998). *Voluntary and involuntary temporary employees: Predicting satisfaction, commitment, and personal control*. Unpublished manuscript, Ohio State University.

Westin, P. (1981). *Whistleblowing!: Loyalty and dissent in the corporation*. New York: McGraw-Hill.

Wheeler, L., & Miyake, K. (1992). Social comparison in everyday life. *Journal of Personality and Social Psychology, 62*, 760–773.

Wheeler, L., & Nezlek, J. (l977). Sex differences in social participation. *Journal of Personality and Social Psychology, 35*, 742–754.

Wheeler, L., & Reis, H. T. (1991). Self-recording of events in everyday life: Origins, types, and uses. *Journal of Personality, 59*, 339–354.

Williams, K. B., & Williams, K. D. (1983). Social inhibition and asking for help: The effects of number, strength, and immediacy of potential help-givers. *Journal of Personality and Social Psychology, 44*, 67–77.

Williams, K. D. (1997). Social ostracism. In R. M. Kowalski (Ed.), *Aversive interpersonal behaviors* (pp. 133–170). New York: Plenum Press.

Williams, K. D., Bernieri, F., Faulkner, S., Grahe, J., & Gada-Jain, N. (2000). The Scarlet Letter Study: Five days of social ostracism. *Journal of Personal and Interpersonal Loss, 5*, 19–63.

Williams, K. D., Cheung, C. K. T., & Choi, W. (2000). CyberOstracism: Effects of being ignored over the Internet. *Journal of Personality and Social Psychology, 79*, 748–762.

Williams, K. D., Govan, C., Croker, V., Tynan, D., Cruikshank, M., & Lam, A. (in press). Investigations into differences between social and cyberostracism. *Group Dynamic: Theory, Research, and Practice*.

Williams, K. D., & Karau, S. J. (1991). Social loafing and social compensation: The effects of expectations of coworker performance. *Journal of Personality and Social Psychology, 61*, 570–581.

Williams, K. D., Shore, W. J., & Grahe, J. E. (1998). The silent treatment: Perceptions of its behaviors and associated feelings. *Group Processes and Intergroup Relations, 1*, 117–141.

Williams, K. D., & Sommer, K. L. (1997). Social ostracism by one's coworkers: Does rejection lead to loafing or compensation? *Personality and Social Psychology Bulletin, 23*, 693–706.

Williams, K. D., Wheeler, L., & Harvey, J. (2001). Inside the social mind of the ostracizer. In J. Forgas, K. Williams, & L. Wheeler (Eds.), *The social mind: Cognitive and motivational aspects of interpersonal behavior* (pp. 294–320). New York: Cambridge University Press.

Williams, K. D., & Zadro, L. (1999, April). *Forty years of solitude: Effects of long-term use of the silent treatment.* Paper presented at the meeting of the Midwestern Psychological Association, Chicago.

Williams, K. D., & Zadro, L. (2001). Ostracism: On being ignored, excluded, and rejected. In M. Leary (Ed.), *Interpersonal rejection* (pp. 21–53). New York: Oxford University Press.

Wortman, C. B., & Brehm, J. W. (1975). Responses to uncontrollable outcomes: An integration of reactance theory and the learned helplessness model. In L. Berkowitz (Ed.), *Advances in experimental social psychology* (Vol. 8, pp. 277–336). San Diego, CA: Academic Press.

Yuille, J. (1988). The systematic assessment of children's testimony. *Canadian Psychology, 29,* 247–262.

Zadro, L., Walker, P., Williams, K. D., & Richardson, R. (2000, February). *The psychophysiological effects of being ostracized.* Paper presented at the 10th World Congress of Psychophysiology, Sydney, Australia.

Zadro, L., & Williams, K. D. (1998a). *Effects of ostracism versus arguing in a role-play experiment.* Unpublished manuscript, University of New South Wales, Sydney, Australia.

Zadro, L., & Williams, K. D. (1998b, April). *Riding the "O" train: A role-play exercise to examine social ostracism.* Paper presented at the Society for Australasian Social Psychology, Christchurch, New Zealand.

Zippelius, R. (1986). Exclusion and shunning as legal and social sanctions. *Ethology and Sociobiology, 7,* 159–166.

Zuckerman, M., Miserandino, M., & Bernieri, F. (1983). Civil inattention exists—in elevators. *Personality and Social Psychology Bulletin, 9,* 578–586.

Index